Warriors *and* Falcons

Life Sketches of 100 outstanding Kashmiri Doctors

Dr.Rumana Makhdoomi (Srinagar)
Prof.Faroque A Khan (New York)

PARTRIDGE

ISBN:	Hardcover	978-1-5437-0927-8
	Softcover	978-1-5437-0926-1
	eBook	978-1-5437-0925-4

Cover page photo

Kashmiri doctors of yore who graduated from the King Edward Medical College Lahore. Front row: Dr. Ghulam Mohammad Qureshi, extreme left; Dr. Hafizullah, third from left; Dr. Ali Jan, extreme right. Standing: bespectacled Dr. Ghulam Rasool.(Courtesy of Dr.Kawoosa)

Print information available on the last page.

To order additional copies of this book, contact
Partridge India
000 800 919 0634 (Call Free)
+91 000 80091 90634 (Outside India)
orders.india@partridgepublishing.com

www.partridgepublishing.com/india

Dedicated to

The spirit of all Kashmiri doctors who lived for the patients and died serving the profession!

The angel of history wears all expressions at once.
What will you do? Look, his wings are aflame for you.

Agha Shahid Ali (The veiled suite)

Preface

We have heard tales from our parents and grandparents about the practice of medicine in Kashmir. Some of them appear to be too magical to be true! While those are tales nonetheless, the history of modern medicine in Kashmir started with British missionary doctors and continued with the local doctors who were trained in England and served in the state. It is not easy to collect the stories of individual contributors, but my job has been made relatively easy by Prof. Gulzar Mufti, who has written a detailed account about the evolution of art and practice of medicine in Kashmir. I thank Dr. Mufti for his wonderful work.

Kashmiri doctors have done a remarkable job everywhere they went. We are filled with pride when we hear the tales of their accomplishment. Back home in Kashmir, they have braved the odds fighting illiteracy, poverty, and conflict. They have kept the candle of medicine burning through Government Medical College Srinagar, which, in spite of constraints, continued to train doctors who were truly world class. Government Medical College Srinagar has become a mother institution that leads from the front to supply doctors to all the regions of Jammu and Kashmir and many prestigious institutions of the world.

Kashmir has produced too many heroes in medicine who have contributed here and abroad. It is not easy to pick up a mere one hundred, sum up their role, and give a gist of their contributions. It is difficult to segregate them as legends and more difficult to write about each such legend. I undertook the task of writing the profiles of a few Kashmiri doctors in a local newspaper to highlight their contributions. Later on, an idea struck me as to why write about just a few—why not a bigger number, say, 100? I was also impressed by the work that nonresident Kashmiri doctors were doing abroad, making us proud of their achievements. Then I thought it would be interesting to write about their contributions too. I shared this idea with Prof. Faroque Ahmad Khan from New York, who, to my great pleasure, agreed to help me with the profiles of Kashmiri doctors who had contributed to medicine in the US. He also agreed to be the coauthor of the book that would bring to the fore the contribution of Kashmiri doctors whether from Kashmir or outside Kashmir. That was way back in 2016. Now the question, Who to put in the list? Prof. Faroque Khan and I sent emails to all the doctors known to us, put our request for nominations on the social media, and waited for the response. There was hardly any response. How Dr. Faroque chose his list, you will know about it elsewhere in the book. While Professor Faroque finished his part of the story quickly, I struggled with my part . . .. . . Many Kashmiri doctors about whom I wanted to write had left this world, and they had no one in Kashmir who would tell me about them. There were no written records about them. Similarly, I struggled to know about Kashmiri Pandit doctors; while some volunteered with the information, some did not want to be disturbed.

In this tough job, my worthy teachers did a remarkable work to help me. Professor Allaqaband was a great source of information; he involved himself wholeheartedly in this project. He contacted people on my behalf so that I would get the desired information. I showed many rough drafts to him to check the authenticity of the information I would obtain from many sources. His astounding memory and his clear recollection of many incidents helped me greatly. The book is as much as his effort as mine. Prof. Muhammad Yousuf (professor and ex-HOD Medicine, GMC Srinagar) also helped me to connect with many of his contemporaries about whom I wanted to know more.

While I was tempted to put many doctors in the list, I had to rely on some very dedicated professionals who scrutinized the list I had made and actually compiled the list for me. Dr. Ajaz Koul of Medicine at SKIMS did a lot of hard work in this regard for me. Some of my colleagues suggested a few names who were real contributors but had been left out. When the list was made, I did not manage to get the profiles of all in the list. Some refused, some avoided me, and some didn't respond. Writing about those frustrating moments will make another book . . . So my collection of outstanding doctors from Kashmir will have deficiencies . . .

It has not been my intention to grade these legends but to gather information about them so that we as medical professionals would look up to them and get inspired by what they did. The book took a long time to be ready. I had my share of sad moments when I was not able to connect with people who could help me, and there were some who promised to help me but did not. "No matter what your pace is, your pace will be dictated by the pace of others" was the lesson I learned during my tryst with finding the profiles of the doctors I wanted.

In this task, Dr. Zorawar Singh from the Department of Pharmacology GMC Srinagar was really helpful. He was helpful to get the profiles of many doctors from his circle. Prof. Ajaz Koul of General Medicine and Infectious Diseases, SKIMS, and Prof. Abdul Qayoom Dar of Anesthesiology, SKIMS, helped me greatly with their suggestions and recommendations greatly aiding in compiling this book.

My list includes Kashmiri doctors who served in Kashmir and practiced allopathy. The list has some exceptions for example Dr. Durrani—I just couldn't skip him. He was so much more Kashmiri than most of us are. Again, I have not included doctors of basic sciences but dared not skip Prof. Taffazul Hussain . . . when you read the profile, you may agree that his name could not be left out.

I am indebted to Dr. K. K. Kaul, who provided some well-preserved and interesting photographs of his father, Dr. Gwash Lal Kaul; Dr. Bashir Ahmad (ophthalmology) for helping me with the profile of Dr. Harbajan Singh; Dr. Ismail Quadiri; Dr. Khurshid Guru; and many others with their suggestions and help. Dr. Fazal Q. Parray helped me with the profiles of Dr. Mahmooda Khan and Dr. Nisar Chowdri.

My coauthor, Prof. Faroque A. Khan, served as a constant stimulus for me. He always thought the work was doable even when I was sure at one point of time that I couldn't just do it. He kept on pushing me to do this work. My family, especially my mother, my sisters, my brother, my nephews, my nieces, and my in-laws, have been helpful. Kamil, Hadia, and little Ilhan deserve special thanks. Dr. Besina deserves special thanks too for her kindness and companionship.

My husband, Dr. Nayil Khursheed, wanted me to complete this project and did all he could to accelerate its pace. My daughters, Maryam, Madeeha, and Fatima, cooperated with me and were a source of support and encouragement. Fatima and her witty quotes and jokes really pulled me up when I was low.

My father has been my inspiration always . . . his death shattered me, but I learned gradually to live with his memory. He taught me to be bold and responsible; my love for history and politics is because of him. While writing this book, I felt a great void, as he was not there to edit it or correct it.

Many thanks and congratulations to all those who are profiled in this book. My apologies to all those whose profiles have not been included here. There is a scope to have one more book with one hundred more profiles. Hope someone takes up this task.

Dr. Rumana Makhdoomi
MBBS, MD, PDF
Srinagar
17-07-2023

Preface

The book *Warriors and Falcons*, describing the bios of one hundred doctors who helped establish and nurture the health-care system in Kashmir over the past one hundred years, is a great and priceless contribution made possible by the patience, diligence, and perseverance of Dr. Rumana Makhdoomi. My thanks and appreciation for her outstanding effort. It's been a long process with multiple highs and lows. Dr. Rumana first contacted me in 2016, and I was delighted to offer my help particularly in nominating the physicians who had settled in the United States and have made remarkable contribution both professionally and in helping the larger community.

As a graduate of the first batch of Government Medical College (GMC) in 1964, I was privileged to have worked with the early pioneers and the flag bearers—for example, Drs. Ali Jan, Ghulam Rasool, Girdari Lal, G. Q. Allaqaband, S. N. Kaul. Reading the book draft, I was impressed and learned about the early pioneers like Dr. Gwash Lal Kaul and Dr. G. L. Vaishnavi and was impressed by the great contribution they made in introducing treatment and management of diabetes and many other public health measures. Of great interest to me was reading the details outlined by Dr. Rumana Makhdomi as to how she was able to obtain the original CVs and detailed bio certificates of these individuals who had left this world.

GMC and its role: To digress a bit, when the GMC was started in 1959, there was a fair amount of skepticism in the larger community about the scope and quality of future GMC graduates. In retrospect, the GMC has turned out to be an anchor, the mother ship—for providing health-care professionals over the past fifty plus years. I believe the secret of the initial success of this new medical school was in hiring out-of-state senior retired teachers and selecting students on merit basis—teachers like Dr. B. S. Kahali in physiology and Dr. Ayar in anatomy and others who followed. I still recall the weekly quizzes given by Dr. Kahali.

Personally, I admire and have great respect for the GMC alumni and others who stayed in Kashmir during a very turbulent period and continued to provide care to the very vulnerable population. Some of us decided to train and settle in USA/UK for a variety of different reasons. Many of us have continued to try and assist in helping improve the infrastructure of health care in Kashmir. It's been a challenge. Two personal examples I can recall: (1) For reasons best known to the authorities in Kashmir, a proposal to start a state-of-the-art hospital in Kashmir by the nonresident Kashmiris from Middle East and USA was not allowed by the JK government. (2) In 1987, the Islamic Medical Association of North America applied for and was denied permission to host its first international convention in Kashmir.

As one of the nonresident Kashmiri doctors who decided to stay in USA, I have hosted many GMC alumni in the hospitals I was associated with. I recall with fondness the visit of late doctor Surendra Nath Dhar when he visited with me for several weeks at Queens General Hospital in New York and attended the pulmonary service of which I was the chief. I encouraged Dr. Dhar to attend the daily ward and ICU rounds. After one such experience lasting several hours in our respiratory ICU, I asked Dr. Dhar about his impressions. His response stuck with me. Paraphrasing, he stated, "You folks provide retail medicine, and we provide wholesale medicine." Dr. Dhar was and Dr. G. Q. Allaqaband played a great role in shaping this hospital. Dr. Ajit Nagpal, a young dynamic professional, created a dream hospital that could compete with the best hospitals in the world. The commitment of Dr. Nagpal to the work that was assigned to him is a dream desire for all founders. The peak to which SKIMS would reach was blunted by the turmoil that brought with it chaos and disorder. Extremely dedicated professionals worked in trying circumstances to keep the lamp of SKIMS glowing. All credit to those professionals who worked with dedication trying to hold together SKIMS at a time when SKIMS needed them the most! Many such professionals who stayed back and worked under pressure serving their own people are a part of this book. I could not include all—my apologies to them—but some whose CVs might look ordinary put up an extraordinary show; I regret I am not able to bring out their work in a better way in this book.

SKIMS came up as a gateway to research. It was difficult to imagine high-quality research coming from a disturbed area landlocked by the Himalayas. The research papers in Lancet and NEJM from SKIMS by Prof. M. S. Khuroo spoke about the level of dedication that he and his team had for science and medicine. Dr. Khuroo inspired many youngsters to do quality research. Dr. Abdul Hamid Zargar became a master endocrinologist and researcher; he and others brought Kashmir on the research map of the world. Some master surgeons from SKIMS too did exemplary work and came up with work that was second to none in the world. It was surprising that in the times when mind and body refused to maintain cohesion, these men of mettle could carry out such outstanding research and quality work! Look at the work they did and the circumstances in which this work was done. Any analogy anywhere in the world would surprise me. The work was really worth a Nobel in medicine!

A generation of brilliant doctors followed who could get accommodated anywhere in the world but chose Kashmir as comparing the patient and workload in Kashmir with New York City. During my regular visits to Srinagar, I made it a point to visit and share my X-rays, talks, and other teaching material with Dr. Dhar and his team at the chest diseases hospital. It was a mutually beneficial experience. Over the years, others and we have hosted many physicians from Kashmir for short-term visits and training.

Let me conclude by saying that this book is a much-needed and uplifting story of the Kashmiri doctors who have brought the health care provided by missionary doctors a century ago to the present state-of-the-art level. My congratulations and compliments to all the people who made these contributions. In closing, let us also remember the contributions of physicians like Dr. Erna M. Hoch, a Swiss psychiatrist who devoted time and energy from 1969 to 1987 in changing and upgrading the psychiatric care in Kashmir; and Dr. Jagat Mohini, who, along Dr. Onkar Nath Thussu, established the Rattan Rani Hospital, which developed a special expertise in women's health issues. I recall a few times when I had to drive my mother to Rattan Rani Hospital for treatment; this hospital had established a great reputation in delivering quality care for women.

Finally, another note of thanks and appreciation for Dr. Rumana Makhdoomi for creating this unique book and also a note of appreciation for all who provided much-needed support to her.

Dr. Faroque A. Khan
MB, MACP
Chairman, Interfaith Institute of Long Island
New York
16-06-2023

CONTENTS

A Kashmiri Doctor

(Journey through pain and uncertainty)

While all else could close in an atmosphere of tension and turmoil, the hospitals in Kashmir could not afford to shut their doors to the people. For a doctor working in Kashmir, turmoil has been almost a constant companion. The doctors in Kashmir had to deal with injuries caused by bullets, pellets, and blasts besides dealing with the whole epidemic of psychiatric diseases consequent to mental trauma. Thankfully, the doctors working here did not fail their population. Every crisis was managed effectively, though no doctor working during peak years of turmoil had ever been trained for what he was treating . . . Doctors sacrificed their time and comfort, compromised their own security, and worked hard. They restored man's faith in humanity and medicine. Most doctors suffered braving the challenging times that would collapse the best health-care systems of the world. All doctors working in those times need to be complimented for how they worked under pressure and pain. There are stories of exemplary work, exceptional courage, and tortuous suffering that went unheard and unpublished. No gallantry awards were given, and no certificates of appreciation were distributed. In such a scenario, every doctor is a hero. How can I quantify the work of one or a hundred? How can I pick and choose one and leave the rest? How can I call one doctor as outstanding and not appreciate what the other did? I cannot do that . . . My apologies to all those brave hearts whose stories remain untold.

Kashmir has seen disorder and disarray to the extent that no one cared as to who worked and who did not. The people who worked, they worked only under the influence of their conscience fearing Almighty God. I am glad many doctors served the people fearing God even when they could have chosen to be indifferent and no one would have questioned their indifference. I have witnessed and worked with doctors who did their duty to perfection even when they could have chosen to do otherwise. One such dedicated doctor has been Dr. Abdul Majeed Ahangar from medicine (SMHS), who is a hero for me. His unselfish work during turmoil to which I am a witness (I have written about it in detail in my previous book *White Man in Dark*) has really impressed me. How many heroes and superheroes have worked and are still working in Kashmir, away from the limelight, I really don't know.

When your outside is burning and inside is in pain, how do you practice medicine? Kashmiri doctors have faced peculiar situations during turmoil. And they have braved the difficult situations and upheld ethics. When in the line of your duty you have to declare your own son dead, what code will you follow? Dr. Poswal in the line of duty had to declare his son dead. The book is dedicated to the spirit he displayed. When you have to remove bullets from a professor's eye with whom out of respect you could never maintain an eye contact, which ethics will you follow? Doctors at SKIMS displayed the patience and courage while removing bullets from Dr. Jalal's eye What when you intubate your life partner who received a bullet injury on his way to the hospital? Dr. Farida Ashai intubated her husband just before he breathed his last. What when before declaring unfortunate news of death to the old and weak parents of a boy who received a stray bullet, you are yourself inconsolable? What when you cannot decide whose life to save first—a man with three tiny daughters or a young man gasping for breath? I know we need to credit each one for what one did. We will need a lifetime to put into the limelight those stories of compassion and valor that doctors of Kashmir exhibited amid crises—and let the world learn from them.

Actually, what has been narrated above is a tale of nearly thirty years . . . it was not how allopathic medicine started in Kashmir. It started with British doctors and a few Kashmiri doctors who dared to study medicine in India and abroad to lay foundations for a system that would withstand the test of the times. Dr. Gwash Lal Kaul, Dr. Vaishnavi, and Dr. Ali Jan challenged an era of ignorance, poverty, and superstition to lay foundations for a rational approach to the health-care-related issues of Kashmiris and replaced superstition with pure science. Hence, they are the leaders who made the switch over possible without resistance and anger. They are our heroes and we owe our gratitude to them. Another group followed who worked further on the foundations that these leaders had laid. They included many prominent physicians and surgeons of their times who were all trained abroad but worked in Kashmir to expand the health care and to lay foundations for more hospitals and a college where medicine would be taught.

The Medical College at Srinagar proved to be a boon for Kashmir. Best minds were shaped by the best in the profession to give to Kashmir and the world an exciting breed of competent professionals. These pass-outs did a lot of good to their own community and stood tall anywhere in the world as the best-trained doctors. All those who were behind this mission need to be complimented. Many generations of medical professionals and the entire community are indebted to those who worked for the establishment of a medical college in Kashmir.

Sher-i-Kashmir Institute of Medical Sciences (SKIMS) was a well-conceived superspecialist hospital and provided superspecialist services to the people of Kashmir. Dr. Ali Jan their destination. Dr. Khurshid Iqbal, Dr. Parvaiz Koul, Dr. Nisar Tramboo, Dr. Nisar Chowdri, and others stayed back to work in Kashmir and contributed towards health care. No doubt they were inspired by the works of their colleagues and teachers who acted as torchbearers for them.

In spite of expansion, the health care in Kashmir is in need of a total overhaul. The system has to get better, it has to make provisions for the brilliant to scale heights, and it has to come out of the old hierarchy system. It has to distinguish between performers and nonperformers; it has to address adhocism and invest heavily in brilliant people who can make a difference to health care. I remember three brilliant doctors who had their superspecialization from the best institutions of India, and they were working on an ongoing contractual arrangement at SMHS Hospital. Neither could they grow in the system nor could the subspecialty that they were aiming to develop. However, they still worked to inspire. Brilliant work by Dr. Bilal Khan, Dr. Parvez Zargar, and Dr. Hayat Bhat. The trio should have been professors in any institution, but they continue on contractual assignments to our dismay. Loss is theirs and ours, but patience is just theirs!

COVID-19 pandemic again tested our doctors and the robustness of our health-care system. The job was done very well. The doctors did not shy away from their duty, and Kashmir's hospitals had the lowest mortality rates. Well-organized teams worked in cohesion and focused on preventive and curative aspects of the pandemic. Six doctors lost their lives. The book is dedicated very much to them also.

The doctors we are producing are brilliant. The numbers are huge too. Kashmiris seem to be inclined (genetically or emotionally) toward medicine . . . so we have a chance to produce world leaders. Our predecessors have done a splendid work; our contemporaries are doing great too. The stories of these hundred men and women should inspire all of us and the generation next to do better!

The Legends

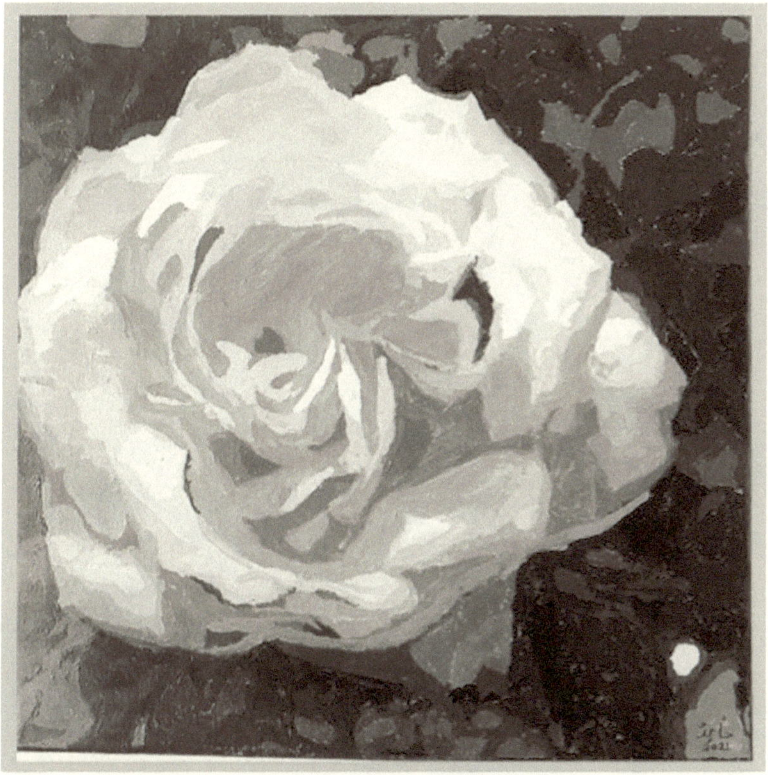

Art by Dr. H. A. Durrani

The Legends

(The arrangement is alphabetical)

1. Dr. Ali Muhammad Jan
2. Dr. Bilqees Jamila
3. Dr. Brij Mohan Bhan
4. Dr. Farooq Ashai
5. Dr. Fazal Rehman
6. Dr. Ghulam Qadir Allaqaband
7. Dr. Ghulam Rasool
8. Dr. Girdhari Lal Kaul
9. Dr. Girja Dhar
10. Dr. Govind Lal Vaishnavi
11. Dr. Gwash Lal Kaul
12. Dr. Hafizullah
13. Dr. Hamid Ali Durrani
14. Dr. Harbhajan Singh
15. Dr. Mahmooda Khan
16. Dr. Manzoor Ahmed
17. Dr. Mehrajuddin Munshi
18. Dr. Mohammad Maqbool Mir
19. Dr. Mohammad Sultan Khuroo
20. Dr. Mohammad Yousuf
21. Dr. (Col.) Saligram Kaul
22. Dr. Surendra Nath Dhar
23. Dr. Syed Naseer Ahmad Shah
24. Dr. Syed Zahoor Ahmad
25. Dr. Wazira Khanam

Dr. Ali Muhammad Jan

A legend of legends!

Writing the profile of one of the most efficient and most popular clinicians of Kashmir is not easy especially when you did not breathe in the same era, so you rely on the stories from his students, his contemporaries, his family, and, most importantly, his patients and admirers. Ali Jan is history, is memory, is inspiration, is skill, and is pure magic. No one can compete with him; no one can stand next to him in popularity and faith. There have been physicians and surgeons in Kashmir with a greater contribution to health care and medical education, but I am sure they cannot match the popularity and faith Dr. Ali Jan enjoyed.

Anyone who writes about the history of medicine in Kashmir will have no option but to give a special space to Dr. Ali Jan. Dr. Ali Jan cannot be ignored if we talk about the evolution of a system in Kashmir over which he uncontestedly presided.

Before I introduce Dr. Ali Jan, here is an excerpt from the Facebook post of Shri Avtar Mota, a critical analyst who writes widely about the culture and history of Kashmir. He writes, "In Rainawari, we had Ram Joo Handoo's chemist shop near Jogi Lanker bridge. He claimed himself to be an RMP. My father had an abiding faith in Ram Joo's degree, diagnosis and prescriptions. He would often tell me . . . *Aem Chha Ali Janus saet Hadooni Kaem Kermechh.*" He further adds, "My father believed that Dr. Ali Jan was the ultimate that modern medical sciences could provide to Kashmir and any person associated with him could never be ordinary. This led him to believe in Ram Joo Handoo's medical practice and prescriptions. He would lay more stress on Ram Joo's association with Luqman of Kashmir, Dr. Ali Jan."

Dr. Ali Muhammad Jan (Fazili) was the son of Mr. Ghulam Rasool Fazili, born at Gojwara, Srinagar, on September 3, 1914. Dr. Ali Jan, as popularly he was called, did his MBBS from King Edward Medical College, Lahore, in 1937. He was an outstanding student who earned the following medals at King Edward:

1. Nelson Reghbir Singh Golden Medal for being the most distinguished graduate of King Edward Medical College (1937)
2. Dr. Rahim Khan Gold Medal for standing first in the final MBBS
3. Neil Memorial Silver Medal for standing first in surgery
4. Sentea Memorial Silver Medal for standing first in midwifery and gynecology
5. Gold Medal in pathology
6. Gold Medal in forensic medicine

In spite of his brilliant academic background, he was posted in remote villages of Jammu province and started as a medical officer in charge of the eradication of venereal diseases. Dr. Jan had to move on foot from village to village in Doda and Udhampur. Sometimes, he would move in the hilly areas on a pony. He was posted as district medical officer, Baramulla, Anantnag, and Gulmarg. He worked as tuberculosis officer and superintendent, Chest Disease Hospital, Srinagar.

After a time of tough postings, Dr. Ali Jan restarted his academic activities with a DCH and MRCP (Edinburgh) in 1950 and 1951, respectively. He finished honors in record time. Dr.

Ali Jan, upon his return from the UK, rose to the position of a physician specialist at SMHS Hospital and retired as a professor of medicine in Government Medical College, Srinagar.

Dr. Ali Jan was a multidimensional personality and a skilled clinician. Prof. Mohammad Yousuf Bhat, ex-HOD Medicine, Government Medical College, Srinagar, worked as his house surgeon and has the following to say about Dr. Ali Jan: "Dr. Ali Jan was totally committed to his patients and would keep a track of them for years. He was a disciplined clinician. He would always listen to his patients carefully many times clinching the diagnosis just from the history. He would always talk to the patients and attendants and ask the right questions which would fetch him the answer. He would use the right key for the right lock. He would examine the patient himself and despite being busy, he had no assistants to write his patients' names and addresses, to take their BP, pulse or temperature etc. for him. His prescription was wholesome with an address and his phone number printed on it. He would write a brief relevant clinical history and the tentative clinical diagnosis. He was respectful to his friends and colleagues. He would never disrespect anyone or call loudly anyone in the ward whatever the nature of one's mistake would be."

Prof. Syed Naseer Ahmad Shah was a colleague of Dr. Ali Jan and in many quarters was seen as his rival. However, in his opinion, "Dr. Ali Jan was my colleague and a role model. He was never jealous of another intelligent person in the department. He was a different doctor and a different person. While examining his patients, he used to forget everything else. The patient was his first priority. What held him apart from the rest was examining the patients and coming to diagnosis with the limited facilities we had at that time."

Dr. Ali Jan was the founder and president of the Rotary Club and Tuberculosis Association of Kashmir. He rendered free medical advice programs in remote villages through the Rotary Club of Kashmir. He contributed toward shaping medical education and research and was instrumental in laying the foundation of a state-of-the-art superspeciality hospital in the form of Sher-i-Kashmir Institute of Medical Sciences. He was the vice chairman of the Governing Body of SKIMS, Soura, and chairman of its Apical Selection Committee. Dr. Ali Jan was a member of the Health and Family Planning Advisory Committee of Jammu and Kashmir State.

Dr. Ali Jan was conferred Padma Shri in 1975 for his meritorious services in health care and medical education. Dr. Ali Jan, though a busy practitioner, was an avid reader of the literature and history of Kashmir. He loved Kashmiri Sufi poetry and music. He was fond of Indian classical music and loved listening to Urdu gazals. He was fond of Beethoven, Mozart, and Chockowsky. He kept himself abreast with national and international news and updated his medical knowledge with journals and books. He would be seen with the latest copy of *BMJ* by his side. Dr. Ali Jan was fun loving and would retreat often to Pahalgam on weekends and enjoy sightseeing and fishing.

Dr. Jan's students and colleagues call him a disciplined and a practical clinician who would always examine a patient to his satisfaction and would never prescribe any drug without a clear indication. He would never order an investigation without reason. Prof. A. Rouf Mir, a well-known nephrologist in the US, talks about Dr. Ali Jan's principle regarding charging fees from his patients. He says, "Dr. Ali Jan would charge fee from all his patients whether known to him or not known as he believed a free prescription had no value in patients mind." He would never refer incurable and terminally ill patients outside the state.

Dr. Jan never exploited his position. Though his friendship was sought by the powerful, he never asked for any favors. In fact, he quit his job early without aspiring for power or position.

Dr. Ali Jan died of pancreatic cancer in a US hospital and, as per his wishes, was flown to Srinagar and buried in his ancestral graveyard. The irony was that without the help of modern gadgets, he had diagnosed his own disease too . . . The master clinician died peacefully on October 31, 1988.

Before I close, I cannot ignore a beautiful tribute written by Prof. K. L. Chowdhury, a clinician who worked with Dr. Ali Jan at SMHS Hospital. In his article on Dr. Ali Jan, he writes, "There was a physician who was neither a researcher nor a missionary nor a community activist. He was an astute clinician . . . . . .He never compromised with quality, abhorred mediocrity and set a trend that the doctors of J&K still follow. It was to write a brief clinical note of the patient on the prescription, followed by the medication he prescribed. It was the briefest clinical file of the patient, a guide for others with whom the patient might land." He further says, "I did not see him performing any miracles but I saw perfection in him. He was a keen listener, a keener observer, quick-witted, highly intuitive and he possessed that extra-sense—the common sense that made him the miracle man." Quoting the patient's desire to be examined by this miracle man, Dr. Chowdhury says, "I remember patients falling prostrate in front of his car and not allowing him to move unless he agreed to examine them." Dr. Ali Jan's prescriptions mattered and were preserved like amulets by his patients. Quoting an incident about his grandmother whose pocket was picked on a wedding and she cried foul not for all the valuables she had lost but for the valued prescription of her beloved doctor,- Dr. Ali Jan,. His grandmother had to be taken again to the clinician in whom she had faith and the prescription rewritten. That was the only thing that could pacify her. Dr. Chowdhury, in an emotional piece decades after the death of his beloved clinician, says, "I cannot forget his mannerism, his soft speech, the shrug of his neck nor his intelligent looks and his sharp intellect." He religiously preserves one of the prescriptions that he retrieved from one of his friends in Jammu. The prescription was a prized archive of a legendary doctor circa 1973. It was preserved passionately with Dr. Chowdhury.

Dr. Ali Jan left behind institutions, many able and competent students, satisfied patients, and a legacy, which makes all clinicians proud. There cannot be another Ali Jan; that is not my view but the viewpoint of the population he treated and impressed. When a Kashmiri woman wishes great for her doctor kid, she says, “May God give you daste-shafa like Dr. Ali Jan.”

(With special thanks to Ms. Nowsheen Fazili, Dr. A. R. Mir, Dr. M. Y. Bhat, Mr. Avtar Mota. Useful information was taken from articles written by Dr. Javid Iqbal and Dr. K. L. Chowdhury.)

Dr. Bilqees Jamila

A champion you can't defeat!

I went into the chambers of a very busy gynecologist and obstetrician, and as I was waiting, I had a look around the impressive walls of her clinic, and on one of the walls, I saw a familiar face smiling at me. When the doctor (herself a retired HOD of Gyne and Obs) entered the chambers, I asked her as to why she had kept that photo hung on her walls. She smiled and said, "I feel safe and secure under her, and her presence gives you confidence. Since I couldn't get her to my clinic, I kept her picture so that I would get positive vibes." Her answer surprised me; I salute the teacher and the taught. The taught for the respect and the emotions, and the teacher for what she is—even after becoming a master in her subject, the student felt the need for the protective presence of her teacher around her. The teacher is Dr. Bilqees Jamila—she represents the ultimate that a doctor could deliver to her society.

I have known Dr. Bilqees as one of the most impressive teachers in Government Medical College, Srinagar. Her captivating looks, her firm voice, her wit, her ability to lead, and her capability to deliver had no match—this when I was a student in Government Medical College almost thirty years back. And this woman never took a leave from the active life that defines her. At almost eighty years of age now, when you try to contact her and chase her in a private hospital, the first table in the OR is set for her. She exerts her mind, heart, and years of experience into the skilled surgeries that she performs at this point of her life. She regularly conducts her OPD and sees patients, treating them, advising them, and counseling them—for all that ails them. She is the charming nightingale of Kashmir. Dr. Bilqees Jamila—the untiring face from the Gynecology and Obstetrics map of Kashmir that refuses to give up, that refuses to fade away!

Dr. Bilqees originally belonged to a remote village of South Kashmir, – Manzgam, and her father settled in Srinagar in connection with a job. In Srinagar, they lived in Drugjan (Dalgate). Dr. Bilqees did her matric from a local school and FSc from Women's College, Maulana Azad Road. Dr. Bilqees was the only daughter among four brothers, and her father encouraged her to study and do well in life. Her parents gave her more attention than her brothers. This did not pamper her but gave her extra confidence to do better in life. Dr. Bilqees had the honor to be the student of the first batch of Government Medical College, Srinagar, selected for MBBS in 1959.

In his article "My Days in GMC Srinagar" (*Greater Kashmir*, September 6, 2020), Dr. Mirza Ashraf Beig, recounting his days in GMC Srinagar, says, "On the first college Annual day in 1962, the college cultural body arranged a fascinating program in Tagore Hall. Dr. Bilqees Jamila, a third-year student then sang a song;

Aey jazbay dil ghar main chahoon
Har cheez muqabil aajayay—
Manzil ki taraf doo gam chaloon
Tou samney manzil aajayay.

The singer at the climax of her youth and prime of her beauty then has proved her mettle. She is one of the most successful gynecologists of the state. True to her oath and mission she proved herself to be what she dreamt to be." After her MBBS, Dr. Bilqees did her housemanship in gynecology and obstetrics and her postgraduation in the same subject in 1973. She worked under the patronship of two pillars of gynecology and obstetrics in Kashmir—namely, Dr. Girja Dhar and Dr. J. A. Naqshbandi. She regards both these women as the ones who have deeply inspired her. Dr. Bilqees was inducted into the faculty at Government Medical College only six months after her postgraduation. From the position of lecturer, she was promoted to various levels and finally became a professor. She became the head of the Department of Gynecology and Obstetrics in 1997 and retired from her position in 2000.

The Lal Ded Hospital of the '90s was a challenging place to work in. Understaffed and overburdened with peripheries collapsed, women had only Lal Ded Hospital to look up to. Dr. Bilqees stood there like a rock with her team and "delivered" the best that could be delivered under those trying circumstances. Lal Ded Hospital has a history of rising from the "deluge" and setting an example for the rest. Dr. Bilqees has been instrumental in setting that "standard" for this hospital. The staff at Lal Ded Hospital have braved odds and faced guns but never shut their doors to the hapless patients from all over Kashmir. We should give due credit to Dr. Bilqees for her role during those times.

While Dr. Bilqees worked in gynecology and obstetrics during the most difficult time of Kashmir's history, she did not stop delivering the best to the health care. Name a procedure she has not had success with, name an intervention that she did not try her hand at – this all when Kashmir was burning! Dr. Bilqees is a strong supporter of women's rights and the education of female folk. She works with many NGOs including the Voluntary Health Association of India to treat patients for free and distribute free medicines among patients. She has been vocal against female feticide and spoken against the practice of blaming women for fertility issues.

Dr. Bilqees loves to work and spends generously on charity. She has a very supportive family. Her husband is a pediatrician, and she has two sons, both doctors who live with their families abroad. She visits them frequently and loves to enjoy her time with her grandchildren.

When asked what made her so popular among people and why she continues to work even now, she had this to say: "I have worked very hard in my life. I used to be the first to reach the hospital and first to scrub so that I would get an opportunity to assist Dr. Girja and learn from her. I would keenly observe her and learn from her. I would move from ward to OR and OR to OPD, and work wherever I was needed. I would not have learnt so much had I not dutifully followed Dr. Girja and Dr. Naqshbandi. With age, you acquire more experience and your decisions become better, I do surgery better than I did 30 years back. I will work, till I can and when I can't I will stop."

Dr. Bilqees is happy and satisfied when she handles a difficult case. She loves it when she sees her patients being discharged from the hospital without any complications. One of the most memorable moments of her life has been when she conducted surgery on a woman who had an abdominal pregnancy, and decades later, when she had forgotten the case, the lady came to her OPD with her daughter, who was pregnant (she was the same child who had been delivered by Dr. Bilqees as a case of abdominal pregnancy)! A gratifying moment she proudly recalls when she conducted the delivery of this young woman!

Dr. Brij Mohan Bhan

Love him for he did not leave you!

When Srinagar was burning in the turmoil of '90s, an old surgeon in the vicinity of GMC Srinagar was examining his patients with care and compassion. This man was affluent, had no need for money—but was still running a clinic for the benefit of his patients. There was fear and uncertainty in Kashmir, and it had little to offer a man who had already reached the pinnacle of his career and retired from his services as the professor and head of the Department of Surgery, Government Medical College, Srinagar. His love for Kashmir kept him glued to it when most of his family members and members of his community left Kashmir. When his son asked him to leave his home, he confidently replied, "I have spent my good days with Kashmiri Muslims and I have no difficulty in spending my bad days with them." He would reassert that Kashmir is the birthplace of his ancestors, and he would love to live in Kashmir and serve the people of his motherland.

This son of soil braved the odds and kept the spirit of brotherhood and "service before self" alive. He was none other than Dr. Brij Mohan Bhan, a surgeon of eminence who served the people of Kashmir all his life. Dr. Bhan was one of the founding fathers of GMC and helped create a place where young surgeons were trained and their dreams were shaped into reality. I have never met him, I have never been taught by him—but even when I was a student of GMC, the imprints he left on the operating rooms of SMHS and its staff were evident as his students who taught us surgery would often mention him with respect and hold him in high esteem because of the profound impact he had in their training and nurturing.

Dr. Brij Mohan Bhan was born on July 16, 1931, in Gilgit. He did his MBBS in 1954 from Gujarat with a distinction in gynecology, ophthalmology, anatomy, and social and preventive medicine. Back home in Kashmir, he worked as an assistant surgeon in SMHS Hospital under Dr. Fazal Rehman. Subsequently, he did his FRCS from the Royal College of Surgeons of Edinburgh (UK) in 1959. He worked as a senior house officer, Ortho and Accident Surgery, in Coventry and Warwickshire, Coventry, England, under Dr. A. J. Watson. He was conferred FICS from the International College of Surgeons, Chicago (USA), in 1968. He was the founder member of Collegium Internationale Chirurgiae Digestiuae Rome (Italy) and founder fellow of the International Medical Sciences Academy, New Delhi. Although Dr. Bhan was a general surgeon, he was interested in gastroenterological problems. He was a keen researcher who worked on echinococcosis, Kangri cancer, ascariasis, etc. More than ten postgraduates completed their postgraduation under his mentorship.

Dr. Altaf Hussain, the eminent pediatrician of the valley, who was a student of first batch of GMC, has the following to say about Dr. Bhan: “Dr. Bhan was associated with the GMC right from its inception. After obtaining FRCS, he started his career in the GMC as a Lecturer in Anatomy in Aug 1959. He taught us Histology. Apart from being a competent teacher, he treated his students with great affection. When the first batch passed the first professional MBBS, we moved to study clinical subjects including surgery. Dr. Bhan joined the newly established department of surgery as an Assistant professor in 1961 and eventually rose to be the HOD surgery. He taught the first batch for all five years of our stay at the college----- the first 2 years of anatomy and the next 3 years of surgery. He is the first state subject to join the faculty of GMC. He contributed enormously to teaching, training and research activities in the dept of surgery, most of the leading surgeons of the state are his students."

Prof. Faroque Khan, famous pulmonologist from New York, who was also a student of the first batch, describes Dr. Bhan as "a young enthusiastic soft spoken faculty member, always well-dressed who showed great respect towards us which was reciprocated. I always had a great deal of respect for him, particularly in the manner he presented himself and the manner in which he dealt with the students—a true professional and a role model."

Prof. K. J. Qazi from Buffalo remembers Dr. Bhan as "a young energetic surgeon with relatively thick and large glasses, always immaculately dressed in suit and tie. His eyes were sharp and piercing which intimidated students and house staff. He was a little chubby with an easy smile which made him more adorable. He was sharp, inquisitive and had a stinging sense of humor. He treated patients and their families with respect which was not always the forte of surgeons at the time. He was an excellent teacher who commanded the attention (and respect) of the audience. I always enjoyed his jokes and light-heartedness. And, he was a great conversationalist."

At a time when Dr. Bhan could have chosen to work abroad, he chose the bicycle shed of GMC to teach not his speciality surgery but basic anatomy. The fact that he taught students for all five years with teaching classes lasting one to two hours speaks volumes about his dedication and commitment to medical teaching and education in Kashmir. Dr. Bhan's colored diagrams depicting anatomic details would impress his students and leave a lasting impact on their memory. Some of his illustrations, as his students recall, were better than the textbooks.

As a colleague, Dr. Bhan was cordial and cooperative. Prof. Mehmooda Khan, the renowned surgeon and former head of the Department of Surgery, GMC Srinagar, says, "On a personal front, I found Prof. Bhan was very cordial and kind to his junior colleagues and never interfered with the working of the other units in the Department. He would treat all with great respect and listen to the concern of his junior doctors and try to solve whatever problems they had. On the professional front, Prof. Bhan was a great and skilled surgeon. He gave his best to the patients and to the Kashmiri community. His patients had great trust in him, and reposed full faith in him to take care of all their health issues."

Dr. Hamid Band, in a Facebook post applauding this great surgeon, says, "His figure illustrating the subject on the blackboard and explaining everything in exquisite detail is unforgettable. I owe one of the greatest lessons to him. As an intern and second assistant during surgery, I was asked to hold two retractors and I did so cross-handed. He simply asked me to never cross-hand in surgery. I knew for sure, surgery was not my future."

Prof. Allaqaband, who has known Dr. Bhan for more than fifty years, rates Dr. Bhan as "a thorough gentleman, an excellent teacher and a very good clinician whose greatest quality was that he stayed back during those turbulent years serving patients." Dr. Bhan has been loved by all. This great son of soil deserved many medals and honors.

Dr. Bhan lives in the hearts and minds of the people of the valley. Dr. Bhan's legacy is preserved through skilled surgeons of international repute that the valley has produced—one of them is his brilliant son, the world-famous CVTS surgeon Dr. Anil Bhan. Out of so many incidents that Dr. Anil has to narrate about his father, this one really sends chills down one's spine: "When I was studying in Medical College, he had operated on a patient at the Srinagar Nursing Home and this patient had a gastrectomy and was bleeding. This patient's blood group was matching mine and he picked me up from home and took me to the blood bank. After collecting my blood he rushed to the hospital to transfuse and the patient did well after that."

Dr. Bhan braved Parkinson's disease for a long time and died peacefully with his family members around him in Delhi. He was married to Shiela Thussu -a soft hearted woman who supported Dr. Bhan through his trials and triumphs.

Dr. Farooq Ashai

A genius of sorts!

Dr. Farooq Ashai was born in Ashai Kocha, Fatehkadal, Srinagar, in 1938 to Mr. Ghulam Hassan Ashai and Taja Beebi. He belonged to a well-to-do and educated family known for their contribution toward education and community service. Dr. Ashai received his schooling from MP School, Srinagar. He studied in SP College and was a position holder in Matric and FSC exams. Dr. Ashai did his MBBS from Amritsar Medical College and was exceptionally bright. He did his MS in orthopedics from Patna Medical College, Bihar, under Dr. Mukhpadya, known as the father of orthopedics in India.

Dr. Ashai did his senior residency in Milwaukee, USA, and joined GMC Srinagar in 1964 as an assistant professor. He was deputed to Iran for two years by the government of India and worked there in a well-established hospital of Mashad.

Dr. Ashai upgraded the Department of Orthopedics at GMC Srinagar from a branch of general surgery to a full-fledged postgraduate orthopedic department. He was instrumental in creating separate Bone and Joint hospital at Barzulla with a separate ALC (Artificial Limb Center) Department. He was a versatile surgeon who started hip and knee replacement surgeries, arthroscopy, spinal fusion, anterolateral decompression of the spine, and improved the existing techniques. He treated all forms of trauma, especially the epidemic of trauma during early

1990s, which comprised of thousands of cases with blast injuries and bullet injuries. He would remain in campus to be available for patient care 24-7 when mass casualties would report to the hospital.

Dr. Ashai has authored a textbook of orthopedics for undergraduate students on common fractures and has published many papers in national and international journals. He organized an orthopedic conference in Srinagar in the early 1980s, which was a great success. He worked as a professor and HOD of Orthopedics and director of Artificial Limb Center (ALC), GMC Srinagar, for nineteen long years. He was a successful administrator and was able to handle the affairs of an important hospital in very critical times. Dr. Ashai was an excellent teacher, a master orator who taught in a very simple and easy language. His students loved him, and his lectures.

Dr. Ashai was a talented surgeon who pursued varied hobbies. He was a great lover of Indian classical music and Kashmiri folk songs. He himself used to play musical instruments like *tabla*, violin, and harmonium. He loved to interact with students and was actively involved in cultural programs of Silver Jubilee of GMC Srinagar. He was a great lover of nature and loved to go for trekking, water sports, and skiing. Landscaping was his passion too.

Besides being one of the famous orthopedic surgeons of North India and an excellent teacher, he had a mechanical mind as well. He started safe nonpollutant kerosene and gas room heaters (German technology) to replace old unsafe wooden *bukharis* of Kashmir. This time, these kerosene room heaters are used in all the cold places of India like Ladakh, Himachal Pradesh, areas of West Bengal, and Sikkim. The factory is now run by his son Zia Ashai- a mechanical engineer.

Dr. Ashai was a very humble and down-to-earth person. He always helped poor, needy, and downtrodden patients of far-flung areas of J&K. He was an active member of Voluntary

Medicare and used to go to far-flung villages to reach out to the needy patients along with other members of his team.

His family remembers him as a dependable head of the family, a caring husband, and a loving father. His students and staff remember him as an inspiring, clean-hearted soul with a broad vision. He was a well wisher of all his friends and relatives. He always wanted a peaceful and a lasting solution to the Kashmir problem without any bloodshed. Dr. Ashai tragically fell to a bullet just outside the hospital where he worked. He died in the same OT where he saved many lives. His wife intubated him, and his students tried to resuscitate him . . . all in vain. The gentleman left behind a devastated family and a traumatized staff on February 18, 1993, at 5:30 p.m. It took them decades to reconcile to the tragedy. More traumatic was the fact that the culprits could not be nabbed!

Dr. Fazal Rehman

A disciplinarian to the core!

I waited a good five years and contacted many people from Srinagar and Jammu to have a detailed information about Dr. Fazal Rehman. However, the information I got from the doctors and the people around did not add more to the information that is present in Dr. Mufti's book (*Kashmir in Sickness and in Health*, Partridge Publishing, pp. 197–198). Dr. Fazal Rehman was born in Mirpur in 1904. JK Medical Council website lists him at serial number 2 with an MBBS from KE Medical College, Lahore, in 1928. It further mentions him as an assistant surgeon, Grade Ist SMHS Hospital, and medical superintendent (MS) and surgeon at SMHS Hospital (the year of registration is mentioned as 1958). Dr. Fazal Rehman was awarded the Fellowship of Royal College of Surgeons (Edinburgh) in 1945. He was one of the first ones to acquire a postgraduate qualification in surgery.

Dr. Fazal Rehman worked as a surgeon specialist and superintendent at SMHS Hospital. Known for his discipline and punctuality, he made a model hospital out of SMHS Hospital. He would take morning and late-night rounds to the wards and stand with the matron of the hospital at the gates and watch the staff coming inside the hospital. Dr. Mufti says in his book that Dr. Fazal Rehman would never shout at people, but his looks would send a wave of fright and the wrong would instantaneously be corrected. Not only was the bedding of the inpatients sparkling, even beds were polished and cleaned. SMHS has yet to see discipline of that caliber and cleanliness of that order. The long-retired professors of GMC who were students those days fondly remember his contribution towards discipline and punctuality that he enforced at SMHS Hospital.

Dr. Fazal Rehman was a highly skilled surgeon who would never start his list late. He was a man of few words. He was an accurate and a safe surgeon, very meticulous in his job, knowing what he wants and getting exactly the same results. He would focus on asepsis and postoperative wound care. He was a master general surgeon and is regarded as the father of surgery in Kashmir.

Dr. Fazal Rehman was well built and well dressed, always took long walks, and actually walked from his home to his workplace. After his retirement, he left Srinagar with his wife, Dr. Iqbal Sawhney, and not many heard about him after this.

Dr. Ghulam Qadir Allaqaband

A teacher of teachers, a witty clinician!

There has been a doctor who has been associated with health care and medical education of the state so intimately that any description of health care and medical education in the state would be incomplete without making a mention of him. His clinical skills, teaching acumen, administrative capabilities, public influence, and image—all that he has accomplished would be a dream for any doctor working anywhere in the world. He has brought honor, glory, respect, and dignity to the profession of a doctor in Kashmir. It is not possible to sum up the contributions of Dr. Allaqaband toward health care and medical education in Kashmir because he has not only been associated closely with the birth of major medical institutions in the state but also contributed to medical education as a dedicated and committed master of clinical skills who merged science with art. He has influenced generations of doctors that Kashmir has produced.

Dr. Allaqaband was born in a below-average middle-class family in Kalaidoori Mohalla (Downtown), Srinagar. His father's name is Ghulam Hassan Shah (Allaqaband), who died two months before Dr. Allaqaband was born. Bright, inquisitive, and efficient, he was destined to be a leader from his early years. He received his schooling from Hamdaniya High School, Nawakadal, and did his matriculation from University of

Kashmir. He did his FSc from SP College and went to pursue his MBBS from Madras Medical College. As a student, he was taught by the best of the teachers who were impressed by his intelligence, sharp wit, and iron will to excel. He passed his MBBS examination with honors in 1959 and was influenced by his professor of medicine, Dr. R. Subramaniam. After his return from Chennai (then Madras), he was posted as a house surgeon in pediatrics at SMHS Hospital in 1960 and worked under Prof. Ali Jan, who was an "astute clinician and a hard task master." He was also posted with Prof. Naseer Ahmad Shah, who was very communicative and jovial.

Dr. Allaqaband qualified for the ECFMG examination and obtained a residency in the USA, and he left for the USA in 1960. After spending two years in New York and Johns Hopkins Hospital in Maryland, USA, he went to the UK to complete his postgraduate studies and qualified for MRCP London and MRCP Edinburgh in his first attempt—a unique thing those days, especially for a doctor from an underprivileged land. During his stay abroad, he worked in prestigious institutions like Brompton Hospital and the Institute of Chest and Heart Diseases in London.

Dr. Allaqaband came back to Kashmir and joined as an assistant professor of medicine in Government Medical College, Srinagar, in 1964. Prof. Ali Muhammad Jan had become a role model for Dr. Allaqaband when the latter joined the Department of Medicine. It is of note here that a young and bright clinician who had been trained in the best institutions of the world had found a role model in a clinician back home—rightly so, it speaks of the charisma and standing of Dr. Ali Jan as a clinician and an academician.

Dr. Allaqaband became the professor of medicine in 1969 and then the head of the Department of Medicine in 1980. In 1980, Professor Allaqaband became the administrator of associated hospitals of the valley. He worked on this post for six years, and during this period, the condition of most of the hospitals in Kashmir improved, and new hospitals were added. Hundred-bedded Women's Hospital became five-hundred-bedded Lal Ded Hospital, new Bone and Joint Hospital under the leadership of Prof. Farooq Ashai was established, Children's Hospital got expansion, and a new "Casualty Block" was constructed at SMHS Hospital. Apart from his administrative capabilities, his primary role as a physician and a teacher won him admirers among his students and his colleagues. Professor Allaqaband is rated as one of the best teachers by none other than the legendary Professor Khuroo, the famous hepatologist from Kashmir. Calling Dr. Allaqaband a "living legend," Professor Khuroo, in his tribute to the great teacher, says, "Dr. Allaqaband had several characteristics which qualified him to be an excellent teacher. His time schedule was to the dot. He had a wide knowledge of clinical medicine and was keen to impart this to his students. Contrary to our initial impression we found him approachable and he was always ready to interact with students, look at even personal problems and give advice for a solution. This made him a popular teacher amongst a wide student base." Dr. Allaqaband has been a very demanding teacher and did not settle for anything but the best from his students; no wonder, he with the cooperation of his colleagues, made Government Medical College a hub of knowledge and learning. It was under his careful guidance that the academic atmosphere in Government Medical College, Srinagar, was nourished and doctors of Kashmir were trained to be leaders of health care in the world. Dr. Allaqaband has always "practiced before he preached." In any discussion on any odd disease, on any odd day, Dr. Allaqaband would be the most well prepared, the most accurate, and the most meticulous of all clinicians. His keen eye would always pick up a finding invisible to the most, and his knowledge of diseases and their behavior would surprise any theorist. His rounds, case discussions, and mortality meet presentations have been unique and are the lessons that his students remember for a lifetime.

Dr. Allaqaband played a vital role when a tertiary care center at Soura was thought of. Together with Prof. Ali Jan, he advised and assisted the planners about the facilities to be made available at the Sheri-Kashmir Institute of Medical Sciences. He served as a vice chairman of Governing Body SKIMS and SKIMS Apical Selection Committee after the death of Prof. Ali Jan and contributed greatly towards making SKIMS a state-of-the art health-care institution and helped in recruiting competent faculty to the SKIMS.

Professor Allaqaband took over as principal of Government Medical College in 1992 and retired in 1994. It was a difficult time for any administrator as there was turmoil all around. He braved many odd situations but stayed firm in his resolve to serve Kashmir and its patients. He kept his clinic open in the worst of the situations and continued to work in a physician's role when most people at that stage would have preferred a hassle-free postretirement life. He doesn't shy away from books or turn away a patient. He, at this stage of his life, makes it to most of the medical conferences, seminars, or discussions held in Kashmir. Not only this, but he also has a wholesome involvement in everything that surrounds him. Dr. Allaqaband is sought in every spiritual *majlis*, in every seminar on ethics and religion, and is well respected in all social circles and loved not only by his patients but also by his students, colleagues, and his well wishers.

Dr. Allaqaband has played a very important role as a social activist. He has cared for the poor and downtrodden and openly spoken and acted against the social customs and called for a ban on "food wasting," advocating austerity, especially at the time of marriages. He is deeply religious and is influenced by Hazrat Sheikh Hamzah, the Sufi saint of Kashmir. He loves Iqbal and admires his vision of an ideal Muslim. While most of us just look at the superficial meaning of Iqbal's verses, Dr. Allaqaband seems to have lived his life as Iqbal's "Shaheen."

Floods of 2014, which hit Srinagar, devastated his clinic and home, but he stayed back assisting his people in those trying times through the organization "Care Kashmir," which he found for helping the deprived and poor of his land.

Dr. Allaqaband extended his generosity beyond Kashmir. His three children, all doctors, groomed by him, are well-known names in medicine in the US. His daughter Sumaira is a family physician, and her husband, Dr. Imtiaz Mekhri, is an ophthalmologist. His second daughter, Sabiha Raouf, is a well-known radiologist working as the chairperson of Radiology, Jamaica Medical Center, and her husband, Dr. Suhail Raouf, works as the chief of Pulmonary Medicine at Lenox Hill Hospital. His son Dr. Suhail Allaqaband is a well-known interventional cardiologist working in Milwaukee, Wisconsin. His daughter-in-law Masarat Mushtaq, a qualified software engineer, has opted to be full-time mother and affectionate wife. His wife, Sardara Parveen, has been a woman of substance supporting Dr. Allaqaband in all the challenging endeavors that he undertook.

Dr. Allaqaband sees his life as a challenge full of trials and tribulations, which he has led to his satisfaction. The greatest influence on his life has been the personality of Prophet Muhammad (saw). And faith in Allah is what keeps him going! He is proud of his humble background, his affectionate wife, and his bright children. Dr. Allaqaband has led a successful life and helped to build foundations of health care and medical education in Kashmir. His deep affection for his people is reflected in the untiring service that he has rendered to them.

Dr. Allaqaband has influenced physicians of all eras in Kashmir. His teaching skills and his understanding of medicine makes him a legend. His mind is sharp, his memory is awesome, and his skill to diagnose and treat people is unmatched. He has now taken it upon himself to educate masses about common

Dr. Ghulam Rasool

A skilled surgeon

Dr. Ghulam Rasool was born in 1912 in Srinagar. His father was Mian Muhammad Iqbal. Dr. Ghulam Rasool passed his FSc from SP College, Srinagar, and completed his MBBS at KE Lahore–Punjab University (1933–1938). He was married to Ruqaya on September 15, 1939.

After graduation from KE Medical College, Dr. Ghulam Rasool was unable to get a job in government service in the J&K State. He joined a missionary hospital, which is the current Drugjan Chest Hospital, and worked with Dr. Waras, who stimulated his interest in surgery. An unexpected opening in J&K Service led to his joining the J&K Service, but this did not last. He lost this job and once again went back to missionary hospital. Finally, for the second time, he joined J&K Service and worked at SMHS Hospital, which I am told at that time was in a different location in Lal Mandi, Srinagar.

Dr. Ghulam Rasool was then transferred to Skardu, and, after an arduous journey on horseback, Dr. Ghulam Rasool, his young wife, and three children reached Shardu, where he worked long hours and obtained great surgical skills and speed with limited support and the unskilled staff that he had to improvise—for example, he performed C-section on a patient with a house knife, scissors, and silk thread. The woman survived and used to visit him for many years after that.

After one year in Skardu, Dr. Ghulam Rasool was transferred to Gilgit, and his family wanted to visit relatives in Srinagar before leaving for Gilgit—that was August 1947. The conflict over Kashmir resulted in the establishment of a line of control, the division of Jammu and Kashmir State, and Dr. Ghulam Rasool's life, like so many others at that time and afterward, was changed forever. Had they not come for a family reunion to Srinagar, they would have been in Gilgit, and employees in Gilgit at that time became part of the Pakistan Civil Service.

He was sent on deputation to the UK by the Government of Jammu and Kashmir and obtained his FRCS in 1957. He was the first one from Kashmir to do so in the surgical field. After his return, Dr. Ghulam Rasool and his contemporary, Dr. Girdhari Lal, became the two leading surgeons in Kashmir—competitors who respected each other greatly and ruled the surgical wards 15–20 in SMHS.

As a surgeon, Dr. Ghulam Rasool was up-to-date, innovative, and a fast operator. He was the first one to report "Kangri cancer"—unique only to Kashmiris. His gastrectomy procedure was a treat to watch, as was his surgery on the thyroid. His assistants always remembered his deep, penetrating, and fixed glare of his bright eyes that showed through his thick glasses. His special interest in thyroid had earned him the nickname "Hashimoto." I remember, as a surgical clerk, watching in awe as he removed a huge hydatid cyst of the liver in a young woman from Ladakh under local anesthesia. Because of his speed, he was able to perform twelve to fifteen surgeries a day. He was blessed with a healing hand, and his patients made a miraculous recovery.

The two surgical leaders soon had to face the reality of having to deal with the challenges posed by the beginning of the new "GMC." There were new bosses to deal with—Professor Khanna was the new chair of Surgery, and Dr. Ghulam Rasool was the associate professor. It must have been hard on them. However, Dr. Ghulam Rasool rose to the challenge and eventually became the HOD of the Surgical Department. His tenure at SMHS was marked by the cadre of young staff who took a deep interest in the field of surgery, and many of them developed into leaders in their own fields. Dr. Ghulam Rasool was responsible for the idea of having a separate bone and joint hospital, pediatric and women's hospitals, and was involved in the initial planning of the Soura Institute as well.

Dr. Ghulam Rasool was a man of simple habits. He, for many years, used to ride to SMHS on his bicycle, and, on occasion as a medical student, I drove past him. Eventually, a family car was purchased, and it was always a sight to see—Dr. and Mrs. Ghulam Rasool and their six children riding in the car, a Fiat. Dr. Ghulam Rasool's driving skills, however, were not at par with his surgical skills. Dr. Ghulam Rasool was very much involved in his professional work. Managing or being involved in the affairs of the house was not in his personality. His wife did that job superbly. Then there was the issue of his temper. He had, as we would say in the States, a short fuse, and smart employees learned to keep their distance during these outbursts. As an administrator, he was hardworking, honest, and a strict disciplinarian who took a keen interest in every aspect of hospital affairs. During his tenure, the SMHS was spick-and-span, visiting hours were respected (once, he turned out his own son, who was visiting his friend in the hospital off hours), and food was of high quality (once, he beat up the milkman who had added water to milk).

He was not very astute politically and did not curry favors with his "bosses," for which, on several occasions, he paid a heavy price. His children performed exceptionally well in academics, and when they got involved in political life as students, Dr. Ghulam Rasool had to pay the price. He was twice transferred to Jammu because of the political activism of his son Aijaz and daughter Abida.

After over thirty years of distinguished service, Dr. Ghulam Rasool retired on August 19, 1973, and he lived a retired life for over two decades. This time was spent mostly with his children, who, by then, had settled in several parts of the world—Zahida, a pediatrician, in New York; Arfa, a radiologist, in New York; Abida, a physicist by training and a businesswoman by vocation, in Saudi Arabia; Rabia, a pathologist, in New York; Aijaz, an engineer, in Kashmir; and Ayaz, a urologist, in New York, who inherited his dad's surgical skills. Dr. Ghulam Rasool was married fifty-five years to Ruqaya Rasool. He left this world in 1994.

In summary, Dr. Ghulam Rasool led a productive, meaningful life. He made major contributions to the medical profession. In the Islamic tradition, it is mentioned that a person who leaves behind a pious child who prays for the deceased parents or an institution of learning will continue to be rewarded even after his death. Dr. Ghulam Rasool certainly did that . . . He left behind a legacy and an ocean of goodwill. Most importantly, he left behind a devoted family who continues in the traditions he left behind.

(Prof. Faroque A. Khan)

Dr. Girdhari Lal Kaul

A surgical genius!

Dr. Girdhari Lal Kaul was the son of Shri Gana Lal Kaul and the younger brother of Dr. Gwash Lal Kaul. He studied at SP College, Srinagar. He did his MBBS from Lahore in 1930 and FRCS from Edinburgh in 1958–59. He was one of the pillars of surgical practice in the valley and worked for the benefit of the poor and needy (*Glimpses of Kashmir*, R. K. Sopori).

Dr. Gulzar Mufti, in his book *Kashmir in Sickness and in Health*, calls Dr. Girdhari Lal Kaul a well-nourished Kashmiri man and further describes him in these words: "Girdhari Lal was more like Sir Lancelot Spratt of Doctor series of the films, a man larger than life who always arrived with an entourage of people ahead, round and behind him." He further says, "He was a general surgeon who could tackle anything, be it orthopedics, abdomen or neurosurgery. Many years later, I saw him lift depressed fractures of the skull, and perform open reduction of fractures and bone grafting and yet he could demonstrate and teach a classic open removal of the prostate (Freyer's prostatectomy). Gall bladder removal was his favorite operation. He was a generous man who loved good food and living." Dr. Kaul was a chain smoker who smoked Gold Flake incessantly.

Dr. Mufti has narrated an incident in his book in which Dr. Girdhari Lal's capability to handle stress and to help a panting younger colleague by his innovative surgical expertise is beautifully described. He helped him to find the appendix by modifying the incision he had made and walked away confidently to the surprise of the youngster calling it "Kaul's incision."

In his practice, he sometimes faced competition with his physician brother Dr. Gwash Lal as patients would be swapped between the two brothers by people; if the patient wouldn't get well with one brother, he would be taken to another. Dr. Girdhari Lal Kaul was a keen golfer and died in 1987.

Dr. Girja Dhar

The woman with a mission!

The dark night had set in, and there was a young assistant surgeon in her twenties, bubbling with enthusiasm and energy, looking after the maternity ward of SMHS Hospital. Three of her patients were sick, in fact in shock needing fluids and blood transfusion. The young doctor had a limited supply of intravenous fluids and blood but used all resources she had and saved three precious lives. As the night passed by and the morning sun smiled at her, she was eager to tell her story to her seniors and to get a pat on her back. Nothing of that sort happened; she was rebuked for having used all the fluids and blood, as whatever was in store was supposed to be used for the next day's patients who were to be operated upon. Her senior rebuking her on morning rounds said to her, "I am operating tomorrow. What do I use if my patients need fluid and blood? My patients might die tomorrow on the table." The witty and enthusiastic young doctor replied, "Madam, your patient might die tomorrow, but the ones I looked after would have been dead already." Her reply surprised her senior and her own self too. How did she get the courage to do what was right and then defend her decision to save three lives?

A few days later in her OPD, this young doctor was perturbed to see three young women who were disowned by their families. After consulting her seniors, she was asked by her seniors to write in their OPD cards that their condition was inoperable and advise some placebos. These women were suffering from a condition named vesicovaginal fistula, which was an embarrassing situation where a woman had an abnormal connection with the bladder resulting in dribbling of urine and offensive smell. These women had become social outcasts for their odor and stench. Each time they would come to the OPD, it was painful for her to see these devastated women, physically disabled, who had no hope of a future family or a reproductive life. The young doctor would be upset and wanted to do something for them. She would frequently ask herself why there were so many such cases in Kashmir and what could be done to prevent their occurrence. She knew if the antenatal care was good and trained medical professionals conducted deliveries, fistulas could be prevented. For patients already suffering from the disease, she wanted relief. She wanted to help them, learn new techniques wherever those were available, and apply them to the distressed patients back home. She chose to fly to the UK and learn new techniques in the most advanced centers to help these patients and to upgrade the standard of care available to patients with obstetric and gynecological problems in a remote place that was her home. This doctor lived her dream. She was Dr. Girja Dhar, the woman of grit and determination who was instrumental in giving Kashmiri women the first maternity hospital, which till date has been a benchmark for the treatment of gynecological and obstetric-related problems in Kashmir.

Dr. Girja Dhar was born into a middle-class Kashmiri Pandit family in Safa Kadal, Srinagar, on May 25, 1934. She received her early education from a government girls' school in Downtown Srinagar. She would never boast but called herself a mediocre student, who was more interested in sports than studies. She received her MBBS from King George Medical College, Lucknow. She served for a short while in Srinagar, but with an urge to perfect herself and help distressed women back diseases and health issues confronting people through videos and Facebook posts. The legends of medicine and allied specialities who have worked with Dr. Allaqaband or have been taught by him inherit his analytical skills and his methods to reach a diagnosis. Dr. Noor Ali, the famous neurologist, proudly accepts this!

home, she went to the UK, earned FRCS and MRCOG, and came back to Kashmir five years later in 1964 and served as an assistant professor of gynecology and obstetrics at Government Medical College, Srinagar. She married Dr. Syed Naseer Ahmad Shah, a clinician of repute, known for his contribution to medicine in Kashmir. The exposure she got in UK hospitals helped her to face the challenges awaiting her in Kashmir. Back home, she literally chased all those socially outcast women with vesicovaginal fistulas and successfully corrected their ailment with surgical intervention. She had learned the art of repair from one of the experts in the UK named Dr. Chessarmoir, whom *British Medical Journal* (1977) described as "a great gentleman; a man who did more than anyone living today to save the lives and relieve the miseries of women." Getting trained under him gave her much-needed confidence. She not only corrected the physical ailment of her patients but also helped them to go back to their families and rehabilitated them socially. Most of these women were otherwise abandoned by their families. Dr. Girja would fondly remember her patients by name and helped a few of them to find employment and have an independent existence.

Dr. Girja reframed the guidelines for antenatal care in her department. She ensured that patient care met international standards. She was a tough taskmaster who would never compromise on hygiene, asepsis, and careful monitoring of patients. She was a skilled surgeon and had a great clinical acumen. Lal Ded Hospital was her brainchild. It flourished under her wings. As the head of the department, she was instrumental in training undergraduates, and also trained generations of gynecologists and obstetricians who served not only in Kashmir but also worked in every nook and corner of the world. The quality of postgraduates in gynecology and obstetrics was of a high standard as they were getting trained under the watchful eye of Dr. Girja Dhar and her other colleagues.

While the entire Kashmir remains indebted to Dr. Girja for establishing and improving gynecological and obstetric care in Kashmir, she played a bigger role as an administrator in the midst of turmoil. She took over as principal and dean, Government Medical College, Srinagar, from Dr. Syed Zahoor Ahmad and continued in this position till 1992. She was the principal of GMC Srinagar when everything was in a disarray. When all the educational institutions of Kashmir Valley were closed, GMC Srinagar was the only institution working. She took a very bold initiative of keeping the college open when it was more convenient to let it be closed. Curfew passes were issued to students and staff, and special buses would ply for them. All hospitals remained operational, and the emergency staff was provided accommodation and food within the hospital. Examinations were held regularly, and teaching continued uninterrupted. Existing staff was taken into confidence to compensate for the deficiency that resulted because of migration. She taught the world how medical education can continue amid turmoil and how doctors can continue to be churned out amid the chaos. In her overenthusiasm to help medical education and health care, she risked her life. She exhibited boldness and sanity when it was needed the most.

After her retirement, her administrative ability was tested further when she served as the chairperson of JK Public Service Commission and JK Women's Commission. She was actively involved in philanthropy and gave a lot back to the community, which showered her with love and affection.

When we look at the enthusiasm with which our young girls take up medicine as a profession, we remember the likes of Professor Girja and Prof. Mehmooda Khan, who led a caravan of medical professionals showing a path that women had not dared to tread, fighting the taboos, lighting up the candles of knowledge, and pushing the brave and bold toward perfection.

Dr. Girja belonged to a class who served their community selflessly, not making fortunes, not building empires, but leaving behind a legacy of commitment and dedication, leaving behind institutions of excellence that were nurtured with the sweat and blood of the dedicated lot. Her life is a lesson. There is a lot one can do for one's community—even when the odds are against you! Along the banks of Dal, she breathed her last on July 13, 2018, barely a few months after her husband's death. She is survived by her daughter, Dr. Tina Anjila Shah, who lives in the UK with her husband and son and fondly rekindles the memory of her parents by organizing health camps, orations, and awareness talks in the honor of her illustrious parents.

PS. I met Dr. Girja a year before she died, and she spoke to me in detail about her life and mission. She seemed satisfied with her life, but before I left her, she expressed concern about the rising number of cesarean sections and the horrifying number of hysterectomies in Kashmir. Someone, kindly take a note!

Dr. Govind Lal Vaishnavi

The great founder!

It was an amazing discovery for me. I thank Facebook for helping me discover the founding father of health care in Kashmir—namely, Dr. G. L. Vaishnavi. I had read in books about him, but there were hardly any credible details about the era in which he worked and the role he played as an expert doctor and administrator. Miracles of modern technology leave you amazed! While searching for Dr. G. L. Vaishnavi on the internet, I saw a post on Facebook by a young artist, Pragnya Wakhlu, who had posted a picture of her great-grandfather—namely, Dr. G. L. Vaishnavi. I quickly jumped onto the post and messaged Pragnya.

Day one, no response. Day two, no response . . . I thought I would just get a hold of the picture and nothing else. Nearly two weeks later, I again checked the Messenger. And this time, to my delight, there was a response. She wanted to know why I wanted the details about her great-grandfather. I stated my purpose of writing about him in my book. She kindly connected me to her mother, Anu Wakhlu, who sent me a treasure. All respect to the one who has written those precious words and all respect to the ones who have preserved them and regards and love to the ones who sent them to me. There were nearly a century-old papers—photographed with care and sent to me in my email. A brief account of the contributions of Dr. Vaishnavi and his biodata. This is perhaps the first properly made CV of a Kashmiri doctor. The CV deserves a place in our archives.

Dr. G. L. Vaishnavi was born in November 1899 at Srinagar. He was the son of Thakurjee Vaishnavi. He lost his mother very early and graduated in medicine from Punjab University in 1925. He joined the Kashmir government service in early 1925 and went to Great Britain in 1927 for postgraduate training in surgery and training in the diseases of the eye, ear, nose, and throat. He did FRCS from Edinburgh in 1930 and returned to Kashmir after successfully completing the training. He worked as a medical officer, Saddar Hospital, for three years and was promoted to the level of chief medical officer in 1935. He worked as an eye, ear, nose, and throat specialist, Saddar Hospital, Srinagar, for two years. In 1941, he became assistant director of medical services and held the post of "Palace Surgeon" till 1943. He was appointed as director of medical services, Jammu and Kashmir—a post that he held till 1950. He was responsible for the technical supervision of all the civil and military hospitals of the state. There was hardly a field where he did not exercise his influence and control. In addition to this, he was in charge of public health, jails, and even meteorological departments of Jammu and Kashmir. He was responsible for the implementation and expansion of many schemes pertaining to the working of medical and health departments of the state.

As a chief medical officer, he formulated the scheme of district medical administration. He prepared a scheme for rural sanitation. He managed many epidemics and formulated control measures for managing cholera, typhus, and other epidemics ravaging Kashmir. He managed immunizations and inoculations. In 1935 and 1937, about 75 percent of the valley's population was inoculated against cholera under his supervision, thus creating a record. Under his supervision, the existing hospitals in Srinagar and Jammu were expanded, and the bed capacity was increased. The then viceroy Lord Wavel, when he inaugurated the hospital, praised Dr. Vaishnavi for his work. He expanded medical and health departments from curative and preventive aspects. Although Dr. Gwash Lal Kaul and Dr. Vaishnavi were contemporaries, Dr. K. K. Kaul, Dr. Gwash Lal's son, has the following to say about Dr. Vaishnavi: "He was my specialist in childhood for my chronic Otorrhea. He did his Diploma in Otorhinolaryngology and DOMS from England, he joined the service early and was permanently senior to my father. Their relations were cordial though they were seen as rivals."

Dr. Vaishnavi was one of the first to frame a plan by which dispensaries and health units were opened at a distance of five miles radius in the whole of Jammu and Kashmir and equipped them with the necessary machines and trained medical staff. He was responsible for the creation of posts of epidemiologists for Jammu and Kashmir so that epidemics spreading in Jammu and Kashmir could be handled in a scientific manner. In his tenure as director medical services, he got an "Infectious Disease Hospital" sanctioned by the government. Under his directions, lunatic asylum was named the mental hospital at Srinagar. He was also responsible for the establishment of Preventable Diseases Bureau at Srinagar and Jammu, respectively. Dr. Vaishnavi was responsible for launching antivenereal disease drive and expansion of TB hospital from twenty beds to one hundred beds. He was responsible for reorganization of jails in Jammu and Kashmir and compilation of Kashmir Jail Manual.

In 1950, he was appointed as assistant director, General Health Services, government of India, New Delhi, and held the charge till 1954, when he was selected as chief medical officer, Calcutta Port Trust. As assistant director, General Health Services, he prepared the administration report of Health Government of India. He was also dealing with the administrative affairs of Medical Council of India, Dental Council of India, Indigenous System of Medicine, and medical departments of all the centrally administered areas of India. He was also involved in constitution of medical examination rules and framing rules of medical boards. Dr. Vaishnavi can thus be termed as the most influential and most powerful medical administrator of his time who had a pan-India influence. He retired from this post in 1957 and was reemployed by the Jammu and Kashmir Government in 1960 to improve the administration at SMHS Hospital and worked directly under the health minister of the state. He served in this capacity till 1961, took retirement, and died in New Delhi on March 31, 1977. He was seventy-eight.

Dr. Gwash Lal Kaul

A Qalandar physician!

I have heard about him from my parents and teachers but did not know how to trace his roots as I wanted to write in detail about this son of the soil who was the first MRCP from Kashmir. My only source about Dr. Gwash Lal was a few articles on him by his doctor son, Dr. K. K. Kaul. Incidentally, I came across a book too by Dr. K. K. Kaul titled *When My Valley Was Green*, which gave a detailed account of his family, the times he lived in, and his work in Kashmir as a qualified physician with a Western degree. Building a rough draft based on the articles and the book, I sent the draft to Dr. Allaqaband, and he pointed out a few mistakes and asked me to get into contact with Dr. K. K. Kaul. He purchased Dr. Kaul's book and got in contact with him before I could contact him and told him about my initiative. Dr. Kaul was kind enough to send me a few articles about Dr. Gwash Lal Kaul, which provided me with a great deal of information about him. He sent me a few old memorable photos of his father and himself. I could not have asked for more!

Dr. Gwash Lal was born in 1900 at Fateh Kadal, Narpirastan, Srinagar. He was the second of six brothers and graduated in 1920s from King Edward Medical College in Lahore. In Lahore, as his son recounts, he would often visit Sir Muhammad Iqbal. He had great love and respect for Dr. Iqbal and sometimes would wait patiently for his attention as Dr. Iqbal would be in his deep thoughts unaware of his presence, but later when he would see him, he would feel apologetic toward him. There was a bit of Kashmir in Dr. Iqbal too as his ancestors were Kashmiri Pandits of the "Sapru" dynasty, and he would welcome Dr. Gwash Lal.

Dr. Gwash Lal was the first Kashmiri physician and one of the few in the country to qualify and obtain the MRCP from the prestigious Royal College of Physicians, London. On return from England, he was appointed as medical officer, Civil Hospital, situated at Hazuribagh, serving as the senior physician and physician to Maharaja Hari Singh in 1931. His contemporaries at that time were Dr. G. L. Vaishnavi (an ENT specialist) and Dr. S. L. Karihaloo (a specialist in Chest Diseases Hospital, Srinagar).

Dr. Gwash Lal was the most sought-after physician of his time. Dr. K. K. Kaul has written about a book by Mr. Arif Baig in Urdu titled *Niyari Yaadein* in which he has dedicated one chapter to Dr. Gwash Lal Kaul. I was told that Dr. K. K. Kaul's son, who is a professor of pediatric gastroenterology at Cincinnati Medical Center in United States, and Mr. Baig's grandson incidentally met at a hospital, and while discussing their common origin, junior Dr. Kaul came to know that Dr. Baig's grandfather had written a chapter in a book about Dr. Gwash Lal. He handed over a copy of the book to Dr. Kaul. The book is beautifully written in chaste Urdu, and Dr. K. K. Kaul was kind enough to share the chapter about Dr. Gwash Lal with me. Mr. Baig seems to be a fan of Dr. Gwash Lal and was greatly impressed by his knowledge and clinical acumen. Mr. Baig talks about the use of unconventional approach by Dr. Gwash Lal at times that cured many of his patients. Mr. Baig narrates the story of a relative's child who was diagnosed as having a perforated appendix, and Dr. Gwash Lal surprised everyone by asking the child to be put in an ice-filled tub. The boy is said to have recovered after this treatment.

Dr. Gwash Lal was a multifaceted personality who was in love with Urdu and Kashmiri poetry and would be seen in the company of seers and saints. He had a passion for Kashmiri Sufiana music and was fond of Mohammad Abdullah Tibatbaqaal, the santoor master; Sanaullah Sahib, the rabab master; and Pandit Satlal, the sitar maestro. Sonabab or Swami Sonakakji once asked Dr. Gwash Lal to carry firewood on his head and walk through a busy market, apparently to teach him the value of humility and to shun his ego forever, which he did gladly.

Though there is a lot of information in the book about his spiritual pursuits, not much information is there about his role as a physician specialist. Dr. K. K. Kaul has narrated some interesting anecdotes about his father when he was a physician to Maharaja.

Dr. Nazir Ahmad Dhar, however, in his article about the treatment of diabetes in Kashmir, says, "In early 40's, leading London trained physician returned to the valley named Dr. Gwash Lal, Dr. Gwash Lal understood diabetes very well and introduced blood sugar monitoring in addition to urine testing in SMHS Hospital. Dr. Mir Ali Muhammad Captain joined him in SMHS Hospital. They hospitalized the 'sugar' patients to monitor blood sugar with insulin and diet control and educated them about diabetes as little was known about diabetes those days. It would not be wrong to say that they were the first diabetologists of Kashmir. In late '40s during the tenure of Dr. Gwash Lal 'Hoaki-si-li' as the diabetes was called that time was replaced by the new English name of 'sugar' rather than diabetes" (*Greater Kashmir*, 2015, Dr. Nazir Ahmad Dar, "History of Hoaki-si-li in Kashmir"). However, this information was refuted by many of the older physicians who were of the opinion that Dr. Gwash Lal did not work at SMHS Hospital but at a hospital in Nawakadal. Prof. Ashraf Mir, the son of Capt. Ali Mohammad, also gave the information that his father worked with Dr. Gwash Lal.

Dr. Gwash Lal used to dress up like an Englishman in a three-piece suit. His way of clinical practice was largely influenced by English education and culture. He was perhaps one of the first to "cure" vitamin B deficiency by the use of Kanz, made from washing rice in a big earthen pot with added Ajwain, muth, and peppermint. Dr. Gwash Lal was one of the costliest doctors of his time, charging Rs 5 as a consultation fee (*Pen Pricks*, October 12, 2020).

Dr. Gwash Lal, one of the first physicians of Kashmir, needs to be remembered for his role in introducing the art and practice of medicine in a place that hardly had any doctors. His work on diabetes and vitamin deficiencies cured by locally available cocktails is indeed a work worthy of mention. Dr. Gwash Lal Kaul has been described by Dr. Gulzar Mufti as the first Kashmiri to introduce and establish the speciality of General Medicine in the valley and was perhaps the first Kashmiri "physician specialist."

Dr. Hafizullah

An admirable Hakim!

Dr. Hafizullah was born in Srinagar in 1917 in the family of Hakims. His father, late Hakim Ahmadullah (Amma Hakim), was a well-known legendry Unani physician. He was the most famous *hakeem* of his time and was also the chief *Unani* physician to the Maharaja of Jammu and Kashmir. He had an elder brother, Dr. Qudratullah, who had done his degree in Unani medicine and was the principal of Unani College Srinagar but passed away at a young age.

Dr. Hafizullah had his schooling from Islamia High School, Srinagar, and did his FSc.from SP College, Srinagar. He obtained his degree in medicine (MBBS) from King Edward Medical College, Lahore, affiliated to the University of Punjab in 1939. After completion of his studies in Lahore, he joined as a medical officer in the State Health Services and was posted in the famed dispensary at Mahrajganj, Srinagar. He worked in various other places in Srinagar and also as a health officer of Srinagar Municipality. He also worked in the Tangmarg Hospital and Sanatorium, where he developed an interest in treating patients of tuberculosis. After serving in the State Health Services for ten years, he went to England to pursue his training in medicine He worked in England for some time and went to the USA for a fellowship in pulmonary and chest medicine in Delaware, USA. On his return to Kashmir, he was appointed as a specialist in

Chest Disease Hospital, Srinagar, where he was elevated as the medical superintendent. He started his practice in Zainakadal at his home and would see patients at Dalgate as well.

Dr. Hafizullah had a passion for serving poor patients. He was one of the first doctors of the state to go after Tuberculosis the killer disease of that time and aimed to defeat it. He was totally committed to his patients and would keep a track of them and listen to them carefully and passionately. He took the initiative for the establishment of TB clinics at Kupwara, Watal Kadal, Anantnag, and Tangmarg. He was an active member and an important office bearer of the Tuberculosis Association of India, besides being a member of the expert committee on tuberculosis program at the Ministry of Health, Government of India. He represented India at the International Expert Meeting in Rome in 1960 and the WHO World Congress in Geneva as a part of the Indian delegation in 1961. He was instrumental in completely revamping the patient care services of Chest Disease Hospital and provided surgical facilities in the hospital. He was closely associated with the establishment of Government Medical College, Srinagar, and was an excellent teacher. He was responsible for elevating the Chest Disease Hospital to the level of one of the best hospitals for chest medicine in North India. He provided mentorship to doctors after their specialization, and they would find it a privilege to work in the said hospital. Dr. G. Q. Allaqaband, Dr. R. K. Zutshi, and others worked at Chest Disease Hospital under the mentorship of Dr. Hafizullah. For some period, he was transferred to Jammu Chest Disease Hospital. When he returned to CD Hospital, Srinagar, he was also assigned the responsibility of planning and starting of the chest and tuberculosis care as the state tuberculosis officer.

Dr. Hafizullah passed away at a young age in an airplane crash over Banihal Pass in 1966. On his sad demise, the entire Kashmir plunged into gloom. Kashmir mourned a doctor who would treat with care, passion, sympathy, and love. He had left his people too early . . .. . He is remembered for his contribution as a chest specialist and for being humble, polite, and caring for poor patients. His clinical diagnosis was accurate and his teaching beyond doubt excellent. He not only was a great chest physician but also had achieved an enviable social stature, as he was a household name in Kashmir. He would keep himself updated with the latest advances in medicine and would apply this knowledge in patient care. Dr. Hafizullah received wide fame as a specialist not only in Jammu and Kashmir but also in Northern India.

(The profile is contributed by Dr. Muzaffar, ex-director, Health Services Kashmir, his nephew.)

Dr. Hamid Ali Durrani

A lover of art!

I had been introduced to Dr. Durrani during my student days when he would take our clinical class in medicine and teach us history taking and clinical examination. Well-dressed, soft-spoken, and sophisticated, he would also talk to us about the common gastroenterological problems in Kashmir and about his research on gastric cancer. In my postgraduate research on gastric cancer, I came across a few credible widely quoted papers by him on the pattern of gastric cancer in Kashmir. For many years afterward, I did not hear about him. My interest in Dr. Durrani was rekindled as I sought to know about his contribution to health care in Kashmir. One of my dear professors got in touch with him, and he agreed to give me his CV. I received a neat two-page handwritten note in my WhatsApp one fine morning summing up his work primarily in gastroenterology at SMHS Hospital, Srinagar. I know Dr. Durrani lived in an era when CV making was not much in vogue. Excited to see his note, I asked a question, "What are your interests, sir"? He wrote back, "Field cricket, brush painting, Urdu poetry, gardening and photography . . .". Just as everybody else has . . . . . .I thought, and I forgot about it till the next morning arrived . . ..

And it was a brighter and better morning! I received innumerable photos of flowers, extremely beautiful paintings depicting birds, flowers, and trees, in addition to hundreds of photos related to his work and involvement in the activities at Government Medical College, Srinagar. I had found a treasure house, I thought. My friends, my colleagues, and my family—all of us were excited to have a wholesome treat. What surprised me the most was the fact that the paintings he sent were made in COVID time (2021) and some in 2022. Imagine a man painting birds and flowers at an age when most of us lose interest in life. Also, Dr. Durrani is not a painter by profession but by passion. I was lost for words. He asked again, "Shall I send you my poetry?" "Why not!" I replied. The ultimate arrived with the arrival of his couplets, his *Nazams* and *Ghazals.* Written in chaste Lucknowi Urdu, I turned to Urdu experts for interpretation. This overflow of creativity at this age was enough to make a hero out of Dr. Durrani for me till I remembered I was writing about his contribution to health care . . .

Dr. Hamid Ali Durrani was born on March 7, 1934, at Ballia, UP, to Mr. Nadir Ali Khan Durrani and Hamida Begum. He did his matric in 1948 from GHS, Ballia, and studied further at Lucknow Christian College. He was bright and talented and sought admission at the prestigious King George Medical College (KGMC) for MBBS in 1952, which he completed in 1956. He completed his MD in internal medicine from KGMC, where he met his future wife, Dr. Massarat, a beautiful Kashmiri girl pursuing her studies at KGMC. He joined the faculty at SMHS Hospital, Srinagar, in 1966 as an assistant professor. He rose to the level of professor and retired as the professor and chief of Gastroenterology, SMHS Hospital, in 1992.

Dr. Durrani became one of the most active and most sought-after faculty members of GMC. In his handwritten note, he says, "While studying at Lucknow, Dr. Girja Dhar and myself were exposed to extracurricular activities which made a big change in our lives and we introduced such activities for our students at GMC. Srinagar. We received tremendous support from Principal GMC. Prof. Naseer Ahmad Shah, resulting in the formation of CASS Union (Cultural, Academic, Sports and Social Union). This gave the students a handy platform to exhibit their talent in diverse fields. The student's response was excitement and exuberating." If we trace the archives of GMC Srinagar, Dr. Durrani is an essential part of all the celebrations, functions, and sports activities of an era when GMC Srinagar was known for these activities.

Dr. Durrani is credited with introducing gastroenterology and endoscopy to Kashmir. He says, "The story of Gastroenterology and endoscopy starts with the heritage endoscope with the light bulb at the tip." Dr. Durrani received fellowship in gastroenterology from the US and one-year fellowship in gastroenterology from the University of Toronto, Canada. Dr. Durrani was instrumental in organizing a National Conference on Gastroenterology in GMC Srinagar, which was a great success. In 1984, Dr. Durrani was actively involved in organizing the "Silver Jubilee Celebration of GMC" that lasted for a week.

His love for his Kashmiri doctor wife, Dr. Massarat, brought him to Kashmir, and he fell in love with Kashmir and its beauty. He worked hard for uplifting the standards of education and extracurricular activities at GMC Srinagar. He runs his private clinic in Srinagar and continues to see the patients there. His children are settled in the US, but after the death of his dear wife, he continues to visit Kashmir and lives in his home. When one of his friends asked him, "Durrani Sahib, why don't you stay with your brothers and other sibs in Lucknow and Aligarh?" In his gentle voice, he replied, "I love Kashmir, cannot stay away from it for long. This is my home." We know that GMC Srinagar has been his second home . . . Dr. Durrani expresses his gratitude to all in these words: "I put on record my gratitude to my colleagues in the department of medicine as well as in other departments. Their gentle advice and warm affection was always available to me and this gave me the impetus to perform with greater zeal" (*KASHMED* 2011 Memoirs). Every painting of Dr. Durrani is inspired by Kashmir and its beauty; every couplet he writes is inspired by his love for its people . . . as he looks at the sprouting flowers of his garden every season with love and passion—Dr. Durrani proves that he is a Kashmiri for sure.

Dr. Harbhajan Singh

A man with a keen eye!

Dr. Harbhajan Singh was born on August 8, 1911, in village Kanihama, District Baramulla. He had his early education at Baramulla and Srinagar. After passing his FSc, he joined King Edward Medical College, Lahore. He completed his MBBS in 1936. Being among the top six graduates, he was appointed as a house surgeon in the Department of Eye, Ear, Nose, and Throat in New Hospital, K. E. Medical College for a period of one year. In 1939, he proceeded to England and did his postgraduation in London, obtaining diplomas in Eye and ENT.

He was appointed as a clerical assistant in Moorefields Eye Hospital and ENT Hospital, Grays Inn, London, and worked there till 1941. Thus, during the period of the Second World War, he was in London. He returned to India and was appointed as eye and ENT specialist at Jammu in 1942. In 1949, he was selected as a civil surgeon in Himachal Pradesh. He was persuaded by Sheikh Mohammad Abdullah, the then prime minister of J&K, to return to the state to serve its people. In 1950, he rejoined the Kashmir Medical Services, and thus began the era of establishing the subspecialties as distinct entities from general surgery.

Dr. Harbhajan Singh pioneered Eye and ENT surgery and was an outstanding surgeon and a clinician par excellence. It was under his aegis that the specialties of Eye and ENT were established in the state. He headed the Eye and ENT Department with distinction till his retirement in 1970. He also served in various administrative capacities including superintendent, SMHS Hospital, SMGS Hospital, and principal of AMT School.

He continued to practice his profession and then was taken into the Council of Ministers by Sheikh Mohammad Abdullah in 1977. He held the charge of minister of state for health and medical education till 1981. He greatly contributed toward health and medical education in Jammu and Kashmir. He resigned in 1981 and returned to his profession. He passed away in 1991.

Dr. Mahmooda Khan

A fragrant rose!

Women do not compete with men in sports. They need not to because their strength, stamina, and potential based on their physiology demand that there are separate events where they compete among themselves. However, in science, skill, language, and maths, there are no separate events for them, no separate competitions, no separate clauses or definitions. Surgery is a science and a skill dominated by men, but women of grit having a passion for surgery do become surgeons more often now than in the past, and some of them excel too. Kashmir is fortunate to have nourished one such surgeon who broke all the glass ceilings to emerge as a falcon of hope. She did not rest becoming a star but embraced a galaxy on her horizon.

Leave aside her contribution to medicine in general and surgery in particular—she toiled for what was impossible those days (these days too it is not frequent) to be a leader in surgery. My words are not sufficient to describe her class, her style, her touch, her skills, her passion, her ambition, her targets, her control over emotions, her innovations—dedication and commitment to surgery as a subject is a tall mountain climbed and claimed by her that her successors in Kashmir are yet to fathom. No one can dwarf her achievements by calling her "the best woman surgeon," but I know most surgeons who have worked with her do call her a "doyen of surgery."

Who else but Dr. Mehmooda Khan has this honor? Born on December 23, 1934, in Srinagar, this great daughter of Kashmir graduated from Lady Harding Medical College, New Delhi, in 1956. She was the best outgoing graduate in gynecology/obstetrics but chose surgery as her speciality. She did her house job in surgery at Lady Harding Medical College and worked there till 1960. She had a strong desire to become a surgeon thereby swam against the tide. This strong-willed woman got her willpower from her father, Col. G. A. Khan, who was a colonel in the army. She did her specialist training in surgery from Temple University, Philadelphia, USA, and her FRCS England and FRCS Edinburgh in 1967. She took up locum jobs in various UK hospitals during this period. Dr. Mahmooda Khan worked as a senior assistant professor in Albert Einstein Medical Center, Philadelphia University, USA, from 1967 to 1968.

She returned to Kashmir in 1969 and joined as associate professor in surgery at Government Medical College, Srinagar, and was promoted as a professor in 1974. She headed the Department of Surgery in 1980 and continued as professor and head of the department till 1993. She has operated on all challenging and complex cases in adults and children. She has taught innumerable surgeons the basic craft of surgery. She has been a strict disciplinarian but a very soft human being.

Dr. Mahmooda Khan was the longest-serving head of a major department at Government Medical College, Srinagar. Her student and the former head of the Department of Surgery, Government Medical College, Srinagar, has the following to say about Dr. Mahmooda: "Even a book cannot fully describe the impact of Dr. Mahmooda Khan on the surgical landscape of Jammu & Kashmir. She inspired generations of young doctors to take up surgery (and its sub-specialities) as a career and her contribution towards the development of surgery (and its sub-specialities) in Jammu & Kashmir is outstanding. Dr. Mahmooda Khan was a highly accomplished surgeon whose mastery of surgical skills was a treat to watch. Whenever she would undertake any surgical procedure, she would work it up thoroughly, plan in advance, the dissection was painstakingly careful, meticulous and artistic. Those doctors who had the good fortune of assisting her will testify that those were masterpieces of surgical craft. I wish her operative work had been video-graphed for posterity as a valuable reference and a treasure of surgical skill and mastery of art.

"She was a clinician par excellence and a gifted teacher who would lay special emphasis on proper history, methodical clinical examination analyzing the data scientifically not letting go of common sense. She would pay attention to minor details and dates on OPD tickets and inpatient case records.

"When she was a faculty at Govt. Medical College, Srinagar, the Department of Surgery at that time was studded with surgical stalwarts, but she would stand out as unique. During the period of turmoil in the 1990's, mass injuries flooded the SMHS Hospital but she set up a Trauma Unit and reorganised the department to meet the challenges in a difficult time.

"She would lay emphasis on professional ethics and expected her students and subordinates to be punctual and disciplined the attributes which she herself epitomized; she would mince no words in conveying her displeasure regarding any violation of these."

Dr. Pankaj Kaul, a student of Professor Khan, wrote this irresistible post (Facebook) about Dr. Khan that I copy with permission: "I worked with Prof Mahmooda Khan as her postgraduate trainee from 1984 to 1986, at GMC, Srinagar, Kashmir. If there was one sentence that could encapsulate her medical philosophy, it was this: Do the right thing. She would never cut corners. She was extremely knowledgeable of her subject, would go to any length to provide what she considered the best treatment to her patients, and was intolerant of laziness, ineptitude or lack of effort. Only a few surgeons would meaningfully survive in her Unit, and all of them were fashioned and modeled to her way of working. She was strict, but very fair, and very wary of loud praise. When I put eight copies of my thesis on 'Thermography in Breast Cancer' on her table, for her signature, some six months before the due date, she looked at me and I imagined just a hint of a smile.'

He further adds, "She was a real 'General' Surgeon, who knew orthopedics, neurosurgery, vascular surgery, plastic surgery, in addition to GI, urology and endocrine surgery. As a result, some of the salvages she effected are still remembered by grateful patients, trainees, even some colleagues whose lives she saved."

Dr. Fazal Qadir Parray, professor and head of Colorectal Surgery at SKIMS, forwarded a presentation on Prof. Mehmooda Khan that he delivered in one of the conferences. Applauding Dr. Khan for her surgical expertise and commitment to the subject and her will to inspire surgeons all round, he calls her a "rose"—a beautiful analogy, and I retain this word for her in this profile. This woman of unmatched will, commitment, and dedication has filled surgery with a fragrance that is spread far and wide. In one of the conferences at Srinagar, Dr. Lal, the director of PGI Chandigarh, called Dr. Khan "the queen of Kashmir" which she obviously is!

Dr. Manzoor Ahmed

In a hurry to excel!

Dr. Manzoor Ahmed was born on March 11, 1940, in an affluent family of Anantnag, Kashmir. He received his primary education in a local school in Anantnag. In 1948, when his father, Kh. Nabji, was appointed as governor of Kashmir the family shifted to Srinagar. Dr. Manzoor went to Tyndale Biscoe School, where he continued his education till he passed the tenth class examination in 1954 at the age of just fourteen years. He was academically brilliant. After passing his class twelfth examination from SP College, Srinagar, he proceeded to Indore in 1956 to study medicine at MGM Medical College. He passed MBBS in 1961 from Vikrant University.

He went on to obtain a master's degree in ophthalmology in 1965 from the same medical college. Upon his return to Kashmir in 1966, he was appointed as assistant professor of ophthalmology in Government Medical College, Srinagar. He soon observed that a large number of patients were visiting SMHS Hospital for treatment of retinal diseases like retinal detachment and diabetic retinopathy. Because of the nonavailability of a retinal surgeon, these patients had to go outside the state for such specialized treatment. This prompted him to apply for a fellowship in retinal surgery. Fortunately considering his academic achievements, Government of India selected him to undergo fifteen months' retina fellowship at the

University of Essen, Germany, in 1971. In view of his command over the German language, he was assigned the patient care and got the opportunity to work under the supervision of the world-renowned retinal surgeon, Prof. Mayer Schwakrath, the inventor of the retinal laser.

He was offered a lucrative job in Germany, which he humbly declined as he wanted to come back and serve his own community. From Germany, he proceeded to London for a course in contact lens fitting at the prestigious Moorfield Eye Hospital. When he returned to Kashmir in August 1972, he was promoted as associate professor. He was assigned to develop a retina clinic at SMHS Hospital. His efforts soon started to show results as retinal surgeries for retinal detachment were being performed routinely in the hospital. In India, there were just a few retinal surgeons, and Dr. Manzoor was one among them.

In 1974, he was promoted as the professor and the head of the Department of Ophthalmology at the age of just thirty-four years. He has the distinction of being the youngest professor ever in the history of GMC Srinagar. He soon worked t to upgrade the Department of Ophthalmology, SMHS Hospital, Srinagar. He equipped the department with the latest equipment like a fundus camera, xenon arc photocoagulator, photo slit lamp, applanation tonometers, etc.

Observing that prevalence of exfoliation glaucoma was very high in the valley, and many people were losing their eyesight as this type of glaucoma would not respond to medication. He went to the University of Klon, Germany, for a glaucoma fellowship in 1975, where he mastered latest trabeculectomy surgery for glaucoma. Apart from patient care, undergraduate teaching improved with the use of audiovisual presentations. In pursuit of excellence, he proceeded to the USA in 1977 for training in advanced cataract surgery. He visited some of the best eye hospitals in the USA like Bascom Palmar Eye Institute, Florida, and Albert Einstein Medical School, New York. Before coming to Srinagar, he purchased an operating microscope, microsurgical instruments, and intraocular lenses, as they were not available in India.

Dr. Manzoor implanted the first intraocular lens in India at SMHS Hospital. By using an operating microscope, fine suture material, and intraocular lenses, he revolutionized cataract surgery as patients no longer needed to wear thick glasses, and their vision was restored to near normal. Soon, the Eye Department of SMHS Hospital was the center of attraction among ophthalmologists in the entire country. Ophthalmologists from AIIMS, PGI, and other prestigious institutes started visiting the Eye Department for short-term training in micro eye surgery under the guidance of Dr. Manzoor. He was invited to numerous conferences and workshops to impart lens implantation training to doctors.

To eradicate preventable blindness, he played a vital role in the establishment of a mobile eye unit in GMC Srinagar. He himself led this unit to visit far-flung areas and performed eye surgeries at the doorstep of patients in such areas where eye care was not available. He was appointed as an adviser on ophthalmology to the government of Jammu and Kashmir.

During the summer of 1979, a leading advocate of Mumbai required cataract surgery, and someone suggested Dr. Manzoor from Srinagar as no ophthalmologist was implanting an intraocular lens in Mumbai. The patient came to Srinagar and was successfully operated by Dr. Manzoor. In fact, Dr. Manzoor made arrangements for the patient to stay at his residence. After this, Dr. Manzoor was invited to Bombay to perform cataract surgery. For many years after that, Dr. Manzoor would visit Mumbai every winter and perform eye surgeries there. Some of his patients included RBI governor, leading businessmen, and sportsmen.

Dr. Manzoor had observed that no doctor was implanting intraocular lenses for Fuch's heterochromic cyclitis anywhere in the world. He started implanting lenses in such cases successfully, and his work was recognized the world over and was published in the textbook of intraocular lens implantation by Dr. John Alpar. Dr. Manzoor was keen to start corneal surgery in Kashmir. In 1988, he proceeded to Singapore National Eye Hospital to learn the finer aspects of corneal transplant surgery.

It was due to his untiring efforts and personal intervention that the Medical Council of India inspected the facilities in the Department of Ophthalmology, GMC Srinagar, and granted permission to start postgraduate courses in 1989. Dr. Manzoor's desire was to establish a private hospital where patients from all walks of life would be provided the highest quality but affordable eye care. To fulfill this desire, he opted for premature retirement in 1989 at the age of forty-nine years after government service of twenty-four years.

He received a setback to this project as turmoil started in 1990. During the tough times of the turmoil, Dr. Manzoor continued to render his services sometimes at the cost of his life. He operated upon many patients who had received firearm injuries. In 1997, he was finally successful in establishing his own eye hospital, Valley Eye Hospital in Wazir Bagh, Srinagar.

Dr. Manzoor was an excellent sportsman and a sports lover. He was an excellent cricketer, tennis player, bridge player, and golfer. He represented Jammu and Kashmir as a wicketkeeper in the interstate Ranji trophy cricket tournament and captained Vikrant University tennis team. He had the distinction of performing a rare feat of "hole in one" in golf at Kashmir Golf Club. Dr. Manzoor was a life member of All India Ophthalmological Society and continued to be the managing committee member of this elite society for many years. He was the founder and president of the Kashmir Ophthalmological Society.

Dr. Manzoor's students remember him as a competent, strict, highly disciplined teacher who taught with great passion and dedication. Dr. Manzoor passed away on March 3, 2004, just seven days short of his sixty-fourth birthday, after suffering a massive heart attack. His family, friends, the public, and, last but not least, his patients mourned his shocking death. His last rites were attended by thousands of his patients from all parts of the valley. They bid farewell to their "own doctor" with moist eyes.

When Dr. Manzoor wanted to start corneal transplant surgery in the valley, he could not find many people who agreed to donate their eyes for this purpose. He made a resolve that he had to set an example for others to follow. So he willed to donate his eyes. He instructed his son, Dr. Khurshid, himself an ophthalmologist, to carry out the donation in case of his death.

Immediately after Dr. Manzoor's death, his entire family agreed to fulfill his desire for eye donation. Dr. Khurshid, despite being in grief, enucleated his father's eyes with a heavy heart. As the facilities for corneal transplant surgery were not available in Kashmir at that time, the eyes were transported to Chennai, where they were used to restore eyesight in two blind persons. This noble gesture was widely appreciated by the people and motivated many to donate their eyes.

Dr. Manzoor's mission of providing quality eye care is being carried forward by his son, Dr. Khurshid, and daughter-in-law Dr. Seema. They left their lucrative government jobs to start Dr. Manzoor Eye Care Center in Wazir Bagh, Srinagar, as a tribute to him. Dr. Manzoor Eye Care Center has emerged as a leading eye care provider of Kashmir. The center organizes eye camps in far-flung areas, and hundreds of free eye surgeries are performed every year in his memory. Corneal transplant surgeries are today being performed routinely at this center.

Dr. Mehrajuddin Munshi (Qazi)

A man of mettle!

Dr. Mehrajuddin was born in Downtown Srinagar on March 7, 1940. He was the son of late Qazi Jalal-ud-din Munshi. He did his schooling from Islamia High School Srinagar and later studied in SP College, Srinagar. He joined Madras Medical College for his MBBS in 1957. After completing his MBBS from Madras Medical College, Dr. Mehrajuddin went to the United States in 1963 to do his residency in internal medicine. He then went to the United Kingdom for further training, where he completed his membership in the Royal Colleges of Physicians of the United Kingdom (MRCP). Dr. Mehrajuddin, during his initial years of education and training, had a sense of responsibility to society, compassion, and concern for others, and this is what motivated him to become a doctor.

Dr. Mehrajuddin's quest to serve the people of Kashmir took him far away from his home and family for many years in search of knowledge and to gain professional medical education and training so that he could one day return home to contribute as a physician. With this desire, he returned to Kashmir in 1969 and was appointed as an assistant professor, and his first posting was in Government Chest Disease Hospital. He spent his life serving his people as a doctor, teacher, institution builder, and selfless public intellectual, thus becoming an emblem of human dignity, sacrifice, and forbearance. He became a renowned professor of medicine, training multiple generations of Kashmiri doctors at Government Medical College (GMC), Srinagar. He guided dozens of postgraduates in general medicine. He was considered to be a strict disciplinarian and was known for his honesty. He was the head of the Department of Medicine at GMC Srinagar and also directly contributed to the foundation of Jhelum Valley Medical College in 1989 (now SKIMS Medical College), serving as its vice chairperson.

During turmoil because of uncertainty and multiple issues confronting him, Dr. Mehrajuddin went to the United States once again in 1994 and reestablished himself as a specialist and a highly committed doctor. He passed all the exams there and worked as a resident doctor under the students he had trained. This tough and stressful situation would have frustrated any professor, but Dr. Mehrajuddin worked with grace and dignity. He never let his ego ruin his interest in medicine. His motivation was to obtain up-to-date knowledge and skills so that he could put those to use as a practicing physician. Through hard work and dedication, Dr. Mehrajuddin was successful in achieving all these goals. He became an exceptional doctor—putting into practice outstanding clinical skills and living up to all the high professional standards, values, and ethics that patients should expect from their doctor. He did not shy away from learning. He turned distress into opportunity and did his fellowship in geriatrics in the United States.

After facing health challenges and open-heart surgery, Dr. Mehrajuddin decided to return to Kashmir. He also had an irresistible desire to serve his motherland and impart knowledge and skills to the younger generation. He finally returned to Kashmir in 2000. After his return, Dr. Mehrajuddin continued to serve Kashmiris. Dr. Mehrajuddin, according to his colleagues and friends, was influenced by two giants of medicine in Kashmir: Dr. Ali Jan and Dr. Allaqaband. He had quietly imbibed the characteristics of both so far as his practice of medicine was concerned. He was quite like Dr. Ali Jan and prompt like Dr. Allaqaband.

Dr. Mehrajuddin credited whatever success he had as a physician and medical professor to one factor: – his concern and empathy for others and his desire to help mankind. He was acutely aware of the role and responsibility of a doctor in society and the reality that effective medicine must bridge the gap between science and society and that medicine is not mere scientific knowledge of diseases—it is a position of public trust. A doctor must respect the feelings of people and work toward the betterment of society. Dr. Mehrajuddin fulfilled these criteria and truly cared for his people, which is why his patients respected him so much and trusted him. This was also the reason why he expected the very best from the medical students he trained—he wanted all Kashmiri doctors to live up to the highest professional and ethical standards and serve society selflessly.

Dr. Mehrajuddin cultivated an interest in world literature, history, and politics. He dreamed that Kashmir could someday become a shining example in Asia – a hub of science and learning, respected for its hard work, culture, and creativity, enlightened and tolerant society with democratic values.

He was greatly influenced by Albert Camus, the French author whose essays and novels he had read during his student years. His favorite quote was "The only way to deal with an unfree world is to become so absolutely free that your very existence is an act of rebellion." He spent the final years of his life quietly serving society as an intellectual, a doctor, a teacher, a loving father, a grandfather, and a dear friend to many. Dr. Abdul Wahid, professor and ex-HOD Medicine SKIMS, in his Facebook post regarding the man under whom he had worked, writes, "He had stopped seeing patients since long, I went to his home and requested him to resume his private practice. I had two things in mind. First, his patient care was superb and people would get benefited. And second, his prescriptions were inspiring and had a lot of message for medical students and practicing doctors. Keeping these two things in mind, I asked him to start seeing patients again. But he told me that his health condition has caused tremendous weakness in him and he has no strength to read recent advances in medicine, cannot keep pace with the recent developments in medical science and is liable to make mistakes while writing prescriptions. That was the degree of his honesty and uprightness." Prof. Faroque Khan, the renowned pulmonologist from the US, talking about his association with Professor Mehrajuddin, says, "I had a long eventful interaction with Dr. Mehrajuddin. When Arfa and I landed in New York we stayed at Queens Hospital where three Kashmiri doctors—Dr. Shafi, Dr. Mehrajuddin and Dr. Rashid were training. Thereafter I used to visit Dr. Mehrajuddin at SMHS hospital during my frequent trips to Kashmir in 70's and 80's. I met Dr. Mehrajuddin again in 90's at my home in New York. Luckily Dr. Mehrajuddin was adjusted in our program at Nassau County Medical center during a very stressful period of his life. He had to work with and under many doctors from Kashmir whom he had trained at SMHS hospital. He had to take many exams in which he always scored the highest percentile and was an example of 'grace under pressure' thereby setting an example for all of us."

Late September and October was one of Dr. Mehrajuddin's favorite seasons. He loved how the autumn sun would fill the sky with light and cover everything in Kashmir with a golden shroud. Dr. Mehrajuddin ultimately died in his homeland surrounded by his family and among his people, and he was buried according to his wishes in Srinagar, where he grew up, in the soil that he loved. When he spent years away from Kashmir, Dr. Mehrajuddin had a longing for Kashmir and had once prepared himself for the possibility that he might never return to Kashmir. As Kashmir's autumn sun rose in 2017, it covered

Dr. Mehrajuddin's grave with a golden shroud, leaving an era behind that had seen selfless service and commitment from a son who loved his homeland dearly. He was seventy-seven.

The very fact that he is resting at his ancestral graveyard at Malakhah is a testament to Dr. Mehrajuddin's unconquerable spirit and his love for Kashmir.

Dr. Mohammad Maqbool Mir

A hope for the lesser mortals

I attended a conference in Government Medical College, Srinagar, as a postgraduate where Dr. Mohammad Maqbool Mir graced the stage. The president of the Otolaryngological Society of India was also there. He thanked Dr. Maqbool for making otolaryngology simple, precise, and manageable. I wondered about the reason. The reason was his textbook in otolaryngology, which, per the speaker, was read by students all over India. According to him, this simple book had made the job of medical teachers throughout India easy. The audience got up in applause to give Dr. Maqbool a big hand. Currently, the textbook is running its twelfth edition.

Dr. Mohammad Maqbool Mir, the second child of a well-to-do family from Downtown Srinagar, was born in 1936. His parents pushed him to strive and to do better in life. He followed the footsteps of his maternal uncle who, incidentally, was the first Muslim doctor of the valley. He completed his MBBS from MGM College, Indore, in 1958. Dr. Maqbool did his residency in eye and ENT and in general surgery. Dr. Maqbool served as a medical officer in Gulmarg Hospital, Health Center Maharaj Gunj, and Health Center Tral. In 1963, he joined the Department of Otorhinolaryngology and completed diploma in otorhinolaryngology (DLO) in 1965. He enrolled for his MS in ENT from King George Medical College, Lucknow, and completed it in 1965 with honors. In 1969, he did his diploma in medical audiology (DMC) from CMC, Vellore, Tamil Nadu. After getting educated from the best institutions of India, he was inducted as an assistant professor in the Department of Otorhinolaryngology, Government Medical College, Srinagar. Dr. Maqbool was instrumental in starting the postgraduate course in ENT at SMHS Hospital/Government Medical College, Srinagar. Besides authoring the comprehensive textbook of ear, nose, and throat, Dr. Maqbool has authored a textbook on "Syndromes in Otorhinolaryngology" and an MCQ-based book on otorhinolaryngology. Dr. Maqbool has published more than sixty-five papers in national and international journals.

In 1969, Dr. Maqbool organized the first International Medical Conference in Otorhinolaryngology, with Dr. William House from Los Angeles, California, USA, as the keynote speaker (who invented the cochlear implant for hearing loss). This conference must have served as a stimulus for the cochlear implant surgery, which was started in the Department of Otorhinolaryngology, SMHS Hospital, under the able leadership of Prof. Rafiq A Pampori decades later. Dr. Maqbool received visiting fellowship by the Indian Council of Medical Research, New Delhi, between 1969 and 1970. He was awarded WHO fellowship in otorhinolaryngology in the United Kingdom in 1975.

Dr. Maqbool has been an outstanding teacher and was awarded Teacher of the Millennium Award by Government Medical College, Srinagar, in 1999. The North-West Zone of Association of Otorhinolaryngologists of India awarded him in 2004 as a distinguished teacher and able practitioner. Dr. Maqbool retired as a professor and head of the Department of Otorhinolaryngology.

Despite being a busy clinician with a thriving practice, Dr. Maqbool founded the Voluntary Medicare Society (VMS). This society provides free camps for children with hearing impairment and provides them with speech training along with hearing aids. Hearing problems of senior citizens are assessed in camps, and requisite advice and help is provided. This initiative was first started by Dr. Maqbool and his colleagues at Government Medical College together with Dr. Manzoor Ahmed (eye surgeon), Dr. Farooq Ashai (orthopedic surgeon), and Dr. Abdul Ahad Guru (cardiac surgeon). VMS expanded its services by starting Shafaqat Special School for multiple disabilities in 2000, and, since then, thousands of children have been rehabilitated. A vocational training center for children is also being run. Many children have been trained in various skills.

In 2006, an initiative to construct a rehabilitation center for individuals with spinal injuries was undertaken, and, since then, thousands of patients have been rehabilitated. Artificial limbs and splints are provided to the needy. Patients with mental illnesses are provided help in Sawab Center, and Prof. Mushtaq Margoob is guiding the project.

In recognition of his service to the community, Dr. Maqbool was awarded Professor Bashir Ahmad Mattoo Memorial Award of Excellence by Iqbal Memorial Trust in 2006. Recognizing his heroic work, Dr. Maqbool was awarded the Real Hero Award in Health and Disability Category by CNN-IBN.

When asked as to what motivated him to start an NGO, Dr. Maqbool says, “Being an ENT specialist, I used to see patients especially handicapped children in pathetic condition. These children were often isolated, discouraged and treated in a demeaning way by their families and community. Their stories, shattered hopes, broken faces always lingered in my mind and the pain that they felt was one that I carried too. So I decided to establish a complete rehabilitation centre where they could avail facilities ranging from most basic to advanced training.”

It has been a life of satisfaction and purpose for Dr. Maqbool, who, besides being an academician, a surgeon, has contributed immensely to the community.

Dr. Maqbool lives in Srinagar.

The website for donation to VMS is

http://www.voluntarymedicare.org/donations.html.

Inputs: Gyawun, “Meet Mohammed Maqbool Mir: An Angel to Many Differently Abled Children,” March 12, 2017.

Dr. Mohammad Sultan Khuroo

A trendsetter in research!

A brilliant young man from Kashmir rattled the world of medicine with his discovery of a virus responsible for an epidemic that played a havoc in one of the rural areas of Kashmir and affected pregnant ladies predominantly. Devoted to science, ready to take risks with an incessant capacity to work hard, Mohammad Sultan Khuroo did the impossible—he chased the invisible and struck the world in awe . . . An epidemic of jaundice had hit two hundred villages with a population of 600,000 in and around Srinagar, 52,000 patients had been affected by jaundice, and 1,700 fatalities had been reported. This young man's restlessness led him to investigate this epidemic and postulate that a distinct viral subtype (non-A non-B) was responsible for the epidemic, which had a feco-oral route of transmission but was severe in pregnant ladies (Khuroo MS. "Study of an epidemic of non-A, non-B hepatitis. Possibility of another human hepatitis virus distinct from post-transfusion non-A, non-B type." *Am J Med.* 1980 Jun; 68(6): 818–24). This virus was later named hepatitis E virus. History had been created, and Kashmir had gifted a scientist and a clinician of repute to the world!

Dr. Mohammad Sultan Khuroo was born on January 17, 1945, at Kraltengh, Sopore, Kashmir, in an educated and respected family. His grandfather, late Haji Fateh Khuroo (1885–1958), was a scholar in Persian literature, and his Quranic recitation was so impressive as to amaze/immobilize the audience. A handwritten version of the Quran on tree paper available with the family is a religious antique held in respect by generations of Khuroos. His father, Haji Abdul Rahim Khuroo (1922–1995), was a noble man, educated in Persian, and spent most of his lifetime in social work and public good.

Mohammad Sultan did his primary schooling in Government Baba-Yousuf School, passed his matriculation from Government High School Sopore, and completed his FSc (eleventh and twelfth grade) from Government Degree College, Sopore. During this time, he was guided by many upright and competent teachers who taught him discipline and mannerism. Based on his brilliant academic records, he got admission in Government Medical College Srinagar in 1962 to pursue his training in medicine. He graduated from Medical College Srinagar Kashmir, India, in 1967. He had a brilliant career record with a gold medal for the Best Outgoing Student (1962–1967) and nine other awards for distinctions and first positions in basic and clinical subjects. Dr. Khuroo had all the chances to move, train, and work in the West (as most of his colleagues chose), and many Western organizations offered him lucrative offers. However, he stayed back to serve his society as he had been advised by his parents to do so. In 1971, he married Haleema Pandith, daughter of the late Haji Abdul Jabbar Pandith.

Dr. Khuroo completed his postgraduate degree in general medicine (MD) from Medical College Srinagar in 1972 and joined the Department of Medicine, Medical College Srinagar, Kashmir India, as a registrar (till 1974) and then lecturer, Department of Medicine (till June 1976). For further pursuit in knowledge, he joined the Post Graduate Institute of Medical Education and Research (PGIMER), Chandigarh, India, for superspeciality (DM) in gastroenterology. These two years (June 1976 to June 1978) represented a turning point in his career as he hardened his clinical skills, learned medicine as an art to practice and teach, and developed an interest in research to explore the unknown. He was inquisitive, hardworking, and saw every patient as a challenge—each one having something new to learn from. During his training period, he described the syndrome of "hepatic vein thrombosis following pregnancy" and published this work in the *American Journal of Medicine* (1980; 68: 113).

He returned to Government Medical College Srinagar, Kashmir, India, in June 1978. His restlessness to know the unknown, to help the desperate, and to treat the sick led him to the abandoned villages and unexplored alleys where he worked tirelessly to find the causative agent behind the epidemic that was threatening the existence of a community. He knew it was a lifetime chance that he did not wish to miss. The famous French microbiologist and chemist Louis Pasteur said, "In the fields of observation-chances favor a prepared mind," and that is what happened. He discovered "hepatitis E" as a new disease entity and spent his next thirty years exploring the intriguing behavior of this entity. "Discovery of hepatitis E" brought him national and international fame, recognition, innumerable awards, and stamped his position in "history of medicine" as a "discoverer" ("Classic Papers in Viral Hepatitis," edited by Lee and Thomas 1992). Besides spending his time and energy, Dr. Khuroo spent money generated from his private practice to fund research projects on "hepatitis E" (the projects received no funding from any other source).

Sher-i-Kashmir Institute of Medical Sciences (SKIMS) was established as a tertiary care center of excellence in Srinagar. In 1982, there was an acute need of senior physicians of J&K state to join this tertiary health-care facility so that exemplary health-care service facility on the pattern of AIIMS (New Delhi) would be established. Dr. Khuroo, along with a few other committed physicians, joined SKIMS to set the foundations of research, teaching, and tertiary level patient care, which would not only benefit the community but also be a haven for researchers and discoverers.

In 1982, Professor Khuroo joined the chair in the Department of Medicine and Gastroenterology at the Sher-i-Kashmir Institute of Medical Sciences Srinagar, Kashmir, India, and over the next thirteen years established a department par excellence with superb clinical, investigative, teaching, and research facilities. He did not rest but worked passionately for the benefit of his community. This time, his target was *Ascaris lumbricoides.* Ascariasis is a common disease in Kashmir because of the high prevalence of the intestinal helminth in this part of the world. He chased the worm in unimaginable locations, recording its every movement anywhere it went. He soon discovered the disease entity of "hepatobiliary pancreatic ascariasis," a biliary disease that he found to be so common in this community and a cause of so much distress to the population. His publications on this entity in high-impact journals are a treat to read, and the photographic representation of the "Biliary Ascarid (Worm) Invasion" is known to all practicing gastroenterologists of the world. His scintillating lectures on this entity "Death Dance of Biliary Demon" make any audience in the world go frenzy, and all gulp a deworming pill the next moment if they had ever visited Kashmir or India. He presented the health-care problems of a third-world country on scientific forums all across the world, which was responsible for turning the attention of planners toward basic issues of sanitation and preventive aspects of common diseases.

Professor Khuroo built up a strong research team at the SKIMS and did extensive epidemiological studies on peptic ulcer, gall stones, esophageal and gastric cancer, and established the state of Jammu & Kashmir in the epidemiological map as a zone for a distinctive disease pattern. He collaborated with national and international research centers to do basic research on hepatitis E, esophageal and gastric cancer, and biliary diseases. Among these, the National Institute of Health (NIH), Bethesda, Maryland, and the Center for Disease Control (CDC), Atlanta, Georgia, figured on the top.

During his stay at SKIMS, Professor Khuroo did extensive research on varied subjects. With the introduction of proton pump inhibitors (omeprazole) he, through gastric pH studies, proved that the stomach can be made anacidic if omeprazole dose is raised to 80 mg (megadose) per day. For the next six years, he did an exhaustive clinical trial on the role of omeprazole as a "clot stabilizer" for patients with recent peptic ulcer bleeding (commonly known as black motion). In a meticulously planned and well-conducted randomized trial, he proved that omeprazole in this dose (80mg) can prevent rebleeding in this subgroup (actively bleeding) of patients and can be lifesaving in most of these patients. This work was so impactful and outstanding that it found a place in the Bible of Medicine (*New England Journal Medicine* 1997; 336: 1054). Recalling this event, Dr. Khuroo says, "On 10th April 1997 at 4 AM in the morning, I received a phone call and the caller said, 'Mohammad I am the editor of *New England Journal Of Medicine* and I would like to congratulate you and your team for a breakthrough publication this week—Congratulations on a job well done!' I quickly went online and my happiness knew no bounds as I became the first researcher from India to be in NEJM for a study performed in SKIMS." This was a fruitful trial that served as a game changer for bleeding peptic ulcers and saved lives of patients with bleeding peptic ulcers all over the world. The impact of this work in the West was so strong that this paper was discussed in the "Journal Clubs" in every clinical unit in USA and Europe. "World Congress of Gastroenterology" at Vienna invited Professor Khuroo for a special presentation on this subject, and the lecture was attended by over seven thousand delegates. Since then, proton pump inhibitors are the mainstay of medical treatment for peptic ulcer bleeding all over the world, saving millions of lives.

Hydatidosis was another challenge that Professor Khuroo undertook. For centuries, surgeons gave a dictum that hydatid cyst puncture and aspiration should never be thought of or done as it means anaphylaxis and death to the incumbent. In 1991, Professor Khuroo performed what had never been done in medicine before. Through extensive and very careful experimentation, he proved that aspiration of hydatid cysts can be performed safely and in fact is the ideal way to manage most of the hydatid cysts in the liver (now commonly known as the PAIR technique). His first few papers on this subject rose international interest in this form of hydatid cyst management, and an extensive study on six thousand patients of hydatid cysts who had been managed by this technique was published from Southern Europe. In 1997, he completed this work by doing a randomized comparative trial between surgical and PAIR, and, again, this research work found a place in the *New England Journal Medicine* (1997; 337: 881).

This entire journey found innumerable rewards for Professor Khuroo; he traveled as a guest speaker to all major institutions and conferences in the world, received honorary Fellowship of the Royal College of Physicians England (FRCP) and the American College of Physicians (FACP). In 1995, the American College of Physicians conferred the coveted title of "Master of American College of Physicians" (MACP) to Professor Khuroo, a title they give to a few of their own legends.

SKIMS has greatly benefitted from the expertise and dedication of Dr. Khuroo. His research papers elevated the standard of SKIMS and brought it into the limelight. He served as a great stimulating power for his younger colleagues and friends. In his capacity as a clinician, he reset the standards. Dr. Khuroo has an intense passion to impart medical care par excellence to his patients. He has maintained high standards of ethics, morals, and discipline of exemplary nature to diagnose and treat his patients. Besides being a researcher and an excellent clinician, it has been his passion to train and teach his students. Throughout his career, he has imparted intense formal, in-service, and practical training not only to his students pursuing medicine and gastroenterology but also to the technicians, nurses, and residents. It is satisfying to note that one of his students who was a technologist at SKIMS and did PhD degree under his supervision is holding the chair of virology at the world-famous Center for Disease Control (CDC) in Atlanta, Georgia, USA. Many of his students are at senior consultant level at SKIMS and at important medical institutions in the Middle East as well as in Western countries. During his thirty-five years of teaching career, Professor Khuroo guided twenty-one MD/PhD projects and trained a huge group of clinicians in the art of medicine and gastroenterology. He always led from the front. In years of intense curfew and *hartal*, he would use his bicycle to be in SKIMS well ahead of the expected time. He would make it a point to visit laboratories himself, look at cells, and learn from colleagues of other specialities.

At SKIMS, Professor Khuroo held the position of dean of medical faculty (1985–1986) and director of SKIMS (1993–1995). As an administrator, Dr. Khuroo played a great role in the growth of SKIMS. He has been instrumental in formulating the policies of SKIMS right from its inception. As an administrator, Dr. Khuroo worked hard to bring SKIMS at par with the best institutions of the world. He showed a deep interest in the health-care delivery system and worked to find solutions to the problems of health care in general and SKIMS in particular. As dean of medical faculty and director of SKIMS, his contribution in academic activities, infrastructure development, and manpower development has been exemplary. A number of observations and recommendations on the state of health care and its betterment were published in local dailies and sent to health planners for implementation. Although he became director of SKIMS in most trying times, yet it is remembered as a golden period of SKIMS by the society and employees of SKIMS. He has a deep understanding of health-care problems of this part of the world; he has dealt with many and knows best how to tackle them.

In 1995, Professor Khuroo worked as the head and consultant of gastroenterology and liver transplantation at the prestigious King Faisal Hospital and Research Center (KFSH), Riyadh, Saudi Arabia. The positions in this premier institution are open only to the whites (American borne and trained), and Professor Khuroo is possibly the only Indian-trained physician to find a slot on the faculty of the institution. During the ten years he spent as a consultant gastroenterologist and hepatologist at KFSH, he helped to set up a program of liver transplantation in the Kingdom of Saudi Arabia. He worked and published extensively during these ten years and found a special place in the institution, country, and among his patients. Finally, his commitment to his soil brought him back to Kashmir in January 2005.

On his return to Kashmir, India, he established a tertiary Care Digestive Diseases Center in Srinagar. The center continues to indulge in research programs related to hepatitis E, hepatobiliary parasites, and upper GI cancer and is collaborating with national and international organizations. He has published many papers from this institute in high-impact journals. Dr. Khuroo has been associated with SKIMS as an Apical Selection Committee vice chairman, governing body member, and has led the task force against COVID-19 for the entire Jammu and Kashmir and formulated diagnostic and treatment protocol for Jammu and Kashmir.

Professor Khuroo, an accomplished researcher, clinician, and teacher, has broken many myths:

1. For great research, you necessarily need to get trained in the institutions of US and UK.
2. While being a good researcher, you cannot be a good clinician.
3. While being a good clinician, you cannot be a good researcher.
4. Great funding is always the prerequisite for great research.

No amount of fame has satisfied Professor Khuroo. He looks at all the happenings around him with a childlike curiosity and tries to reason with his own mind and then is never tired of asking why and how in each case he sees or each happening around him. He approaches all problems with enthusiasm and energy even at this stage of his life.

Dr. Khuroo has 250 scientific publications and has authored fifteen books and nineteen book chapters. He has an H index of 57. He has figured in Elsevier's global database of highest-cited researchers for 2021 and figured in top 2 percent of global researchers in Stanford University's list of top global scientists for 2020. Some of his publications in journals of repute include NEJM-3, Lancet-6, Ann Int Med-2, Gasteroentrology-4, Gut-4, to name just a few. He has traveled extensively as an invited speaker to deliver guest lecturers in international conferences and as visiting professor to institutions of repute. He is a great orator, with a deep and effective voice, and has the capability to literally move the audience with his presentations and pictures. Masters of hepatology and gastroenterology flock around him in conferences and meets to learn from him; he is the most sought after man for youngsters, who keenly take a selfie with him.

Dr. Khuroo has a lot of regard and affection for his wife, Haleema, and believes his success in life is due to the exemplary dedication his wife has shown toward him. He has three children—all doctors. Dr. Khuroo is a family man who respects his wife to no end, cares for his children no less than any other parent would, and loves his grandchildren dearly.

Dr. Khuroo is a man of extraordinary qualities. Such men are born once in a century. The qualities he possesses are difficult to be embodied in one human being. He is a role model for many in the world and an inspiration for all Kashmiris, especially Kashmiri doctors. May he live a long life and continue to inspire us.

Dr. Mohammad Yousuf

Humility personified!

"I understand there is nothing unusual or extraordinary in the above resume, however, it gives me great pleasure to say that I have served the people of God in general and my own people in particular." Imagine these are the concluding lines of the resume of a professor of medicine, loved and respected by his students so much that most rate him as the best teacher that GMC Srinagar ever had. His colleagues called him soft, his friends called him humble, and his students called him "Marshal." Tall, handsome, and immaculately dressed, this gentleman inspired doctors of all cadres and students of all types. I remember so many who wanted to be like him.

For a third-year MBBS student not used to the environment of the wards, not used to touching patients, not used to hearing the noise and screams Professor Yousuf's clinical class would come as something out of this world-mesmerizing, hypnotizing, fantasizing, all . . . . . .What an ultimate delight his clinical class used to be! That powerful voice would rip apart each veil of inattention, permeate the most insulated minds, and get engraved in each heart and awaken the soul of each "would -be doctor." There are students who say they could repeat Dr. Yousuf's every word taught in the class years afterwards. His theory classes were equally captivating. Extremely aware of what a medical student should know, his class was solid, sufficient, and left behind a sweet after-taste and a cherishing memory. No more hunting for notes and books . . ….

Dr. Yousuf was born on April 16, 1942, in New Theed Harwan. He did his MBBS in 1966 from GMC Srinagar and MD in medicine from the same institution in 1971. He worked as an assistant professor, Department of Medicine, GMC Srinagar, from 1972 to 1983. He was promoted as an associate professor in 1983. Besides being a postgraduate guide to more than two dozen students, Dr. Yousuf headed a unit of medicine comprising of more than fifty patients and worked as a senior consultant. He was promoted as the professor and head of the Department of Medicine, Government Medical College, Srinagar (1997–1999).

Dr. Yousuf has authored four books and published many articles in leading national and international journals. His book titled *Handbook of Medical Emergencies* is widely read by residents and clinicians and is running into its seventh edition. He has compiled "Quarter Century Medical Research in Kashmir" published by the University of Kashmir, India, in 1998, which is based on the compilation of twenty-five years of research performed at GMC Srinagar. He has authored a book titled *God's People in My Life as a Doctor* (1998), based on his own experience as a clinician, and talked exclusively about his difficulties, joys, and aspirations as a doctor dealing with patients and his colleagues. He has talked about how things can be made better by understanding each other and also by cultivating a healthy relation with the patient and his family. He has authored *Disease and Humor*, a handbook on the description of humor displayed by patients and lessons learned by the treating doctors (2012).

I have done housemanship in Dr. Yousuf's unit at SMHS Hospital and found him humane, dedicated, and committed to his work. He would never shout, never rebuke, or never talk ill of anyone in the ward. Doctors, students, and hospital staff would always flock around him. I do not remember an occasion when he would refuse to see any patient. He would always update himself with the latest information available and spread across those pearls of wisdom during the ward rounds.

He would respect the knowledge and wisdom of his juniors and never hesitate to refer a difficult patient to a junior. I remember him sending many of his patients to Dr. Abdul Majeed, his junior colleague, and seek his opinion. He would always encourage a resident, a postgraduate student, or a junior colleague to do better and would go out of way to help. I remember him spending a great deal of time counseling confused and frustrated youngsters—advising them and recommending them to the places where they could do better. His soft nature and humble temperament would sometimes become his weakness as people would take undue advantage and eventually harm him.

As a house physician, I did sometime ask him what made him such a brilliant teacher. His reply surprised me. "I would work very hard on a class, I would practice a lot, read a lot—understand the topic myself and try my best to make it simple." To become a good teacher, never take a student or his knowledge for granted—he would always reiterate that.

Presently, he is a full-time physician working at his private clinic at Polo Plaza and in Brein, Srinagar, Kashmir for six hours a day besides actively participating in various conferences, lectures, and awareness programs of the Cancer Society of Kashmir and updating his knowledge about medicine through the internet to write newer editions of his book of medical emergencies.

Dr. Yousuf is a gentleman, a man known for his integrity, honesty, great temperament, and humble nature. His peculiar smile and his shy nature define him. This is what Dr. Yousuf has to say about himself: "I tried to give my best and always valued my patient as a better person than myself. I made every attempt not to fail in observing medical ethics in letter and spirit. I always shared the best time with my students who contributed to teach me medicine and gave me lessons about life. This process is still a part of my life and something most dear to me. A friend (not wishing to be named) has inspired me to work for excellence. Besides him the source of my strength has been my wife, my children Zeenat and Kousar who have kept my candle glowing."

Dr. Yousuf lives with his wife in Srinagar and has been bestowed with two daughters, both of them medicos, one of them a nephrologist in the US and the other working in Srinagar. He loves his family, especially his grandchildren.

Dr. (Col.) Saligram Kaul

A sober colonel!

Dr. Saligram Kaul, popularly known as Colonel Kaul, was born to Pandit Aftab Kaul Nizamat and Mrs. Devaki Kaul in 1913. The family lived in Brekujan quarter of Habba Kadal, Srinagar. Dr. Kaul was educated at Babapora School near Habba Kadal and then State High School. He studied at Sri Pratap College (SP College) in Srinagar and then completed his medical education at the University of Lahore. Dr. Kaul did his FRCP from London and is listed in its archives.

From an early age, he had been involved with young people who gathered under the name of "fraternity" and believed strongly in the rights of women to be educated and for the widows to remarry. Dr. Saligram Kaul had a distinguished career as an able physician as well as an administrator. He served as principal, Government Medical College, Srinagar, and director of Health Services, J&K, before his retirement in 1973. He was a thorough gentleman and extremely dedicated to the job that he was entrusted with. He was a good administrator and a great academician. He streamlined teaching at Government Medical College, Srinagar, and would spend hours formulating and implementing the roster along with another legend of his time, Dr. D. N. Thussu. Prof. A. R. Khan of Pathology calls Dr. Kaul an extremely dedicated doctor who knew his job very well.

Dr. Allaqaband joined GMC in 1964, while recalling his days in his essay titled "Agony of Adolescence" published in *KASHMED* (2011), he says, "As I presented myself before the HOD of Medicine, he was a sober intelligent academician in the form of Col. S. Kaul. He was pleased to see me and expressed happiness because both of us were members of the same Royal College of Physicians of London, the only two belonging to that college at that time. He had great ideas about the academic development of the department and wanted to enforce the same discipline for which he was trained in the armed forces. He did succeed to some extent but soon took over as the Principal of the college. His field of activity widened and hope was generated for the true academic environment of the college." Professor Khuroo, in his tribute to Dr. Kaul, calls him "a medical giant who taught his students the most difficult art of history taking, palpating the magic box of the human body (i.e., abdomen and listening to the demanding tender human structure namely the human heart)." Dr. Altaf Hussain, the famous pediatrician, in his tribute to Dr. Kaul, says, "Col. S. Kaul first HOD medicine has left an indelible mark on the history of Govt. Medical college. His teaching of history taking and physical examination is unsurpassed in my experience in the east and west. He also taught us bedside manners very rigorously" (*KASHMED* 2011, pp. 93, 105). Dr. Durrani recalls Dr. Kaul's contribution to medicine, acknowledging the fact that he was instrumental in setting up the gastrointestinal division of medicine at SMHS Hospital and worked tirelessly for its growth and development.

Dr. Saligram Kaul is rated as one of the best academicians of GMC Srinagar and one of the architects who build a template upon which generations of doctors were trained at GMC Srinagar. He died in 2005 after a brief illness.

Dr. Surendra Nath Dhar

In a never-ending love with Kashmir!

As a pathologist who looks at lung specimens and biopsies, I would encounter anthracotic nodules with extensive fibrosis in patients belonging to the higher reaches residing in low-ceiling huts. This entity is known as "Gujjar lung." The entity Gujjar lung was first introduced in 1991 by Dhar and Pathania from Kashmir when they noticed miliary mottling and reticulonodular pattern in the chest radiographs of patients belonging to the Gujjar community. These patients were empirically put on therapeutic trials with antituberculosis treatment, but the shadows remained unchanged despite adequate dosage and duration of treatment. Finally, the lung biopsy was done, which revealed the findings of anthracotic nodules, carbon-laden macrophages, and fibrosis. The authors attributed it to indoor air pollution with smoke from biomass combustion, mainly pinewood. This is what Dr. Surendra Nath Dar gave to the medical world—a well-researched entity known as Gujjar lung, the word coined by him (Dhar, SN, Pathania, AGS "Bronchitis Due to Biomass Fuel Burning in North India: "Gujjar Lung" an Extreme Effect." *Semin Resp Crit Care Med* 1991; 12(2): 69–74).

Dr. Dhar did his postgraduation from All India Institute of Medical Sciences, New Delhi, and started his career as an assistant professor in the Department of Medicine in Government Medical College, Srinagar. He served in the Chest Disease

Hospital as an assistant professor and was later promoted as a professor. It was here in Chest Disease Hospital that he proved himself as an ace clinician and excellent researcher. He established himself as a healer for a community where chest problems were rampant. Dr. Dhar retired as the head of the Department of Chest Medicine. Dr. S. N. Dhar did not leave Kashmir even when most members from his community left Kashmir in the peak years of turmoil. He kept on seeing his patients and rendering the service to his community in spite of the difficulties he faced.

His colleagues best describe him: "Dr S. N. Dhar was more than a mere clinician. He had a deep understanding of the socio-cultural, socio-economic and socio-political compulsions of Kashmiris. He stayed back to serve his people even as he was taken hostage during turbulent years. He believed firmly in the principles of medical ethics. He never practiced the so called 'commercialized' and 'mechanized' medicine. He never aspired for power or position of authority. He never resorted to means of cheap publicity. He was a gentleman par excellence who served humanity with humility, love and devotion."

When I feel short of words to describe a legend in our profession, I turn to Dr. K. L. Chowdhury's write-ups about the legends with whom he had spent time. Luckily, I came across an obituary by Dr. Chowdhury published in the web magazine *Shehjar*. Here it goes:

"It may seem unnecessary to speak about his professional attainments for he was a household name in Kashmir, a physician in demand, and the fact that patients had to wait 3–4 months for an appointment with him speaks volumes about his standing. But all that fame and name did not come easy. He worked assiduously, starting from his Safakadal backyard and building up his reputation by competing with the big names of that age. It was just a matter of time for him to take a quantum jump from Safakadal to Polo View, the Harley Street of Srinagar, to rub shoulders with the legends and to become a living legend himself. The final move to Rajbagh, the Shangrila of his practice, was as fortuitous as it was welcome after his release from captivity for 83 days. He held his patients under a spell through his gentle manners, soft speech, clinical acumen, and his captivating charm. It is the combination of these attributes in practice that go by the single expression in Kashmiri 'Shafa,' which he was endowed with in such abundance. He was as courageous from the inside as he was cool on the exterior and never afraid to fight it out and to speak out, not only for himself but others."

Dr. Chowdhury further describes him: "He was versatile—a genial personality, highly communicative and a great conversationalist who had an inexhaustible fund of anecdotes, jokes and puns, with which to hold his audience in thrall. Often he emerged as the centerpiece of a group. His sonorous voice helped him in no small measure in mesmerizing others. He liked music and played the tabla. He could have been a great vocalist with that hypnotic voice of his. But it was not just professional success he wallowed in. He lived a much fuller, richer life with his penchant for outdoor activities, his passion for hiking, his liking for the game of bridge where he took pride in partnering with his wonderful spouse, Dr. Vimla, and his flair as a cricketer. He always opened the innings on behalf of the staff in the Staff versus Students cricket match in the Medical College. Well! That brings me to yet another attribute of Dr. Dhar. He was as good a writer as he was a speaker. The famous memoir of his captivity is a remarkable book, *83 Days: The Story of a Frozen River*. He was a complete person, a man of tastes, an entertainer who threw parties and collected the best people around him, a man without rancor or hatred even for his adversaries, a good friend, and a Family Man."

When he breathed last away from his home in Goa, his colleagues paying him rich tributes were discussing his health problem with deep concern. And it was opined that tuberculosis possibly was the disease that had claimed his life. The disease that he encountered most during his practicing years was possibly the disease he succumbed to.

Dr. Dhar is survived by his wife, Dr. Vimla Dhar. Dr. Chowdhury and Dr. Dhar were not only good friends but also connected to each other through their children. Dr. Chowdhury's daughter is married to Dr. Dhar's son.

Dr. Syed Naseer Ahmad Shah

An institution builder!

This is a life I wanted to talk about, know more about, and write not just a gist but an entire book. Dr. Syed Naseer Ahmad Shah's contribution to health care and medical education in Kashmir is unparallel. As a medical student in '90s at Government Medical College, Srinagar (GMC), I always heard my teachers talk about the "Golden Era" of GMC, and by this, they meant the period when the college was headed by Dr. Naseer. It was an era when GMC Srinagar was living its youthful years and aiming for a top slot at the national level. It was an era of excellence and achievement, an era of competitiveness and growth, an era when science was replacing the tradition, and an era when life was reverberating through medical college. To the college, he brought glory; to the patients, he brought relief; and to the dull and depressed medicos shrunken under the burden of books and skeletons, he brought a life of ease. To the demanding life of a medical student, he added the fuel of sports and the humor of cultural activities, taking care not to compromise his efficiency as a doctor. "Medicine was never so interesting," all those lucky ones who graduated from GMC Srinagar during its "Golden Era" will tell you.

I was not lucky to be his student but would watch him from a distance and hear his words of wisdom when he would come to attend various functions at GMC or SKIMS. A crowd would rosette around him, hugging him, shaking hands with him, and kissing him. When walking through the lanes of SMHS, he would stop to receive young and old with warmth and compassion even when he had ceased to be their boss. I heard him many times addressing doctors, talking about his life, his passion for medicine, and his concern for this community. Of course, the longest-serving principal of GMC that produced stalwarts of medicine manning institutions of repute throughout the world had a lot to talk about. And we had a lot to learn.

For someone interested in collecting profiles of outstanding Kashmiri doctors, I was desperate to meet this legend. I managed an appointment with him and his equally impressive life partner, Dr. Girja Dhar, through Prof. Azra Shah, his niece. As I met this wonderful couple in the beautiful lawns of their home, I could sense an encyclopedia unfold. My memory and my pen were not able to keep pace with all that he had to tell. He told his story his own way—humorously and forcefully.

Dr. Naseer was born on January 5, 1929, in an official quarter in Booniyar (Baramulla), where his father, Ahmad Ali Shah, was posted as forest range officer. Dr. Naseer's family has roots in Teetwal village of Karnah; it was part of the Muzaffarabad District in the erstwhile state of Jammu and Kashmir. The family was well educated, and most of his siblings were serving in good positions. He traced his journey from his birth to his tumultuous life as a medical student, getting trapped on the other side of the border when India was partitioned while he was studying at King Edward Medical College, Lahore. Longing for his home, he came back to Kashmir, trying to earn his livelihood as a doctor. There were disappointments here. From here, he went on to the UK. Once there, he completed his MRCP and became the member of the Royal College of Physicians in London. With one more diploma, he became the first qualified specialist in tropical diseases in northern India.

His fascinating account of his years in London would leave you wonderstruck.

And the beautiful part of his life was (as he recounted) his journey back home—serving his community as an able and efficient doctor. If the UK attracts our doctors now, how much more attractive it would it have been fifty years ago? He married Dr. Girja Dhar, who was herself committed to serving her homeland. So he and his wife chose Kashmir, its patients, its pain, and involved themselves not only in caring for its sick but also building institutions where future generations of doctors were trained. He talked to me about his initial years of clinical practice, his years of struggle in his Drugjan clinic, and his success in replacing unscientific with scientific, replacing vague with definite and despair with hope. He talked to me about how he performed an ascitic tap on a distressed cirrhotic patient in his clinic, diagnosed an unsuspected myocardial infarction, and treated medical emergencies with success.

Dr. Naseer took over as the principal of Government Medical College, Srinagar, in 1969 and retained the position for twelve years, till he opted for premature retirement in November 1981 at the age of fifty-two years. His administrative skills aside, he was a visionary who added postgraduation in almost all disciplines and used his personal influence to get MCI recognition for many departments. We need to be grateful to him because not only did GMC Srinagar produce specialists for the entire state but also his efforts turned GMC into a unique institution where leaders for the world's famous institutions were being churned out. It was his vision to have medicine specialized and diversified and to have a network of hospitals around GMC. This dream was realized with time. For the poor and needy of rural areas, he brought health care near their doorstep by starting the Chitranjan Mobile Clinic.

What made Dr. Naseer unique was his student-friendly attitude. When I asked him, "Why were you so popular amongst students?" he remarked, "I looked into their individual and collective problems and tried my best to sort them out. My doors were always open for them and I remembered most of them by their names." His students remember him as a generous, soft-spoken, fatherly figure who would go out of his way to help them. He was caring and helpful to all the students, including the international students who used to come to GMC Srinagar under an exchange program. He even used to buy books for the students who couldn't afford them.

Dr. Naseer raised the bar of the principal of GMC Srinagar. Most of the administrative decisions were taken by the principal, and he was never called to the secretariat. He had absolute powers and would make the selections for MBBS course and postgraduation courses at GMC Srinagar; he also made the appointment of the staff for the hospital and the college. After his retirement, he was appointed as a member of legislative council in 1996, and he held the position for six years; he left it in 2002. He was also awarded Padma Shree in 1984. He left the world on October 11, 2017. The patients who were emotionally and psychologically dependent on him lost their dear doctor and thronged his funeral as he was laid to rest. Dr. Naseer is survived by his daughter, Dr. Tina Anjila who lives with her husband and son in the UK.

When medicine is losing its charm, when money and medicine are synonymous, we need the likes of Professor Naseer to reassure us about the greatness of our mission, the purpose of our lives, and the importance of our patients on whose prayers and faith we thrive. We need the likes of Professor Naseer to make us feel proud of our profession.

Prof. Naseer Ahmad Shah loved his motherland and chose to return here to serve it . . . He did not get the power and position easily . . . . . .but he delivered in whatever capacity he served in. This is the spirit that the present generation of doctors has to inculcate!

Dr. Syed Zahoor Ahmad

A physician gentleman!

There is an annual event at the Sher-i-Kashmir Institute of Medical Sciences in which postgraduates present their research work to the audience. The postgraduates are judged for their presentation and their research. All postgraduates annually look forward to this event as it is here that their skills as orators is tested, their confidence is boosted, their research is subject to critical analysis and their fears are overcome. This event was started by Dr. Syed Zahoor, who, despite the turmoil, made postgraduates present their research work in this annual event at SKIMS. This is a unique event that has continued annually at SKIMS no matter what the odds and constraints the institution faced. Over the years, it has become a defining attribute of SKIMS.

Dr. Syed Zahoor Ahmad has been one of the most qualified doctors who has been trained in the US and UK but chose to come back and serve his own people. He was born in Dooru, Kashmir, and did his MBBS from MGM College, Indore, in 1956. He did his MRCP from London and Edinburgh and his FRCP from London. He was also a diplomate of the American Board of Medicine. He served as assistant professor in medicine from 1961 to 1964 at the University of Pennsylvania, USA; as lecturer of Medicine Guys Hospital, London, UK, from 1964 to

1965; and as assistant professor of medicine at the University of Pennsylvania, USA, from 1966 to 1968.

After serving in developed countries as a faculty member and acquiring knowledge and expertise from there, Dr. Zahoor joined the Department of Medicine, Government Medical College, Srinagar, J&K, India, in 1968 and served as the professor and HOD of Medicine. He served as dean and principal of Government Medical College, Srinagar, from 1981 to 1985. Dr. Syed Zahoor Ahmad was made commissioner secretary, Health and Medical Education, Government of Jammu and Kashmir, and served in this capacity from 1985 to 1986. He served as director and dean, Sher-i-Kashmir of Medical Sciences from 1986 to 1992. In short, there is not a prestigious position that he has missed. In his tenure as principal of GMC Srinagar and Director SKIMS, many departments at GMC and SKIMS started their postgraduation courses. He served as a member of many national bodies, which include member of Medical Council of India from 1981 to 1994, member of Post Graduate Committee MCI, and member of National Board of Exams, New Delhi, from 1983 to 1994. He was also a member of ICMR Committee, India, from 1972 to 1985.

Dr. Zahoor has been a clinician of great repute known for his punctuality and discipline. He was humble and, in spite of acquiring power and position, always been a down-to-earth human being who was in love with his roots and his people. He has been a feminist at heart and encouraged his wife, the revered Prof. Mehmooda Khan, to go against the tide and to excel in the male-dominated faculty of surgery. Prof. Mohammad Yousuf, ex-HOD Medicine, GMC Srinagar, has the following to say about Dr. Zahoor: "Dr. Zahoor was a real academician, who believed in quality teaching, being the first one to introduce a feedback sheet from students about their teachers. As far as his clinical practice goes, he is the only physician in Kashmir who maintained a meticulous record of his patients and he could trace details of his patients even after decades. Unfortunately in the 2014 floods, all records were washed off. Otherwise one could write a book, about the disease pattern and the peculiar cases that he would see." Prof. M. I. Quadiri, the renowned hematologist, says that during peak years of turmoil, SKIMS worked ten times more, and the credit for that work goes to Prof. Syed Zahoor Ahmad, who was calm and upright despite the external and internal stresses. Dr. Quadiri recalls an instance when bullets were kept on his table.

Dr. Zahoor has been a family man who is survived by three children; two of them are doctors, and one is an engineer.

Dr. Wazira Khanam

A tough woman!

Dr. Wazira Khanam was born in Laduwa, Ladora, Baramulla, Kashmir, on April 24, 1939. Her parents were Mr. Hidayatullah Khan and Sayeeda Begum. She was exceptionally brilliant from her childhood and always wanted to do something exceptional. She received her education at Women's College, Srinagar. She broke the stereotype and was one of the very few Kashmiri women of that era to receive training in medicine. She was selected for MBBS in 1956 and did her MBBS from Patna Medical College in 1961. In college, she was considered to be bright and brilliant. She was interested in obstetrics and gynecology and did her MS in obstetrics and gynecology from Patna in 1965. It was a difficult time for a young girl who had lived among streams and mountains to bear the scorching heat of Patna. In those days, travel was also cumbersome and lengthy, but with her interest in medicine, nothing deterred her from her goal. In Patna Medical College, she was greatly influenced by Dr. Kamala Acharya, who was her mentor.

When Dr. Wazira Khanam returned from Patna, she was appointed as an assistant professor at GMC in 1965 and received training in Japan from 1969 to 1970 in gynecologic oncology. She is thus the first gynecological oncologist of Kashmir. She worked under Dr. Girja Dhar and together with her helped in making gynecology and obstetrics a highly skilled and scientific branch at Lal Ded Hospital. She became an associate professor in 1975 and subsequently became the HOD of Obstetrics and Gynecology. As HOD, her achievements were to streamline the teaching and training of undergraduates and postgraduates. Gynecology and obstetrics is a very lucrative branch, and doctors earn a lot of money, but Dr. Wazira had a passion for this subject and never ignored her role as a teacher, surgeon, and doctor in the hospital. She has guided many students in the subject. Her students remember her as a tough disciplinarian and a very noble soul.

She took over as the principal of GMC Srinagar in 1998 during very difficult times. Professor Yousuf of Medicine remembers Dr. Wazira as a very simple and clean-hearted woman. She was very daring too. In the peak turmoil when Dr. Beig (HOD Psychiatry) was very sick and admitted in the SMHS Hospital, Dr. Wazira came all the way from her home in the ambulance during the dead end of the night when the whole area was under curfew to monitor Dr. Beig. As principal of GMC, she had to face a difficult time keeping the hospital running and medical education going. She retired from services in 1998.

She was the first gynecologist to start colposcopy in the valley for diagnosis of precancerous conditions of the cervix, which helped in early diagnosis and treatment. Besides the routine gynecological and obstetric problems, she had a special expertise in fistula repair. Dr. Wazira is a very skilled surgeon who has done very difficult and challenging surgeries and set very high standards for the doctors who followed her.

Dr. Wazira lives with her husband in Srinagar, and her two children are settled in the US; both of them are doctors. One is a GI specialist and another is an internist. She spends her winter time with them enjoying with her grandchildren.

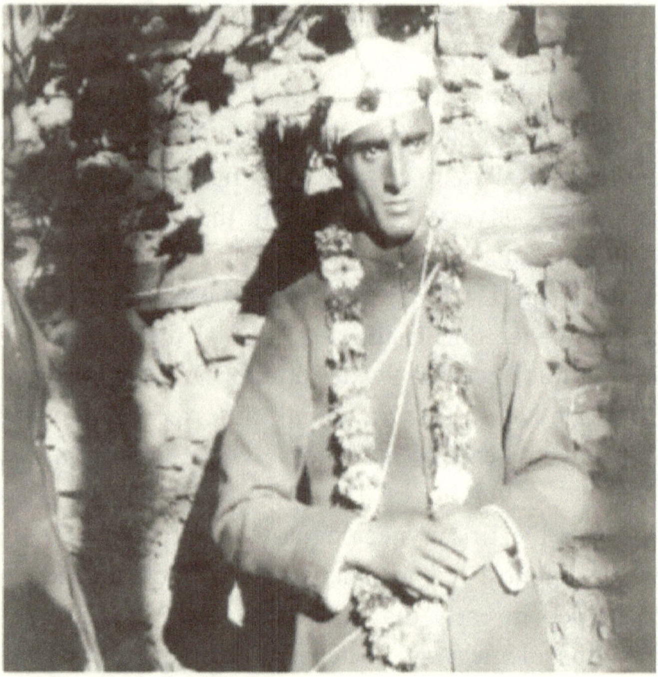

Dr. G. L. Vaishnavi (wedding photo) (1899–1977)

1.	M.B.B.S.	Punjab	1925
2.	D.O.M.S.	London	1929
3.	D.L.O.(R.C.P.S)	London England	1929
4.	F.R.C.S.	Edinburgh	1930
5.	F.R.F.P.S.	Glasgow	1930

He was elected as follow of the Royal Society of Tropical Medicine and Hygiene England (F.R.S.T.M.& H) in 1930

B. PROFESSIONAL EXPERIENCE.

Worked as:-

1. Medical Officer Sudder Hospital, Out-patient Department, Srinagar, for about 3 years.
2. Eye, Ear, Nose and Throat Specialist for about two years, Sudder Hospital, Srinagar.
3. Senior Medical Officer Incharge Sudder Hospital, Srinagar for about 4 years.
4. Chief Medical Officer for about five years in Jammu and Kashmir Prévinces
5. Palace Surgeon for about two years.
6. Director Medical Services, His Highness' Government Jammu and Kashmir State. Technical Supervision of all Civil and Military Hospitals for over four years.
7. Consulting Surgeon to Rattan Rani Charitable Hospital, for two years, 1948-1950.

C. ADMINISTRATIVE EXPERIENCE.

1. Chief Medical Officer and Superintendent of Jails and Asylums, Jammu and Kashmir Government on 750-50-1000 P.M. for about five years.
2. Assistant Director Medical Services, Jammu and Kashmir Government on Rs.1000/-plus Rs. 100/- P.M. as allowance for about one year.
3. Director Medical Services and Inspector General of Prisons, Jammu and Kashmir State on Rs. 1500/- P.M. with permission to have private practice for over four years.

As Director of Medical Services he was incharge of the Civil and Military Medical, Public Health, Jails and Meterological Departments of Jammu and Kashmir State.

During the tenure of this service as Chief Medical Officer, and Director Medical Services, he sponsored a number of schemes for the expansion and working of the Medical and Health Departments in the State.

(a) — As Chief Medical Officer, he formulated the scheme of District Medical Administration, which was sanctioned by the Government. He also prepared a scheme for rural sanitation. In the field of epidemic control apart from the implementation of other administrative means, he organised and managed mass cholera, typus and other inocculations. In 1935 and 1937 about 75 % of the total population was inoculated against Cholera ...

CV of Dr. G. L. Vaishnavi (possibly the first well-made CV of a Kashmiri doctor)

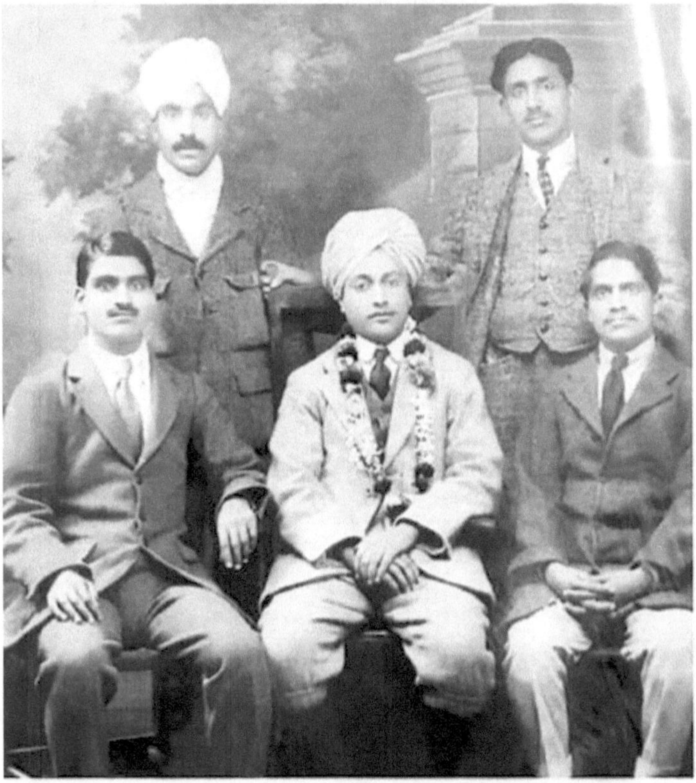

Dr. Gwash Lal Kaul (standing right) with Dr. Vaishnavi (sitting left). Photo courtesy of Dr. K. K. Kaul.

DR. G.L. Vaishnavi, M.B.B.S.(pb.), F.R.C.S.(Edinbourgh), F.R.F.P.S.(Glasgow), D.L.O.(R.c.P & S)(England), D.O.M.S.(London), F.R.S.T. M & H.(England).

Born in November, 1899 at Srinagar. Graduated in Medicine from the Punjab University. Joined Kashmir Government Service in early 1925. Went to Great Britain in 1927 for higher post Graduate training in Surgery and deseases of Eye, Ear, Nose and throat. Returned in 1930 after successfully completing the training. Was promoted to the post of Chief Medical Officer in 1935. In 1941, he became Assistant Director Medical Services and held the post of Palace Surgeon till 1943, when he was appointed as Director Medical Services, Jammu & Kashmir Government, which post he held till 1940. In 1950 he was appointed as Assistant Director General Health Services, Government of India, New Delhi and held the charge upto July 1954, when he was selected for the post of Chief Medical Officer, Calcutta port Commissioners. He retired from this post in 1957 and has since been practising in Sri Nagar as Consultant Optalmist. and general Surgeon. During his tenure of service in Kashmir Government and at Commissioners for Calcutta Port, he organised and expanded the Medical Departments from bothe curative. and preventive aspects and in Kashmir Government he framed schemes by which dispensaries and health units were framed schemes by which dispensaries and health units were opened at a distance of 5 miles radius in the whole Jammu and Srinagar and equipped them with all necessary equipment and trained staff for the benefits of Urban population. He was re-employed by the Kashmir Government in October 1960 as Superintendant to improve the administration and working of Sri Maharaja Hari Sing Ji Hospital, Sirnagar directly under the Health Minister of the State. After organising and expanding the Hospital to serve the needs of a Medical College, he relinguished the post in October 1961.

He died in Delhi on March 31, 1977. He was 78.

Short bio of Dr. G. L. Vaishnavi

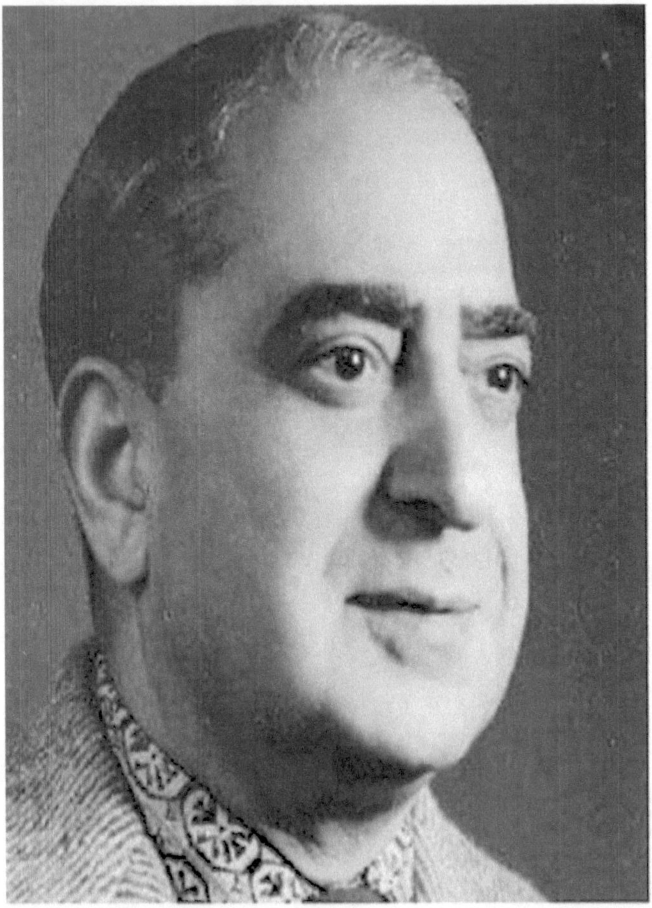

Dr. Ali Jan—the most popular physician of Kashmir believed to be the “Luqman of Kashmir” (1914–1988)

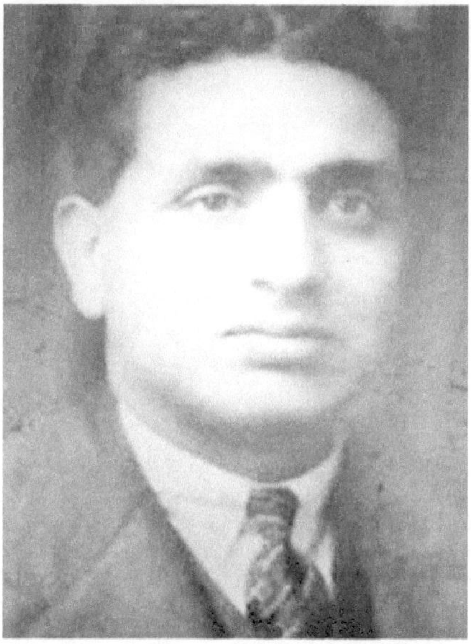

Dr. Gwash Lal Kaul—the first MRCP from Jammu and Kashmir

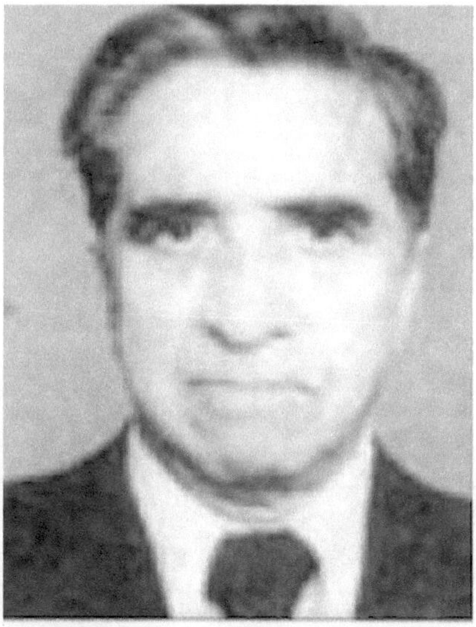

Dr. (Col.) Saligram Kaul (1913–2005)—an excellent clinician and teacher who served as the principal of GMC Srinagar and director of Health Services Kashmir.

GARFIELD G. DUNCAN, M.D.
THEODORE G. DUNCAN, M.D.

PENNSYLVANIA HOSPITAL • 330 SOUTH NINTH
PHILADELPHIA, PENNSYLVANIA 19107 • WALNUT

October 25, 1968

TO WHOM IT MAY CONCERN:

This is to certify that I have had the opportunity of helping to train and of observing the development of Dr. Syed Zahoor Ahmed as a clinician, teacher and clinical investigator during the period from July 1, 1960 to September 1, 1963. During that period Dr. Ahmed had unusually favorable opportunity of teaching interns, residents and fourth year medical students of the University of Pennsylvania. In this capacity he excelled. Returning to my service July 1967 to August 1968 after succeeding in getting his F.R.C.P. both in London and Edinburgh, he prepared for and was successful on his first attempt in becoming a Diplomate of the American Board of Internal Medicine. (Failures to achieve this advanced recognition were as high as 65 per cent while I was a member of the Board.)

During this past year at the Pennsylvania Hospital Dr. Ahmed had increased opportunities to teach and to do clinical research. In these endeavors his capacity equalled those expected of an Assistant or an Associate Professor of Medicine. In a previous commendation of Dr. Ahmed I stated to the effect that he has shown, in many ways in his chosen specialty, that he is qualified for a professorial appointment in a Class A school of medicine. I can repeat this with even greater emphasis since reviewing his accomplishments of the past year. Furthermore I predict a great future for him and that he will be a credit to any medical school fortunate enough to take advantage of the professional contribution he has to offer.

Garfield G Duncan

Garfield G. Duncan, M.D.
Professor of Medicine, University of Pennsylvania
Consulting Physician, Pennsylvania Hospital

GGD:pkf

Dr. Syed Zahoor (LOR)

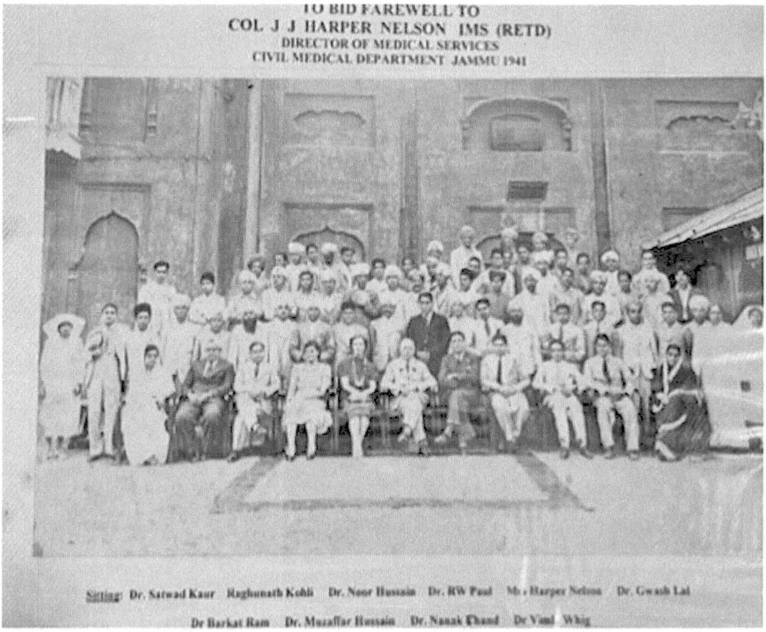

A memorable picture of Dr. Gwash Lal on the retirement day of Colonel Nelson (1941)

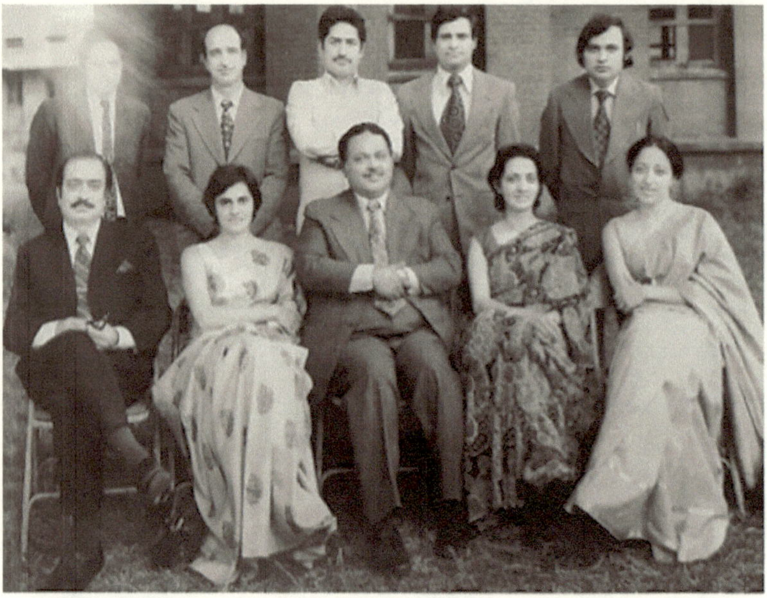

The stalwart teachers and administrators of GMC Srinagar (photo credits *KASHMED* College magazine, 2011). Starting from L to R: Dr. B. M. Bhan, Dr. Girja Dhar, Dr. Syed Naseer Ahmad Shah, Dr. Mahmooda Khan, Dr. J. A. Naqshbandi. Standing, second, from L: Dr. Syed Zahoor Ahmad; fourth, Dr. Manzoor Ahmed.

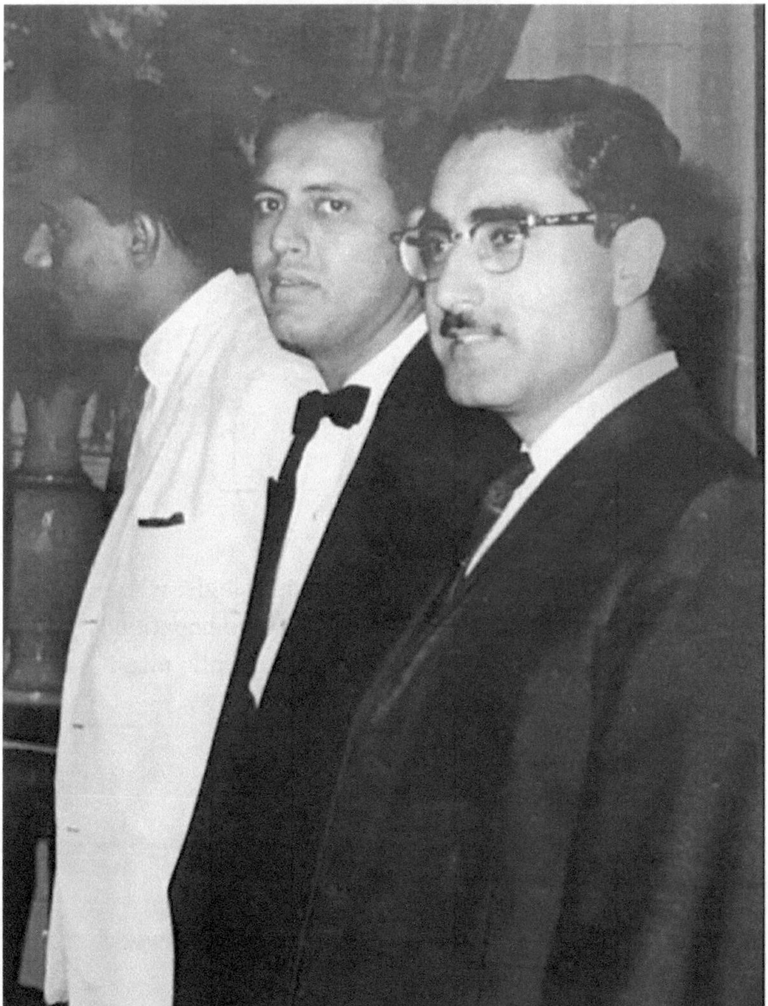

Dr. G. Q. Allaqaband—the master clinician and teacher who has exerted tremendous influence over clinicians of all the eras at GMC Srinagar. Here seen with Dr. Sikand and Dr. Durrani (photo courtesy of Dr. Durrani).

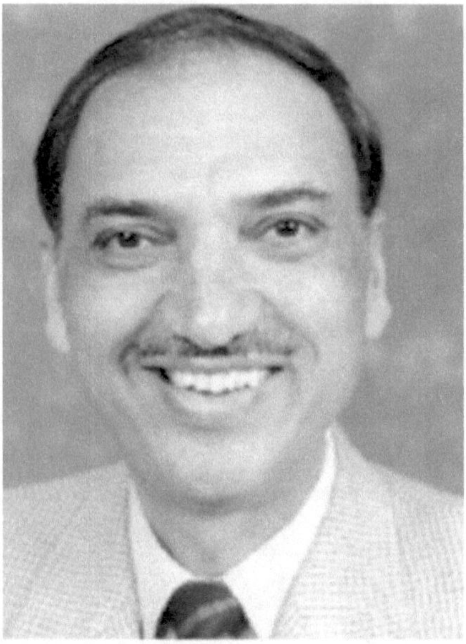

Dr. M. S. Khuroo, the gastroenterologist who performed excellent research on viral hepatitis, hydatidosis, biliary ascariasis, and peptic ulcer.

The
New England
Journal of Medicine

Established in 1812 as the NEW ENGLAND JOURNAL OF MEDICINE AND SURGERY

Volume 336 April 10, 1997 Number 15

Original article

A comparison of Omeprazole and Placebo for Bleeding Peptic Ulcer

Mohammad Sultan Khuroo, M.D., D.M., Ghulam Nabi Yattoo, M.D., Gul Javid, M.D., Bashir Ahmad Khan, M.D., Altaf Ahmad Shah, M.D., Ghulam Mohammad Gulzar, M.D., and Jaswinder Singh Sodi, MD. page1054-1058

Editorial

Therapy for Bleeding Peptic Ulcers

John R. Saltzman, M.D. and J.K. Zawacki, M. D. page 1091-1093

The landmark paper of Prof. M. S. Khuroo in NEJM (1997) with the editorial that changed the management of peptic ulcer.

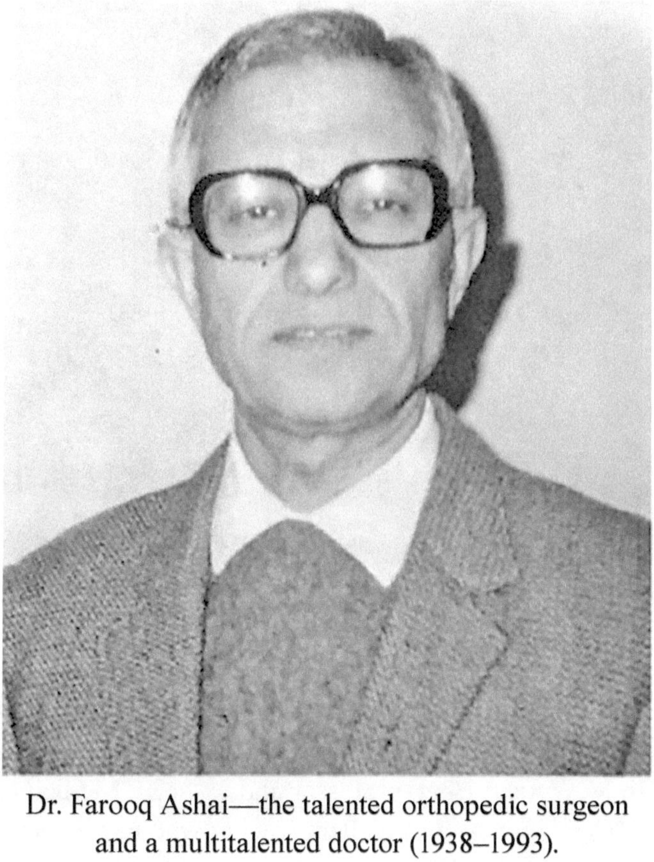

Dr. Farooq Ashai—the talented orthopedic surgeon and a multitalented doctor (1938–1993).

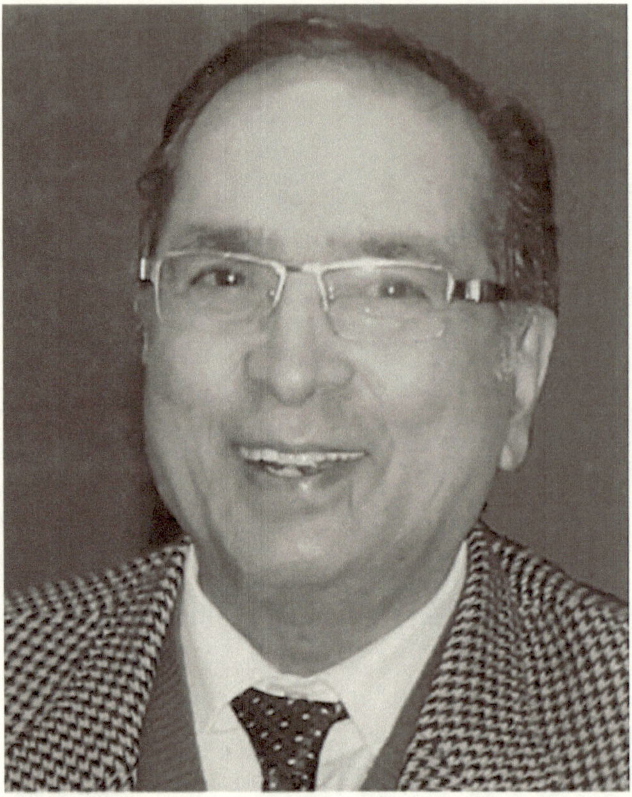

Dr. M. Yousuf Bhat, professor and ex-head, Medicine, GMC Srinagar—an excellent teacher who has inspired hundreds of his students to pursue medicine.

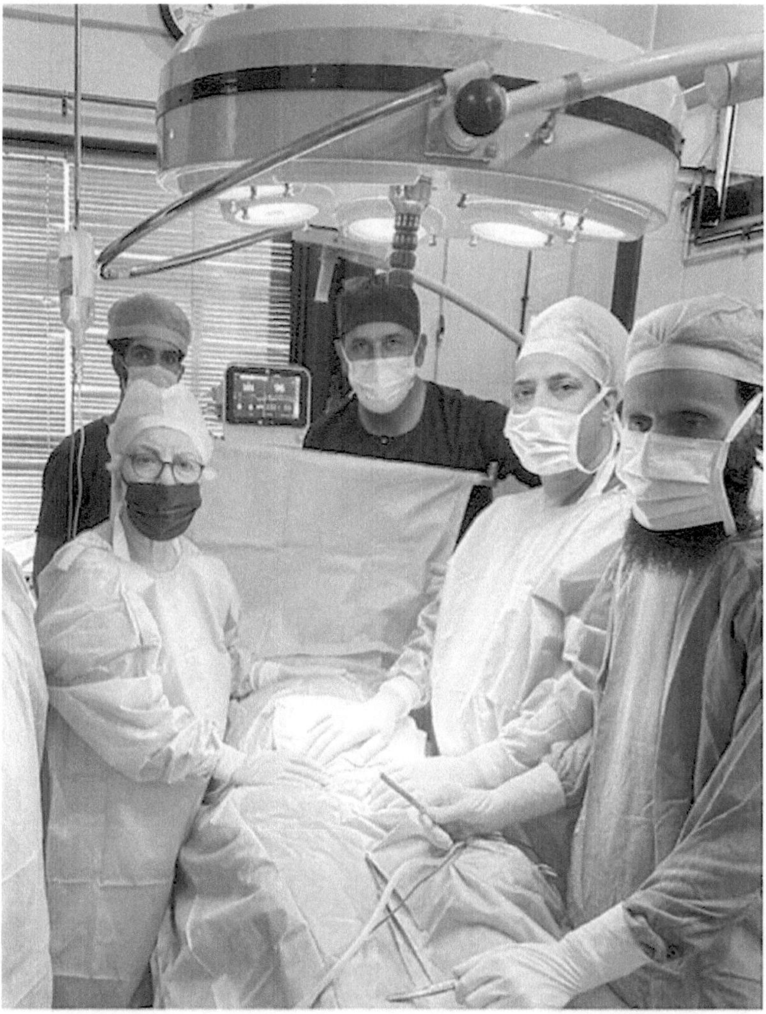

Dr. Bilqees—the versatile gynecologist and obstetrician
who continues to operate—with the theater staff
doing surgery (photo taken on July 7, 2023).

The Pioneers

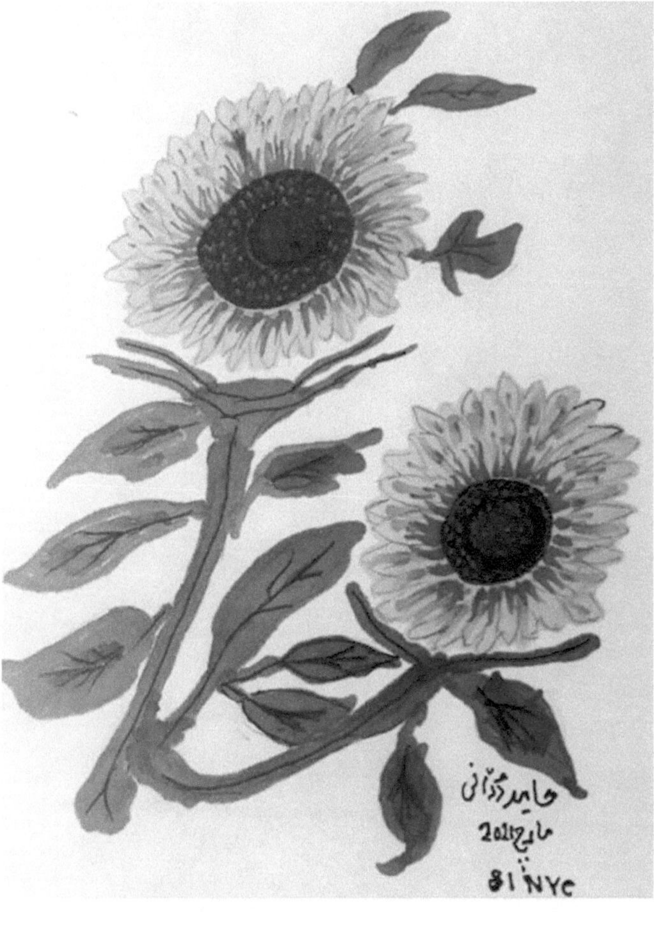

1. **Dr. Abdul Ahad Beig**
2. **Dr. Abdul Ahad Guru**
3. **Dr. Abdul Hamid Fazili**
4. **Dr. Abdul Hamid Zargar**
5. **Dr. Abdul Rashid Khan**
6. **Dr. Abdul Rauf**
7. **Dr. Amarjeet Singh Sethi**
8. **Dr. Bashir Ahmad**
9. **Dr. Ghulam Mohammad Dhaar**
10. **Dr. Ghulam Mohammad Shah**
11. **Dr. (Col.) Ghulam Nabi**
12. **Dr. Ghulam Nabi Kozgar**
13. **Dr. Jagdish Singh**
14. **Dr. Kundan Lal Chowdhury**
15. **Dr. Mohammad Ismail Quadri**
16. **Dr. Mohammed Sayeed**
17. **Dr. Mushtaq Ahmad Margoob**
18. **Dr. Nazir Ahmed Wani**
19. **Dr. Pirzada Abdul Rashid**
20. **Dr. Rafiq Ahmad Pampori**
21. **Dr. Sheikh Abdul Ahad**
22. **Dr. Sushil Razdan**
23. **Dr. T. S. Sethi**
24. **Prof. Taffazull Hussain**
25. **Dr. Zubaida Jeelani**

Dr. Abdul Ahad Beig

Dr. Erina M. Hoch did a remarkable job in Kashmir converting an inhuman asylum into a hospital for psychiatric diseases. Dr. Abdul Ahad Beig helped to build up on the work done by Dr. Hoch and give the subject of psychiatry its due. Dr. Beig is credited with introducing the subject of psychiatry to his students at Government Medical College, Srinagar, and worked hard to remove the stigma from psychiatric diseases. He projected psychiatry as a science and a branch of medicine. He helped to generate interest among his students in the subject of psychiatry so that many pursued it as a career of choice. "Psychiatric ailments had a cause and could be treated and reversed"—he would make this bold statement in our theory and clinical classes in an era when misinformation, disinformation, and ignorance about psychiatric diseases were rampant.

Dr. Beig was an extremely soft-spoken and deeply learned psychiatrist. I had an opportunity to be his student in my MBBS and his house surgeon in Psychiatric Disease Hospital. He was a gifted orator who could explain the most complex Freudian theories in a simple language. He would hold the attention of the entire class and cater to the needs of inpatients and outpatients in the hospital. He was sober and gentle with the most aggressive and tactful and humane toward the most difficult patient. We would accompany him on the rounds and would be surprised to see his attention to the detail and his care for the inpatients. His outpatient clinics were always overcrowded. He would listen to the patients with attention and never lose an opportunity to comfort them. He was the one who recognized the effect of trauma on the psyche of Kashmiris and was one of the first few to stand up to the mental challenges that Kashmiris were facing. He alarmed the society and the government about the "psychiatric epidemic," which was erupting in Kashmir as the conflict was unwinding.

This illustrious psychiatrist was born in Bandipora, Kashmir, on July 8, 1947. His father, Mr. Ali Mohammad Beig, never expected his son to do medicine. Dr. Beig received his schooling from Government Higher Secondary School, Kuloosa, Bandipora, and got admission in Government Medical College, Srinagar, for MBBS in 1964. He went against the tide to be a psychiatrist. He was inspired by Dr. Hoch, who worked in Government Psychiatric Hospital, Srinagar, when he joined there. Dr. Beig liked her way of working and was greatly inspired by her dedication. He was a clinical demonstrator in psychiatry from 1971 to 1973. He pursued his dream of becoming a psychiatrist when he went to PGI Chandigarh in 1973 for his MD in psychiatry, which he completed in 1976. He did his registrarship in psychiatry from 1976 to 1977. He was recruited as a lecturer in psychiatry in Government Medical College, Srinagar, later in 1977. He rose to the position of assistant professor (psychiatry), associate professor, and became a professor of psychiatry in 1993. He became the head of the Department of Psychiatry and died after a brief illness while still in service in 1995. His departure at an early age left not only his young wife and kids orphaned but also orphaned most of his patients who had developed an addiction to him and had become psychologically dependent on him.

Dr. Beig was a life fellow of the Indian Psychiatric Society. He was the pioneer of hypnotism and hypnotherapy in Kashmir. He was given a Lifetime Achievement Award by the Doctors'

Association of Kashmir posthumously in recognition of the distinguished work he did as a psychiatrist.

Dr. Beig had many admirers. He would quietly attend to social and familial issues of his friends, colleagues, and patients. His patients trusted him with their secrets and their mental problems, and most of the times he helped them to come out of the gloom and despair that the circumstances had put them into. He never let anyone down.

Dr. Abdul Ahad Guru

It was 1984. A twenty-five-year-old man, Sofi Ghulam Hassan, from Pantha Chowk, Kashmir, a diagnosed case of a heart ailment, was referred to AIIMS, New Delhi, for open-heart surgery. The man was poor and had three children and couldn't afford Rs 20,000 needed for the surgery, so he sought treatment from doctors back home. On October 1, 1984, a team of Kashmiri doctors headed by the dynamic cardiovascular and thoracic surgeon, Dr. Abdul Ahad Guru, did what seemed impossible—performed the first open-heart surgery in the state of Jammu and Kashmir on this poor desperate man. The surgery was a success and took a tiring nine hours for the young team. The local population was thrilled—there was no need to go to Delhi for open-heart surgery; doctors back home had conquered the heart. Urdu dailies reported the news with great enthusiasm, and a few days later, *Times of India* (October 6, 1984) reported the news about the first open-heart surgery in Kashmir. Congratulations poured from all the corners. The then health minister visited SKIMS personally and congratulated the team leader. The team leader, Dr. Abdul Ahad Guru, was no ordinary surgeon—he had a class of his own; he was bold, innovative, and confident. He founded a department, took first leaps at treating sick hearts, and brought relief to thousands till a mysterious gun took his precious life away.

Dr. Abdul Ahad Guru was born in Seer Jagir, Sopore, Kashmir, on April 13, 1940. He did his MBBS from Bangalore

Medical College, Bengaluru, in 1964. He completed his master's in general surgery from King George Medical College, Lucknow, in 1969. He did his superspeciality training (MCh) in CVTS from AIIMS, New Delhi, in 1978. For a short while, he worked as an assistant professor of surgery in Government Medical College, Srinagar, and proceeded to the USA in 1980 to have fellowship in cardiovascular surgery at Buffalo Children's Hospital. He worked in Milwaukee, Chicago, with the world authority on cardiothoracic surgery, Dr. Denton Cooley (who had performed more than eight thousand surgeries, including one on India's president Neelam Sanjeeva Reddy). Dr. Denton was highly impressed by Dr. Guru's surgical skills and once remarked that he had nothing extra to offer to Dr. Guru as he saw him as an expert cardiac surgeon. His eagerness to treat his own people and to help them brought him back to Kashmir, and he joined SKIMS as an associate professor of CVTS in 1982. He was promoted as a professor in 1984 and held the chair of the Department of Surgery from 1984 onward. Dr. Guru gave up a lucrative offer in the US to build up an institution and establish the Department of Cardiovascular and Thoracic Surgery at SKIMS to help the poor patients back home.

There is an interesting case of subdural hematoma described by Dr. K. L. Chowdhury in his collection of cases where he talks about how courageous Dr. Guru was and how he saved the life of a patient who had been refused treatment from the premier medical center of India. Dr. K. L. Chowdhury diagnosed a case of subdural hematoma at SMHS Hospital (possibly the first such case diagnosed in Kashmir), and the surgeons at SMHS who had no prior experience in dealing with such cases referred the case to AIIMS. A month later, the patient returned from AIIMS without any treatment, but his symptoms had worsened. When the diagnosis was clear after an angiography was done, the senior professor was hesitant to take a risk and looked quizzically at his assistant professor, Dr. Abdul Ahad Guru. Dr. Guru readily agreed to operate upon the patient. Recounting this incident, Dr. Chowdhury calls Dr. Guru "a young dynamic surgeon, always ready to have a go at difficult cases, always ready to try new things." The enthusiastic young surgeon asked Dr. Chowdhury to accompany him to the operation theater, which he happily did. Dr. Chowdhury was impressed to see a burr hole being made and dark fluid (blood) being drained and was a witness to a historical procedure at SMHS Hospital (stories from Dr. K. L. Chowdhury's *My Medical Journey*, compiled by M. K. Raina).

Dr. Guru was an able guide and a keen researcher who worked on hydatid disease of the lung, bronchogenic carcinoma, empyema, valve prosthesis, atrial septal defect, patent ductus arteriosus, and surgical aspects of peritonitis. He had many firsts to his credit. One of his colleagues, Dr. Ashiq Hussain Naqshbandi, has described Dr. Guru as a "bold, courageous and competent surgeon par excellence" (*JK Practitioner* 1996). Prof. Abdul Ahad, former HOD of ENT at GMC Srinagar, describes Dr. Guru as an excellent surgeon, humanitarian, and social worker (*JK Practitioner* 1996). All youngsters who were taught and trained by Dr. Guru found him helpful; in fact, he would teach them with patience and would always ignore their shortcomings. He helped many physicians and surgeons to grow and flourish professionally. He would always ensure to boost their confidence. For his juniors, he was a source of light; for young surgeons, an inspiration; and for his colleagues, a reliable friend and a guide. He was one of the founder members of SKIMS, and in the day-to-day meetings in the institute, his advice and wisdom helped the institute executives to take the decisions and provide for the facilities that helped the institute to attain its peak.

Dr. Guru was known for his philanthropy and his concern for the poor. In spite of his busy schedule at SKIMS, he would be available for free service and consultation at his residence in Barzalla every morning and at his native village on weekends.

He established *Sarais* near hospitals to provide accommodation to families of needy patients who had to come down to towns and cities for treatment. Some of these *Sarais* are still functional. He established X-ray clinics and laboratories at Barzalla and Sopore where various tests were conducted free or at nominal charges.

Dr. Guru loved to dream for his people. He concentrated his efforts to realize his dreams. To this great man goes the credit of establishing Jehlum Valley College of Medical Sciences—the first private medical college of the state making it functional against all the odds in record time. This college, now named SKIMS Medical College, with its attached well-established hospital, is a gift of Dr. Guru to the people, and this college adds 125 doctors per year to the state pool and has several postgraduate departments.

In the early 1990s, when the state witnessed turmoil, Dr. Guru provided financial assistance to the victims of turmoil. He used his own vehicle to reach far-off areas and literally converted it into a mobile dispensary providing medical assistance to the needy amid curfews. To provide emergency treatment to the needy people, Dr. Guru would not hesitate to drive an ambulance himself amid curfew and help to provide medical aid. Dr. Guru was was a competent doctor, a team leader, a philanthropist, and a well-wisher of Kashmiri people.

Dr. Guru was abducted from his place of work, and, the next day, his bullet-ridden body was found near Soura. Nobody owned this cowardly act. Kashmir lost a legend, a doctor, and the poor lost their hope. Guru family is known for its philanthropy and love for Kashmir and its people. Dr. Guru's son in the US is taking further his father's dream of helping Kashmiris. He has done a great deal of work in education and health care—there will be more to come in the future Inshallah!

Dr. Abdul Hamid Fazili

Dr. Abdul Hamid Fazili was born on March 30, 1937, to Mr. Mohammad Sayed Fazili and Sara Begum in Srinagar, Kashmir. He received his schooling from MP School, Srinagar, and did his MBBS from MGM Medical College, Indore (1959). He did his postgraduation (MD) in pharmacology from GMC Srinagar. He served as HOD Pharmacology, GMC Srinagar, from 1971 to 1985. He has been a brilliant teacher who left a lasting impact on his students. His teaching methods were unique, and students would remember what they had been taught for a lifetime.

Dr. Fazili took up many foreign assignments and served as the head of the department, Mosul University (Iraq), and HOD Pharmacology, Benghazi University, Libya. After his retirement, he served as HOD Pharmacology, SKIMS Medical College (JVC), Srinagar.

Dr. Abdul Hamid Fazili was a passionate teacher who made the subject of pharmacology easy and interesting. He taught with his heart and was student-friendly. One of his students who retired as a professor of medicine said that he learned clinical medicine from Dr. Fazili's classes in pharmacology. For instance, when Dr. Fazili taught about the drugs used for the treatment of Parkinson's disease, he would demonstrate the typical features of the disease (tremor, gait, etc.) on himself; the impact of his teaching was so much that the students never forgot the clinical features or the drugs used in Parkinson disease. His granddaughter recalls him having handwritten notes on old-fashioned note books, and he would add up to them from new editions of textbooks. When asked about these notes, he would say, "It is never too late to learn, and I am always a student."

Though Dr. Fazili was an old-fashioned teacher, he had a quest to learn about technology. His daughter-in-law recalls him as a man who was ahead of his times and would always advise his students and family members not to run away from the digital world. The conversations with him would enrich you with knowledge.

Dr. Fazili was a kind and gentle soul who inspired his family, friends, and colleagues with his impeccable manners. He had precious advice to give on parenting and religion besides medicine and life. He was a dignified man, always neatly dressed and always thought good for others. He treated his colleagues and subordinates with love and respect. He would secretly help the people in need and go out of way to address their problems.

As one of his family members told me about him, Dr. Fazili never conformed to tradition; he challenged not only people around him but also himself with an open mind. Dr. Fazili was one of those rare bright lights—when gone, you can feel the remnants even years after it is gone. A feature that described Dr. Fazili was that he was soft and kindhearted permanently. No wonder this great teacher GMC Srinagar and SKIMS-MC is a common denominator in terms of being a "favorite teacher" for all the doctors from these institutions who have benefitted from him.

Dr. Fazili has two sons, Sajad and Irfan, and a daughter, Samia. Sajad is an ophthalmologist, and Irfan is an engineer. His daughter, Samia, is a doctor too. His children and grandchildren remember him for his values and the softness of his heart. His daughters-in-law speak of his gentle manners and caring nature.

Dr. Abdul Hamid Zargar

As the dawn pierces through the mighty snow-clad mountains and illuminates Srinagar, I see men and women, walking and running, singly, in pairs and groups, feeling the morning breeze and cutting through the sharp rays of the sun. A dawn of activity, a dawn of engagement has descended on this population. To one's satisfaction, in these marches and runs early mornings, women outnumber men. What is it that has brought this huge population out to chase the dawn and its beauty? What is it that has pulled people away from their beds, away from their slumber onto the roads and parks early mornings? Is it a concern for health, care for their hearts, a scare of obesity, a worry of disability, or a fear of sudden death? Whatever the reason, it is a pleasure to watch this activity in a valley where people have been sealed for years together in their confines. Someone needs to cheer up, someone needs to be given a credit for bringing out a change in the mindset of our population, and someone needs to be complimented for spreading this awareness among people of all ages . . .

On the outskirts of Srinagar overlooking the Anchar Lake, a huge structure stands witness to the amount of effort that people working under this roof have undertaken to bring about the change that is visible on the roads. There may be many who need to be complimented for what is evident, media might have played a role as well, but ask an old diabetic as he races along the roads at the far end of his life as to what made him overcome his laziness and his disease; his answer would be "Zargar Sahib said so . . ." This health march has become a march of faith for the old man afflicted with a "sweet disease" . . .

Prof. Abdul Hamid Zargar was born on April 12, 1951, in Baramulla Kashmir to Mr. Abdul Rehman and Sara Zargar. He did his MBBS from Government Medical College Srinagar in 1976, MD in medicine from the same college in 1981, and DM in endocrinology from PGI Chandigarh in 1985. He became an assistant professor in the Endocrinology Department at SKIMS in 1990 and later on rose to be the professor and head of the department. He put in nearly thirty years of service at the Sher-i-Kashmir Institute of Medical Sciences and during this time involved himself in patient care research and academics. Call him a physician, an endocrinologist, a diabetologist, an epidemiologist, a thyroid disease specialist, an infertility disease specialist, or whatever; he is a man who took up the challenge of challenging the diseases that had squeezed us, disabled us, and given us all pain and agony. He turned "diabetes the killer" into "diabetes the chiller," recommending constant physical activity, a change in dietary habits; otherwise, our hostile climate and constantly disturbed sociopolitical scenario were enough to give us all that would predispose us to this disabling disease. Recommendations for diabetics were not merely "copied notes" from books but were based on exhaustive and useful research undertaken by Dr. Zargar at SKIMS. The burden of diabetes in this population, the predisposing factors for the disease, the preventive, and the curative modalities were all worked at, and the world of science looked with awe toward this small place for something new and informative on diabetes. Dr. Zargar did debate rare syndromes and genetic aberrations but focused himself on a disease that had threatened our existence.

A modern man is obsessed with the idea of "woman's emancipation," "woman's liberation," etc. but hardly talks about woman's health. Imagine a woman with a slender body, fragile bones, and a depressed look who is sinking in her own pain without relief. This woman does not seem to have a visible disease but just has pains, aches, and fatigue. She has lost herself and lost interest in herself, her spouse, and her children; she is a suffering woman of a suffering family. Dr. Zargar recognized these women who are not uncommon on the countryside as the ones suffering from a disease known as "Sheehan's syndrome." This syndrome became a subject of interest for Dr. Zargar, and he took up the challenge of studying this disease threadbare. These silently suffering women were identified, diagnosed, and treated. Not that these patients were not identified earlier, but Dr. Zargar's research held the disease by its neck . . .

Women suffer from other age-related diseases and specific diseases of bone known as osteoporosis—the preventive and therapeutic aspects of this another preventable disease have a lot to offer to a Kashmiri woman who in her daily slog has ignored her bones . . .. .

Though women form the backbone, children are the hope of tomorrow—imagine the life of a family where a mentally abnormal child is born. Many of these children were rescued in their wombs by recognizing specific deficiencies that lead to mental abnormalities in children. Iodine deficiency was studied on a large scale, recognizing disturbing dimensions of such deficiency in women, children, and adult Kashmiris who are predisposed to such deficiencies because of the inherent deficiency of iodine in our soil. Imagine the penalty we are paying for deficiency of a nutrient, which if restored in diet can prevent huge losses—Dr. Zargar has been instrumental in giving the recognition and treatment of iodine-deficiency disorders a priority slot in preventive health care.

Dr. Zargar headed the Department of Endocrinology at SKIMS and has trained an excellent team of doctors who I am sure will carry ahead the work that he has initiated. Dr. Zargar, before his retirement, climbed up the ladder and became the director of SKIMS.

Dr. Zargar has been a dynamic academician, a researcher par excellence, and a humane clinician. Dr. Zargar has powerful oratory skills and mesmerizes the audience with his speech. A humble doctor of my status cannot write a note on him. But I felt the urge to write—for all to know how a man of extraordinary talent worked tirelessly in the below-average working conditions and came up as a hope for the hopeless patients of Kashmir and challenged the world of medicine with the remark that "excellence can be achieved while treating the ordinary."

I am sure profiling Dr. Zargar has its limitations as I cannot enlist his contribution to the field of community health and medicine in this small space. The work Dr. Zargar has done is no less than what a Nobel laureate does; the community service he has rendered is no less than what Edi has rendered. His commitment to the cause of patient care will inspire many youngsters and draw them toward need-based research.

When Dr. Ali Jan and other legends conceived the idea of SKIMS, I am sure they were on a hunt for people like Dr. Zargar. Legendary Dr. Jan has made a permanent place in our hearts as a doctor who took care of Kashmiri and his diseases at an individual level, but Dr. Zargar has removed the mites from the entire orchids .... There is that old diabetic waiting for his advice, that Gujjar lady with Sheehan's praying for his long life, that boy with obesity whom he helped to become a smart young man, and that childless couple who are now father and mother—my wishes might be corollary, but, nonetheless, I say God bless you. Truly, you are the "doctor of masses."

Dr. Abdul Rashid Khan

Slender, smart, and quick-tempered, Dr. Abdul Rashid Khan is a hero. The whole medical fraternity respects him and knows him. He is a pathologist who is practicing pathology for the last forty-five years in Kashmir. His eye is the eagle's eye, and his knife-sharp brain makes him a darling of all the clinicians. You like him, you hate him, but when a diagnosis is in doubt, you seek his opinion.

Dr. Khan was born on May 25, 1944, to Mr. Ghulam Qadir Khan and Jalila Begum in Chinkral Mohalla, Habba Kadal (downtown), Srinagar. Bright and sharp from the beginning, he went to Government Medical College, Srinagar, in 1962 and completed his MBBS in 1967. The famous hepatologist of the valley, Prof. M. S. Khurro, in his description of Dr. A. R. Khan, his classmate, says, "One who impressed me the most was a tall skinny fellow from Chinkral Mohalla (now legendary pathologist Prof. Abdul Rashid Khan) and every day we walked together from Medical College gate to his home discussing Best and Taylor (Physiology) and Gray's Anatomy. It always astonished me how he had mastered these books including the footnotes." This is when one genius acknowledges the genius of his buddy (*KASHMED* 2011, p. 92).

Dr. Khan moved away from routine; though he excelled in medicine and surgery, he chose pathology as his subject of interest. He received training in cytology, gyne-cytology and, histopathology from PGI Chandigarh and did his MD in pathology from PGI Chandigarh in 1974. He started the gyne-cytology service center at Lal Ded Hospital, Srinagar, in collaboration with Prof. Bilquees Jamila. He set up the Pathology Department at Government Medical College, Jammu, and was its lone faculty member and head of the department from 1974 to 1977. He established histopathology service, cytopathology service, and diagnostic hematology at Government Medical College, Jammu, and would personally go to PGI Chandigarh and collect specimens from there for the museum. Professor Pathania, principal of Government Medical College, Jammu, would always be all praise for Professor Khan and call him an asset privately or in public.

Dr. Khan has served as a professor and head of the Department of Pathology, Government Medical College, Srinagar, and has been a favorite teacher of his students. Besides routine, he has diagnosed the rarest of the rare tumors and pathological curiosities. Dr. Khan is a brilliant histopathologist but loves to do FNAC (fine needle aspiration cytology). Clinicians love his report—which is always crisp and to the point. What he diagnoses on preliminary tests comes out to be the "same" in spite of vigorous IHCs and molecular tests. He has an aptitude for oncopathology especially lymph nodes, gynecology, bone, and soft tissue tumors.

As a postgraduate student of Professor Khan, I have seen him to be a tough taskmaster. I remember when, during my postgraduation, I requested him a leave in view of my marriage, he gave his own microscope to me telling me that I should complete my thesis work at home. I remember taking the microscope home and doing the required work. Dr. Khan has a vast experience of reporting histopathology specimens and biopsies. Besides the work that he did at Government Medical College, Srinagar, he has reported more than one lakh fifty thousand biopsies at his private clinic. He has performed more than one lakh twenty thousand FNACs and helped to alleviate the distress of lakhs of patients. We must look at what the world record for the maximum number of FNACs and reporting of histopathological specimens by a single pathologist is. Dr. Khan maintains a meticulous record of his cases and invariably remembers the names of his patients.

He has published more than fifty papers in international journals and during COVID time authored two books: one on fine needle aspiration cytology of head and neck paragangliomas of which he has the largest series in the world literature. He has also authored a book on FNAC of thyroid and its application in a place with limited resources.

Dr. Khan is a hard-core pathologist who, in spite of opportunities to work in the West (both UK and the US), refused them and happily chose to render his services in Kashmir. Dr. Ali Jan was quite fond of him and wanted him to work at SKIMS, Srinagar, and take care of pathology there. However, the Government Medical College principal refused to relieve Dr. Khan, and he continued his services at Government Medical College, Srinagar. Somehow, he did not join SKIMS, which later on he regretted because pathology at SKIMS was advanced and the academic atmosphere superior. But then, that is what Dr. Khan does—swimming against the tide. When everybody else joined SKIMS, Dr. Khan refused to join it.

Dr. Khan is a lively man who has enjoyed playing cricket, bridge, and loves listening to Gazals. He is always well dressed and has good command over Urdu, Kashmiri, and English. He is a workaholic and works in style, never overcharging, always obliging his friends and colleagues and students with one last glance on the "slides" for a final opinion.

As a postgraduate, I used to ask him, "Sir, you have made the diagnosis, why do you continue to look at the slides?" He would calmly say, "I enjoy the beauty of this slide, I want to treat my eyes with this beauty, and I want my brain to retain it."

Prof. G. Q. Allaqaband sent him two Geimsa-stained slides from FNAC of an upper abdominal mass in 1988. He interpreted the slides as adenocarcinoma of the pancreas. Dr. Allaqaband called him to his chamber and revealed that the slides belonged to Dr. Ali Jan. Dr. Khan was shocked but helpless. The legendary physician was nearing an end, and Dr. Khan was not happy about what he had seen . . .

Dr. Khan is an influential pathologist well known in the pathology circles. He works in his private laboratory still and lives with his wife in Srinagar.

Dr. Abdul Rauf

Kashmir Valley was under a blanket of recognized and unrecognized nutritional deficiency disorders (i.e., iron deficiency anemia, iodine deficiency, vitamin D deficiency, etc.) and many preventable diseases (helmithic infestations, bacterial infections, etc.)—these diseases had assumed an epidemic form and were responsible for the agony of a large chunk of population. Nonstop awareness campaigns and tireless efforts were required to address these diseases. The credit goes to Dr. Abdul Rauf for bringing in various sponsored projects and schemes to the valley whereby these deficiency disorders and preventable infections and infestations were recognized in our population and appropriate preventive and curative measures were taken up.

Dr. Rauf was the principal investigator for the ICMR project titled "Evaluation of National Nutritional Anemia Prophylaxis Program in J&K." He has been the principal investigator for the ICMR project "Double Salt Fortification" and the district nutrition project for the prevention and control of micronutrient deficiency disorders. These projects brought the deficiency disorders to the fore, and corrective measures were employed to address these disorders. He was the chief coordinator for state-level ICDS (Integrated Child Development Services) survey, which is an integrated scheme looking after the health of children and mothers. Dr. Rauf has served as the principal investigator for the ICMR project related to human reproduction research. He has been one of the first researchers/health-care experts to study mortality and morbidity in children as regards their socioeconomic status.

Dr. Abdul Rauf was born in Srinagar on May 29, 1944, to Mr. Ghulam Nabi and Salima Mir. He did his schooling at CMS School Srinagar and his FSc from SP College, Srinagar. He did his MBBS in 1968 from Government Medical College, Srinagar, and MD in SPM (Social and Preventive Medicine) from Government Medical College, Srinagar, in 1973. He served as a demonstrator SPM, Government Medical College, Srinagar, from 1971 to 1974. He was inducted as an assistant professor in the SPM Department of Government Medical College, Srinagar, in 1974, and was promoted as an associate professor in 1981 and as a professor in 1983. He headed the Department of SPM from 1983 to 2000.

Dr. Rauf has been the recipient of many fellowships and has participated in many international seminars conducted in collaboration with WHO and UNICEF. He has been the recipient of a WHO fellowship titled "Epidemiological Services Development and Training" from the Tropical School of Medicine USA for 1987. Dr. Rauf has organized a dozen workshops and conferences in the Department of SPM, GMC Srinagar, which brought the department into the national and international limelight. He has been awarded the Lifetime Achievement Award by the Indian Association of Preventive and Social Medicine in October 2015. He has also received an Award of Honor from UNICEF.

Dr. Rauf has been a postgraduate guide to more than fifteen postgraduates in preventive and social medicine. He has more than two dozen papers to his credit and has presented his work at many national and international conferences. His papers about the problems related to the common man and improving the health-care delivery system in Kashmir Valley became the baseline for framing guidelines and implementing various preventive health programs and guidelines. This included papers related to parasitic infestations in Kashmir, the tuberculosis scenario in the valley, anthropometry in school-going children, and health hazard problems related to the dwellers of Dal Lake. Many of these studies were collaborative in nature and done in collaboration with the Department of Environment, Government of India. He has been an expert in the selection of faculty at AMU, AIIMS, New Delhi, and the Union Public Service Commission. He has been a consultant for the school health project in Kashmir's schools and chairman of a number of committees at GMC Srinagar.

Dr. Rauf is a thorough gentleman who is known for his honesty, integrity, and teaching skills. Dr. Rauf served as the principal/dean of Government Medical College, Srinagar, from 2000 to 2002. He has been one of the visionaries of the GMC Srinagar who has done a lot of work related to its all-around development. He became the principal of GMC Srinagar in turbulent times but held on to the uneasy position with grace. With his gentle mannerism and a helping attitude, he was able to lead the GMC in tough times.

Dr. Rauf is married to Dr. Azra Shah. They have two children: a daughter, who is a neuro-oncologist in the US, and a son, who is a banker Dubai. He lives happily with his children and lovely grandchildren, and the family visits Kashmir often.

Dr. Amarjeet Singh Sethi

Dr. Amarjeet Singh Sethi was the third child of a prominent medico, Dr. Mohan Singh Sethi, who had his roaring medical practice at Lal Chowk Clinic for five decades. Not many children of an era spanning decades have escaped being seen by the father-son duo. He was born on April 20, 1943, and studied at Tyndale Biscoe School. "In all things, be men" was his motto in life.

Dr. Sethi was a very bright student and was admitted to AIIMS New Delhi for MBBS in 1960. He graduated in 1965 and pursued his postgraduation in pediatrics from AIIMS. He was awarded a Gold Medal in 1965 by the honorable president of India, Mr. V. V. Giri. Dr. Amarjeet Singh Sethi was the first pediatrician from the Kashmir Valley to have graduated and postgraduated from the prestigious All India Institute of Medical Sciences, New Delhi. He is also the first doctor from the valley to receive a gold medal from AIIMS. He did his fellowship in pediatric hematology from the US in 1970 and returned to Kashmir in 1974 to help in shaping up the pediatric hospital and to set up his practice in Kashmir. Once recruited into the faculty at GMC Srinagar, he rose to the position of professor and HOD Pediatrics, GMC Srinagar. He was responsible for helping pediatrics be recognized as a separate speciality and would always say, "Pediatrics is not mini-medicine, children are not mini-adults." He was the first one of that era to have publications in prestigious and indexed journals in the early '70s. He was the first pediatrician to introduce proper immunization of children in Kashmir Valley. He introduced pediatric hematology in the pediatric hospital.

Professor Mushtaq (former professor of pediatrics at SKIMS) has the following to say about Dr. Sethi: "Dr. AS Sethi was Assistant professor in 1978 when I was a House Surgeon in his Unit. He started pediatric hemato-oncology in Pediatric Hospital and encouraged all of us to publish papers. He was a great clinician and academician besides being a thorough gentleman. He has contributed greatly to academics and the practical application of immunization program in the Pediatric Hospital."

He supervised the exchange transfusion for hyperbilirubinemia in newborn babies in 1977 for the first time in Kashmir. He started phototherapy treatment in Children's Hospital Srinagar by making a unit, taking help from a local carpenter, electrician, and others. His students described him a great personality. He was a wonderful human being and a great teacher. Dr. Sethi was involved with many charitable organizations, orphanages, and was also the president of the Rotary Club in the 1990s where charitable events were performed.

On a personal front, Dr. Sethi married Ms. Sovinder Sethi in 1969, who was from a prominent business family of Cuttack, Odisha. The couple was blessed with two daughters, Guleen and Pavleen. *Gul* means "flower" in Persian, and *Pav* means "flower" in Russian. One of the flowers (i.e., Guleen) passed away in 1986. The other daughter is a dentist who lives with her husband and two sons in Japan. Dr. Sethi was a scholar and loved poetry. He loved Urdu and Punjabi poetry and would often recite the couplets relevant to the circumstance. He had a great sense of humor. He was fond of pet dogs, fishing, and gardening.

Despite very difficult circumstances, he never left Kashmir and continued to serve its people. The location of pediatrics hospital in the middle of a volatile area did not prevent him from attending to his duties regularly. Whether floods or turmoil, he stood by his Kashmiri brethren through thick and thin. He lived in Gogjibagh, Srinagar, however died in COVID times at his sister's place in Haryana in 2020. His favorite quote was "I know what I want to be, He knows what I shall be."

(The profile was submitted by Dr. Sethi's nephew Mr. Gurpreet Singh Sethi.)

Dr. Bashir Ahmad

Dr. Bashir Ahmad was born in a small village fifty kilometers away from the main city of Srinagar. Despite limited academic opportunities and meagre resources, he managed to get his medical training (i.e., MBBS and MS in ophthalmology) from Maulana Azad Medical College, New Delhi, through sheer hard work and determination. He completed his MBBS in 1966 and MS in ophthalmology in 1970.

He worked for a short period as registrar in Maulana Azad Medical College and its associated LNJP hospital. Seeing the people from the valley moving from hospital to hospital in Delhi, he had an ambition to do something for the people in his own state so that there would be no need for poor patients to go out of the state for treatment, at least in the field of ophthalmology. After returning from Delhi in 1970, he joined Government Medical College and its associated hospitals as registrar and was appointed as an assistant professor in 1974, promoted as associate professor in 1981, and then professor and head of the department. Dr. Bashir had a chance to serve Government Medical College, Jammu, for a short period as professor and HOD. Dr. Bashir did his fellowship training from the Institute of Ophthalmology in Moorfields Hospital, London, in 1984, followed by a fellowship from the Institute of Ophthalmology, Kiryu, Japan, in 1992. He got an opportunity to serve in Iran. In Iran, he was awarded Outstanding Foreign Doctor Award in 1980.

As an ophthalmologist, he did everything possible to upgrade the teaching standard and patient care not only in the Medical College, Srinagar, but also even in the private sector. His zeal to help his own people made him bring the latest equipment for the diagnosis and treatment of eye diseases and set up his own center. This center is a "high-tech eye center" and is equipped with the technology and infrastructure to meet all the routine and emergency investigations and surgical treatment of eye diseases. The center is one of the best eye centers in India. The first intraocular lens (IOL) implantation was performed in this center in 1984. This center was among very few centers in India at that time to have started lens implantation. The latest techniques in glaucoma surgery were started in this center in 1982. Green laser, diode laser, and YAG laser were introduced in the early '90s along with Humphrey visual field analyzer. The corneal transplantation was done at this center in 2005 in association with MM Eye Tech, New Delhi. This center is the only health-care organization in J&K to have received national accreditation (NABH) in 2016 as Small Health Care Organization (SHCO). Dr. Bashir has not stopped at what he has achieved. The center is constantly looking for an opportunity to upgrade the facilities to an international level so that there are no referrals for any patient with any type of eye disease to go out of Kashmir.

Dr. Bashir has received more than a dozen awards from India and abroad. According to Dr. Bashir, the most precious award for him was bestowed upon him by his own students after his retirement in the form of Most Popular Teacher Award, 2015. He received an award by Bakhshi Memorial Committee too. He is a leader who has spoken for himself and his ilk; no wonder he has been a chairman/president of many organizations and committees, including the Medical College Teachers Association, J&K Medical Employees Association, Consultants Rights Society, Kashmir Ophthalmological Society, etc.

Dr. Bashir is a satisfied man who has been an excellent ophthalmologist, a great teacher for undergraduates and postgraduates, and has proved to be an employer by setting up a state-of-the-art eye center in the heart of Srinagar, which has not only decongested the overburdened government hospitals but also provided the facilities for which patients had to go outside the state. Dr. Bashir has trained many budding opthalmologists at his center for the sensitive and complicated procedures for which there are limited facilities in the valley. For the new entrants to the medical profession, he advises that the profession of medicine demands a tremendous amount of hard work, dedication, sincerity, and compromises. Anybody wishing to have a comfortable and luxurious life should not go into this noble profession.

Dr. Ghulam Mohammed Dhaar

Dr. Ghulam Mohammed Dhaar (GM Dhaar), son of Haji Ghulam Hassan Dhaar, was born on April 12, 1935, in the Aali Kadal area of Srinagar City. Having received his initial education in a local government high school, he joined the Sri Pratap College, Srinagar, for his premedical course.

Dr. Dhaar was selected for undergoing undergraduate medical training in Osmania Medical College, Hyderabad, where he obtained MBBS degree in 1959. Upon graduating, he moved back to his home state and joined the SMHS Hospital as a medical officer. Here, he had the opportunity of working with the first-line leaders of medicine in the state, including Prof. Ghulam Rasool, Prof. Ali Mohammed Jan, and Prof. Harbhajan Singh. This was the time when the late Mr. Bakshi Ghulam Mohammed, then prime minister, was personally monitoring the process of opening the Government Medical College (GMC) at Srinagar. After briefly serving the state health services in some of its inaccessible and remotest locations, Professor Dhaar left for Calcutta to join the prestigious All India Institute of Public Health, where he obtained a diplomate in Public Health. Upon his return, he served the Srinagar Municipal Corporation for almost two years as health officer and later as administrator, Srinagar Municipality. Subsequent to this, he was selected for postgraduation in public health at the prestigious King George's Medical College Lucknow, where in 1971 he was awarded MD in the newly created speciality of community medicine. He thus became the first-degree holder postgraduate in community medicine from the state of Jammu and Kashmir.

Upon joining the Government Medical College, Srinagar, as an assistant professor in preventive and social medicine, he rose to become its head of the department. Rising from the ranks, he later served as an associate professor before being designated as a professor in 1981.

In the late 1970s, another important event was taking shape in the medical history of this state: the Sher-i-Kashmir Institute of Medical Sciences (SKIMS) was being conceived. Upon the insistence of Professor Nagpal, the first project director of SKIMS, Professor Dhaar joined SKIMS in early 1981 as head of the Department of Community Medicine. Since SKIMS was in its infancy, Professor Nagpal entrusted him with the additional responsibilities of functioning as additional secretary of medical education, coordinator of manpower development, and member of various selection committees, including the Apical Selection Committee of SKIMS. In 1995, Professor Dhaar finally superannuated from the SKIMS. After his retirement, he assumed the headship of Community Medicine at the SKIMS Medical College, Bemina, till 1997 and later ASCOMS Jammu till June 2000. Presently, he devotes his time to the in-depth study of Islamiyat and the spread of the peaceful message of Islam for eliminating unrest and distress in the society.

Contributions of Professor Dhaar are multifarious spreading over diverse fields of his speciality. In the field of medical education, he is considered a reputed teacher in community medicine having served as an empanelled examiner in undergraduate and postgraduate courses conducted by reputed national medical institutions and universities. As a postgraduate teacher, he guided a number of students in community medicine and allied specialities. He established a multidisciplinary department of community medicine at SKIMS and converted the erstwhile 'Trust Hospital' into a maternity hospital.

Eventually, with the active collaboration of the Neonatology Department, he succeeded in establishing a maternal and child health center, whereby integrated services are being provided to mothers and children. In the field practice area, Professor Dhaar helped establish intensive internship training programs in various blocks.

Professor Dhaar initiated the teaching of preventive and social medicine to undergraduate students of Government Medical College, Srinagar, as per the guidelines of MCI and made it an essential subject for passing the prefinal examination. He also introduced teaching and training of MD postgraduates in community medicine at GMC Srinagar and earned its recognition by the MCI. Dr. Dhaar also introduced teaching and training of MD postgraduates in maternal and child health; this was the first program of its kind in the country that earned MCI recognition.

Professor Dhaar is credited with having established a unique personal health-care delivery system in the state. He served as an inaugural advisor for the introduction of the ICDS and *Rehbar-i-sehat* projects in the state of J&K. In the field of public health, Professor Dhaar contributed meaningfully to the national smallpox eradication program, universal immunization program, and RCH in the affiliated field practice areas. He also contributed significantly in implementing the malaria eradication program in his capacity as a state malariologist.

Professor Dhaar is a keen researcher and a celebrated author. His book entitled *Foundations of Community Medicine* is a complete treatise on the subject extending to nearly a thousand pages. This book was published by internationally renowned medical publisher Elsevier Ltd. Apart from being on editorial boards of different journals, his publications in national and international journals are numerous, having significantly contributed to different areas of community medicine, including epidemiology, primary health care, health administration, and family welfare.

Professor Dhaar took a keen interest in introducing and building professional forums and bodies including the J&K Students Association at Hyderabad, the Medical Teachers Association in the Government Medical College, Srinagar, and Faculty Solidarity Forum at SKIMS. He has also served as an advisor and member of several committees and boards, including the College Council of GMC, the board of studies in GMC/University of Kashmir/SKIMS, Staff and Hospital Council of GMC and SKIMS, Deans Committee SKIMS, Apical Selection Committee SKIMS, and Senior Selection Committee SKIMS. He has also served as a member of governing bodies of such professional associations as the Indian Association of Preventive and Social Medicine, Indian Association of Public Health, Indian Association of Maternal and Child Health, Indian Hospital Association, Indian Institute of Public Administration, Indian Institute of Management (IIM), and Alumni Association of National Institute of Health and Family Welfare.

Dr. Dhaar has been awarded numerous fellowships by international and national professional bodies. He was awarded Lifetime Achievement Award by the Indian Association of Preventive and Social Medicine. Being the first doctor in the state who specialized in social and preventive medicine, who established the departments of community medicine, and who introduced MCI-recognized undergraduate and postgraduate training programs in the subject, Professor Dhaar is acknowledged as the "father of community medicine" in the state of Jammu and Kashmir who served his speciality with utmost dedication, conviction, commitment, and devotion (with inputs from Dr. Irfan Robbani, his son).

Dr. Ghulam Mohammad Shah

Dr. Ghulam Mohammad Shah has been one of the first physicians from his state of Jammu and Kashmir in India. He was born in a remote village, Lalpora, in Kashmir and distinguished himself from an early age by being highly self-motivated and ambitious. He was one of many siblings and eventually moved to the city of Srinagar to pursue his education. He never shirked work and indeed underwent serious financial challenges on the way to his goal of obtaining higher education.

Dr. Shah obtained his Bachelors of Science from J & K University in 1950. Through his hard work and dedication, he obtained admission to MBBS in Agra University and completed his medical degree in 1956. By 1960, Dr. Shah had completed his MD degree in physiology. Dr. Shah also obtained additional training and hematology in Calcutta, neurophysiology in New Delhi, cardiovascular physiology in the State University of NY, Buffalo, and also completed a medical teachers' training course in PGI Chandigarh.

After doing a brief stint in Kashmir as a medical officer in charge of the district hospital and health center, he was appointed as assistant professor in physiology in Government Medical College, Srinagar, Kashmir. Dr. Shah then ascended to the post of professor and head of the Department of Physiology in 1971, and he stayed in that post till 1990. From 1991 to 1993, he was appointed head of the Department of Physiology and dean of the Jhelum Valley College of Medical Sciences and Hospital in Srinagar, Kashmir (now SKIMS Medical College).

All his life, Dr. Shah has contributed by serving in various administrative capacities such as head of the Department of Physiology, principal/administrator at Jhelum Valley Medical College, and acting principal/dean of Government Medical College (on and off) for twenty-three years. Dr. Shah also served as administrator of the Associated Hospitals of the Government Medical College, Srinagar, Kashmir. Dr. Shah has had multiple publications in India as well as in the US, where he completed a research fellowship. During his long and successful life, Dr. Shah has never forgotten his roots and has always contributed heavily to his place of birth, his parents, and his siblings. He has always been extremely generous to everyone he encountered in life, and, regardless of his own economic state, he has helped everyone. During all his struggles and successes, he has been steadfastly supported by his wife, Amina, also a very successful obstetrician and gynecologist. A man of sterling character, a man of principle, steadfast to his purpose in life—that sums up Dr. Shah in a nutshell.

(Contributed by Dr. Suhail Shah, the son of Dr. Shah)

Dr.(Col.) Ghulam Nabi

Dr. Ghulam Nabi was born on January 1, 1909, and breathed his last on October 19, 1994. He was born in Srinagar in a middle-class family and lost his father early in life and was adopted and brought up by his maternal grandfather Dr. Abdul Qadeer.

He recieved his schooling from the Christian Mission School (Biscoe), Srinagar, and passed his BSc from the then Punjab University. He did his MBBS from King Edward Medical College, Lahore (the year is not clear). After passing his MBBS, he joined the Army Medical Corps (AMC) and served as a doctor in far-flung areas of various parts of India, including Jammu and Kashmir, UP, and Punjab.

As part of the allied forces, he was deputed and served the Middle East, in the Persian Gulf during World War II from 1943 to 1945. During this time he worked in Syria (Damascus), Iraq (Basra and Baghdad), and Iran. He spent these two years in the war serving the wounded, the sick, and the infirm.

Here, it is pertinent to mention that his grandfather Dr. Abdul Qadeer also served as a doctor in the Middle East during World War I. In my opinion, this is the only example of a grandfather and grandson from J&K who had the distinction of serving in the two great wars. Both were awarded various medals and honors for their work during wartime. Dr. Ghulam Nabi worked in the AMC till his retirement in 1964.

Dr. Ghulam Nabi was appointed administrator of SMHS Hospital, Srinagar, in 1965, where he continued to work till

1968. He contributed to the administrative affairs of the SMHS Hospital. With his army background and his skill in dealing with the crises, he was able to exercise his influence in the hospital and ensure discipline. In 1969, he was appointed as the administrator of the University Hospital, Aligarh Muslim University, where he worked for eight years. In 1978, he joined the HMT factory in Srinagar as medical officer, where he worked till 1980.

Dr. Ghulam Nabi was a member of the J&K Red Cross Society and worked as the medical officer during 1981–1982.

(The profile has been submitted by Prof. Azra Shah.)

Dr. Ghulam Nabi Kozgar

Dr. Ghulam Nabi was born at Khanquahi Moulla, Srinagar, in 1918. His father, Hakim Mir Ahadullah, was a popular Unani Hakim of that time and belonged to a clan of Unani Hakims; the ancestors trace back to the entourage of Shahi Hamdan, Mir Syed Ali Hamdani.

Dr. Ghulam Nabi had his early education in Srinagar. His father ensured he gets a good education and pursued allopathic medicine. In 1942, Dr. Ghulam Nabi completed his medical graduation from Lahore. Subsequently, he served as a civil surgeon at various places in Kashmir before he was posted at Doda. This was the time when partition was happening. Back home, nobody knew if the family was alive. The eldest child, their daughter (Dr. Nasreen Kaunsar) was about two years old. They had to travel on foot and on ponies to return home. During this difficult time, his son (Dr. Gowhar Ahmad) was born at Barath a place in Doda. After returning to Srinagar, he pursued ophthalmology at Madras in 1953.

Subsequently, he went to Vienna, Austria, for postgraduation in ophthalmology and ENT, which he completed in 1958. Dr. Ghulam Nabi joined SMHS Hospital as a specialist in ophthalmology and ENT and was later inducted into the faculty when MBBS was started in GMC Srinagar. He has been the contemporary of Drs. Ali Jan, B. M, Bhan, Fazal Rehman, Hafizullah, and, later, Drs. G. Q. Allaqaband, Mir Mohammad Maqbool, and Syed Zahoor Ahmed.

He pioneered ophthalmic and ENT services in Kashmir. He has been one of the most sought-after ophthalmic and ENT surgeons in the valley. Besides being a successful medical doctor, he was deeply religious and God-fearing and devoted a lot of time in the affairs of the Khanquahi Moulla shrine. He also served as the trustee of Muslim Auqaf. He left this world peacefully in 2005 surrounded by his family members who loved him dearly.

(The write-up is contributed by Dr. Khurshid Iqbal, son of Dr. Ghulam Nabi.)

Dr. Jagdish Singh

Anatomy is the "first shock" that a medical student receives when he joins the medical training. The fright of dead bodies that you got to befriend, the strong odor of formalin that your sensory organs need to tolerate, the lifeless bones in osteology, and the clueless slides in histology leave you crazy! You need someone who understands your agony, someone who translates this all into a digestible format, someone who cares to teach, who cares to translate, someone who can hold you together at a critical point of entering into a new phase of life where life starts with "dissection." At that intersection, GMC Srinagar had a great anatomist. The lucky ones who were guided by that "doyen" remember him as J. Singh. Dr. Jagdish Singh, or J. Singh, as he is fondly remembered among his colleagues and students, was a renowned anatomist who had the honor of heading the Anatomy Department at both Jammu and Srinagar Medical Colleges and SKIMS (Jhelum Valley Medical College) Srinagar. He was born in 1933 in Baramulla province of Kashmir. Early in childhood, he lost both his parents and was brought up by his maternal grandmother. He received his initial education in Baramulla and Srinagar and his medical training (MBBS) at Amritsar Medical College from 1955 to 1961.

After completing his MBBS, he returned to Kashmir in 1961 and worked at SMHS Hospital in various positions. After completing his MS in anatomy, he worked at GMC Srinagar as a faculty member and eventually became head of the Anatomy Department. He worked in GMC Srinagar till 1981, before taking up this role at Government Medical College, Jammu. Here, he was instrumental in upgrading the department and was head of the department till 1991. He worked hard to bring his departments at Jammu and Srinagar on to the national stage and was president of the Anatomical Society of India. He organized the Indian Anatomical Conference at Jammu in 1983.

Dr. Jagdish Singh is remembered for his passion for teaching, and his students fondly remember him for his analogies in particular in the subspecialty of embryology. He had a great sense of humor and would use it to teach his subject. Teaching anatomy had become the purpose of his life. He would put everything into teaching . . . his mind, his body, and his soul. His research interests were in comparative anatomy, and he widely presented his work at various national level conferences. He inspired everyone around him and left a lasting memory in his undergraduate and postgraduate students. As a professor of anatomy, he was able to shape careers, inspire, and mentor a lot of people who later served the medical profession in various capacities. He was without doubt the best anatomist that Kashmir ever produced.

As a human being, he was always happy to help people around him, treated everyone equally, and is remembered for his simple and principled living. Professor Yousuf of Medicine describes Dr. Jagdish as a man full of life, wisdom, and humor, but all his jokes and puns were centered on anatomy. Dr. Jagdish Singh was well-known in his speciality circles and touched the lives of so many with his energetic demeanor and set up high professional standards. His sudden passing away at an age of sixty-one in 1994 was a great loss to the profession and left an unfilled vacuum.

(Contributed by Jagwant Singh and Dr. Preeti Kour)

Dr. Kundan Lal Chowdhury

Pain

The phantom stalks all the time,
now lurking in the shadows,
now lurking in the mind,
now seizing hold—
Inflicting itself on me
with unerring constancy.

With its invisible armory
It pierces and bores,
crushes and grinds,
saws and hammers,
cuts and tears,
burns and sears,
and delivers lightning bolts,
any place of its choosing,
now forewarning,
now catching me unawares.
(K. L. Chowdhury)

You need to hear and feel the agony of a patient of trigeminal neuralgia. Dr. Chowdhury has aptly described the pain, and experts would agree this poem best describes the pain of trigeminal neuralgia. Dr. Chowdhury was a rare combination of a hard-core clinician and a writer who could spin words in beautiful prose and impactful poetry. Who would write a poem about the pain of trigeminal neuralgia, a poem about dress code of a doctor, a poem about dilemmas and clinician faces when making a diagnosis, or a poem about the flow of blood? Only a passionate clinician with a command over language and rhythm would do that. I came across a lot of material written by Dr. K. L. Chowdhury. Many essays, many poems, many columns related to politics, but most interesting of them all is his descriptive analysis of many cases with detailed case histories, how he reached the diagnosis, and what are the points that people should know about a particular disease in question. These case histories are compiled by Mr. M. K. Raina in the form of a book titled *Stories from Dr. K. L. Chowdhury's* My Medical Journey. The case histories written so well speak about the caliber and the level of this great clinician. Many case histories related to common and rare neurological disorders, neurosurgical emergencies, psychiatric disorders diagnosed by him are meticulously described. Dr. Chowdhury's medical history diary is worth a read as it gives an insight into the medicine practiced in the pre-CT and pre-MRI era in Kashmir. He talks about the first subdural hematoma diagnosed by him and treated by a young and bold surgeon. He talks about the first cerebral angiogram conducted by Dr. Shafat Fazili, the first case of catatonic stupor diagnosed and treated by him, and many more interesting cases. The interesting description of these cases projects Dr. Chowdhury as a clinician who wants to pass on the art of medicine (so fast vanishing now) to the generations of clinicians in future and also educate the masses about common diseases.

Dr. Kundan Lal Chowdhury, or Dr. K. L. Chowdhury, as he was called, was born in Srinagar, Kashmir, in 1941. He was the son of an eminent criminal lawyer of his times, Mr. J. L. Chowdhury. Dr. Chowdhury did his MBBS from Punjab

University (Patiala) and postgraduation (MD) from Delhi University (MAMC). He started his career as a faculty member in Government Medical College, Srinagar. He was an excellent clinician, a wonderful teacher, and a good researcher. Very sharp with an intensely accurate clinical sense and teaching aptitude, he was greatly loved by his students and respected by his colleagues. He did his fellowship in neurology from London and pioneered neurology as a speciality in the GMC Srinagar.

Dr. Chowdhury was greatly impressed by the personality, charisma. and clinical sense of Dr. Ali Jan. Dr. Ali Jan, in turn, valued Dr. Chowdhury's opinion, especially for the cases related to neurology. Dr. Ali Jan would call Dr. Chowdhury as a young bright doctor. Regarding the mutual respect that Dr. Chowdhury and Dr. Jan shared and regarding his interest in neurology, Dr. Chowdhury says, "I was the only faculty member in Medical College Srinagar with an interest in neurology. Though I had no postgraduate degree in the speciality, neurology was my passion. My Professor, the legendary Dr. Ali Mohammad Jan, having recognized my aptitude for neurology, would send the most intricate neurological problems from his private practice to me for examination and discussion with the residents and postgraduates. Tuesday of every week was the neurology day in my chamber in ward 3 of SMHS hospital and very special for me."

Dr. K. L. Chowdhury became a professor of medicine at GMC Srinagar and moved to Jammu in 1990. He was not only a renowned physician but also an acclaimed writer and a social activist. He started charitable work by organizing the doctors of KP Community and provided free medical care to thousands in the migrant camps. Thereafter, he started Shirya Bhat Mission Hospital and Research Center, which provided free multispeciality consultation and treatment to poor and indigent patients and conducted medical camps, surveys, and research. He conducted pioneering work on the "Health Trauma of the Displaced Populations" and coined new terminology like "stress diabetes," "psychological syndromes of exiles," "the 10-12 syndrome," "the metabolic syndrome in 'migrant' camp inmates," etc. and highlighted the adverse effects of environmental and lifestyle changes on a displaced population. Dr. Chowdhury was engaged in multifarious activities as a medical professional, social scientist, poet, and writer.

Dr. Chowdhury wrote many books; his command on English language was immense. His works won him many awards, including the Best Book Award for Excellence in Literature in 2008. His collection of poems titled *A Thousand Petalled Garland and Other Poems* (2003) makes an interesting read.

I am greatly impressed by Dr. Chowdhury's write-up about Dr. Ali Jan and Dr. S. N. Dhar. I am sure no one could have written about them in a better style, and that is the reason I copied his words about these impressive doctors in this book. Many of his writings display his disgust with the happenings in his homeland (some uncomfortable remarks about his colleagues also)—but as a clinician, he hardly had any parallels. His death was widely mourned by his students, who called him a fine clinician greatly influenced by Dr. Ali Jan. He passed away in the US in 2021 after a prolonged illness. He was eighty. His wife, Dr. Leela Chowdhury, and two daughters survive him.

Dr. Mohammad Ismail Quadri

Dr. Mohammad Ismail Quadri is responsible for establishing hematology as a separate speciality at SKIMS and amalgamating laboratory hematology and clinical hematology to help patients with hematological disorders who otherwise had no option but to go for diagnosis and treatment outside the state. Incidentally, SKIMS Hematology was the first department in India where quality control and automation were introduced under the leadership of Dr. Ismail Quadri.

Dr. Mohammad Ismail Quadri was born in Dooru Shahbad in 1950. He did his MBBS from Government Medical College, Srinagar, in 1973. He was very active during his student days at GMC Srinagar and became social secretary CASS Union GMC and organized Fun Fair (Best Organizer Award). He added one more subhead to CASS Union, which was Aid for Poor Students.

Dr. Quadri did MD in the speciality of pathology from PGIMER Chandigarh, India, in 1977. Post MD, he worked as tutor in hematology at PGIMER Chandigarh and during that period helped/guided all trainee technical staff of SKIMS, Srinagar, who were sent to PGIMER for one-year training. Dr. Ali Jan, who wanted excellent laboratory services at SKIMS, had a lot of faith in Dr. Quadri. When staff and students from SKIMS were sent to PGI for training, Dr. Jan would ask Dr. Quadri to monitor their training and would even write letters to Dr. Quadiri regarding various matters pertaining to their training. He would ask him to ensure that the training was complete in all aspects so that state-of-the-art laboratory facilities could be made available at SKIMS. According to Dr. Quadri, Prof. A. M. Jan was the real architect of SKIMS who paid attention to the personnel who would man SKIMS laboratories for decades to come.

Dr. Quadri was the first in India to get MNAMS (National Academy of Medical Sciences–India) in hematology in 1980. He also became the first faculty member of SKIMS selected as a lecturer in hematology in 1981. Dr. Quadri did his PhD in hematology from PGI Chandigarh in 1982. He received Commonwealth Medical Fellowship at Royal Free Hospital London and worked at some other prestigious institutes in England from 1988 to 1989. He joined SKIMS in 1981 (before completing his PhD) and was later promoted to the level of professor and HOD, Hematology/Blood Banking, at Sher-i-Kashmir Institute of Medical Sciences Srinagar. He worked at SKIMS till 1994.

Dr. Quadri developed the Clinical Hematology Department at SKIMS and introduced automation. Dr. Quadri provided clinical services to those who were not properly diagnosed or treated before (i.e., hemophiliacs and leukemic patients). He also introduced component therapy and plasmapheresis. He played a leading role in establishing technical courses like BSc. MLT and MSc. MLT in hematology and other disciplines at SKIMS. As Dr. Quadri worked at SKIMS during peak years of turmoil, the job as HOD Blood Bank, among all other duties, was risky and life threatening.

Dr. Quadri went to Saudi Arabia and worked as consultant/HOD Hematology/Blood Banking Regional Laboratory, Saudi Arabia (Dammam), from 1994 to 2000. On his return from Saudi Arabia, he joined Government Medical College Srinagar as professor/HOD Hematology/Blood Banks and served in that capacity from 2001 to 2009. Dr. Quadri helped GMC Srinagar with its deficient faculty to get MCI recognition for postgraduation in pathology, which was pending for a long time. From 2005 to 2009, he worked as an expert in blood banking for Kashmir/Ladakh Division, and licensed blood banks were established at district and subdistrict levels across Kashmir and Ladakh. During this time, Dr. Quadri was instrumental in framing guidelines for the State Transfusion Council.

Dr. Quadri established his private hematology center in 2001 named Dr. Qadri's Hematology Center and Clinical Laboratory, Srinagar, which is NABL accredited and recognized by the government of Jammu and Kashmir. This laboratory has collection units in the entire Kashmir Valley and is highly rated for its accuracy and issuance of reports in time. It did a wonderful job during the COVID time and provided service to Kashmir in a time of great need. This center has employed many technical personnel, doctors, and other workers. In the time of rampant unemployment, Dr. Quadri's lab has served as a place where employment is generated. Dr. Quadri established an institute in 2014 named Dr. Qadri's College of Medical Laboratory Technology, which is affiliated with the University of Kashmir Srinagar and is an institute in which various laboratory courses are taught.

Dr. Quadri has led a successful life contributing to health care as a pioneer in hematology and through his well-established lab provided state-of-the-art facilities to the people of Kashmir. He lives with his family and children in Srinagar.

Dr. Mohammed Sayeed

Dr. Mohammed Sayeed was born in Jammu, the winter capital of the state of Jammu and Kashmir in 1935. The youngest of four siblings, including a brother and two doting sisters, he lost his father while still a toddler. In 1947, when he was just twelve, his family was displaced to Srinagar during the partition of India. The family lost a flourishing business and was left with only a summer- house in Srinagar, where they lived on a refugee ration. He completed his higher secondary education in the Tyndale Biscoe School and secured a government sponsorship to pursue a medical degree at the Sawai Man Singh Medical College in Jaipur, Rajasthan, from 1954 to 1959. It was during this time that he met Marianne Pinto, the future Mrs. Sayeed. In 1958, he lost his mother, and his brother died the next year, leaving behind a family of ten. Dr. Sayeed had to give up a house job in surgery in Jaipur to take on the responsibility of caring for the family. For the next three years, he was stationed as a medical officer in Keran, a remote village in Kashmir. During this period, he had to work under trying circumstances and with limited resources. He then returned to Jaipur to keep his promise to marry Marianne in 1963.

Dr. Sayeed completed his postgraduate studies in 1967, writing his thesis on the neurophysiology of the urinary bladder. He pursued his interest in human physiology and joined the Department of Physiology, GMC Srinagar. The GMC/SMHS was in its development phase, and Dr. Sayeed helped set up the experimental physiology laboratory as well as the clinical physiology lab and wrote scientific papers on neurophysiology and other topics of his interest over the next ten years. He collaborated with the Department of Medicine to establish an animal lab to conduct clinical experiments and set up a device for recording ECG, EEG, and EMG simultaneously in animals. In 1978, he traveled to the University of Birmingham, UK, on a WHO fellowship to work on human neurophysiology. Subsequently, he taught at the Alfatah University in Tripoli, Libya, from 1980 to 1985. Word has it that his physiology lectures were taped and the lecture notes were copied and passed on to incoming medical students.

Dr. Sayeed's lasting legacy is in the realm of education. He quickly established himself as a revered teacher. He would spend hours preparing each lecture and use overhead projection to display important material. Spending time with students, he would help them understand concepts rather than emphasize memorization. His door would always be open for students to come in and seek clarification. During lab time too, he would be available and help anyone who was struggling. He would make it a point to get to know the students personally, and, years later, when they were ready to graduate, he would still remember them and make sure to congratulate them. He was a good guide for those seeking direction for furthering their career.

Dr. Sayeed was a mentor to many subsequent postgraduate students such as Dr. Mumtaz Goni, who later joined the Department of Physiology. He established himself as a guardian to all the out-of-state students who studied at GMC and opened his home to them on all Sundays and festivals. He organized activities in the CASS union and managed the cultural programs, college fairs, and sports day activities.

His students are spread far and wide in the world, practicing in prominent positions in USA, UK, and various parts of India and Kashmir. As one student describes, "He was an excellent teacher who sought to engage his students by simplifying information. For a bunch of overawed and confused freshmen, that went a long way in calming our nerves and better understanding of complex physiological processes. Revered by students not only for his academic excellence, he was loved by all for his gentle countenance and pleasant disposition. His courteous and solicitous nature made him easily approachable for any perplexities we harbored in our minds. The knowledge a good teacher graciously bequeaths to his/her students nurtures an entire generation. Dr. Sayeed will always live on in the lingering fragrance of his blossoms."

Another student says, "I remember him saying once on the sets of cultural activities when the participants were rehearsing for a drama sequence . . . Keep the scene changing otherwise it looks dead . . . He was a lively person who kept the scene changing till the end, and now he is in our memories. God bless his soul."

Dr. Sayeed also established himself as a wise man in the community as well as among friends and family. People would approach him without hesitation at any time, knowing they will not be turned away. His colleagues, who looked up to him and constantly sought his guidance, loved him. He rose to the rank of professor and was head of the Department of Physiology from 1990 and was principal/dean of GMC until his retirement in 1993. He went on to be the head of the Department of Physiology at Jehlum Valley Medical College (now SKIMS-MC) and became principal/dean of this institution until 1997, when he took up a retired life.

Dr. Sayyed was a supportive husband and a doting and proud father. He derived pleasure in traveling to the US to visit his children and grandchildren. Although not a collector of worldly items, he enjoyed collecting family portraits and took pride in displaying those and talking about his family to anyone lending an ear. Large-hearted by nature, his children describe him as "giving and loving." They recall multiple instances of his charity, perhaps recalling the painful childhood he had spent wanting.

He stayed active until the end when he was diagnosed with metastatic cancer to which he succumbed after a brief period of illness in 2013. He is survived by his loving wife, Dr. Marianne Sayeed (professor of obstetrics and gynecology); son, Dr. Faisal Sayeed (pain specialist in Baltimore, Maryland, USA), and daughters, Dr. Salma Iftikhar (women's health specialist, Mayo Clinic, Rochester, Minnesota, USA) and Zarina Babur (information technology, Mayo Clinic, Scottsdale, Arizona, USA). His nine grandchildren live in the USA and remember him fondly.

Dr. Mushtaq Ahmad Margoob

An era when Kashmir was exposed to intense stress arising out of mass destruction of life and property, crushing fear and uncertainty, the astounding increase in the number of people falling prey to mental diseases coincided with Professor Dutta's (the prof and HOD) retirement and Professor Beg's demise. The result of which was that the Postgraduate Department of Psychiatry shrunk to the status of negligible faculty strength comprising of only two consultant psychiatrists, both lecturers. There was no professor, no clinical psychologist, no psychiatric nursing staff, and no psychiatric social workers. As if it was not enough, it was at the peak of this crisis that a devastating fire nearly destroyed everything in the hospital in March 1996. This most stigmatized place was conveniently called "*Pagal Khana*" and left to itself. It was on the verge of a collapse in the mid-1990s when the government declared its inability to rebuild the hospital for the lack of finances.

Dr. Mushtaq Margoob was watching this fall in pain. The hospital was overburdened with people who sought help. The data from the psychiatric hospital in Srinagar revealed the frightening impact of turmoil on every segment of society and every aspect of life. Against a total number of 1,762 patients in 1990, the hospital exploded with 17,584 patients in 1994. Soon, the number crossed one hundred thousand persons seeking help in a year. It takes people with extraordinary abilities to deal with such a catastrophe—mental in this case. Dr. Mushtaq Margoob used his personal influence and worked with the international medical humanitarian organization Doctors Without Borders (MSF) in 2001, and they rebuilt a portion of the gutted structure of the hospital. Subsequently, another NGO initiated a PIL in the High Court, which was pursued vigorously by a young dynamic advocate without any financial gains or claims that led the state government to start constructing the remaining portion of the hospital almost on the previous pattern and outlay. Dr. Mushtaq was able to get a grant of Rs 2.5 crore from the Union Health Ministry in 2007 that eventually altered the face of the hospital. In 2010, the ministry under the National Mental Health Program granted Rs 30 crore for upgrading the hospital as one of the eleven centers of excellence. Within a few months, the center was adopted as the model for North Indian states, and all the directors and health secretaries of the respective states were asked to attend the specific Regional Training and Sensitization Workshop of the National Mental Health Program by the Union Health Ministry at Srinagar on June 14–15, 2011. The centers of excellence in Chandigarh, Rohtak, IHBAS Delhi, and Rajasthan were eventually set up on similar lines. Rest is history . . . A particular example of how a "center of misery" is converted into a "center of excellence." Dr. Mushtaq was the man responsible for this tremendous transformation. Dr. Mushtaq held the hands of so many miserable patients and built up a place where he and his team would treat them with dignity. You actually need to know and see what Government Hospital for the Psychiatric Diseases was and what it got transformed into.

The man with the grit and determination to fight this crisis, Dr. Mushtaq Margoob was born on October 13, 1955, into a family of poets and intellectuals, being the son of the famous poet Margoob Banhali. He did his MBBS in 1978 from GMC Srinagar and MD in psychiatry from GMC Srinagar in 1985. He was recruited as a lecturer in psychiatry at GMC Srinagar in 1988, was promoted as assistant professor in 1997, became an associate professor in 2002, and, finally, a professor in 2008. He was heading the Department of Psychiatry besides being the medical superintendent of Government Psychiatric Hospital from 2010 to 2013. It was under the guidance and stewardship of Professor Margoob that Government Psychiatric Diseases Hospital was transformed into the Institute of Mental Health and Neurosciences (IMHANS).

Dr. Margoob has nearly forty years of teaching and research experience. He has done extensive work on the psychiatric disorders confronting the population of a conflict zone (i.e., Kashmir). He has brought the psychiatric ailments of this society to the attention of the world. It is rare to find a combination of a busy practitioner, an able administrator, and a researcher who presented Kashmir and its mental issues to the world.

Dr. Margoob has published his research in journals of national and international repute. He has published extensively on post-traumatic stress disorder (PTSD), especially childhood PTSD. He has worked on obsessive-compulsive disorder (OCD) and the treatment modalities for "treatment-resistant OCN." He has published very interesting studies related to the role of spirituality in psychiatric diseases. His study "Disaster Situations: Pir, Faqir Psychotherapist, the Psychosocial Intervention of Trauma" is a widely quoted research paper related to the role of faith healers in understanding psychiatric problems. Dr. Mushtaq advocates that mental health professionals in Eastern cultures must propagate the bio-psycho-socio-spiritual model in their approach to psychiatry so that treatment technique like "spiritually augmented cognitive behavior therapy" is formally incorporated into the management of patients with mental-health-related issues. A genuine faith healer and a psychotherapist share in the community similar experiences of balance between inner and outer life.

Dr. Mushtaq Margoob has been instrumental in bringing to the fore the problem of drug addiction and substance abuse in Kashmir. He is the founding director of SAWAB, which is the acronym for Supporting Always Wholeheartedly All Broken-Hearted and is the innovative voluntary psychosocial community care and research outreach initiative in Kashmir started by him in the early 1990s. It was a one-man mobile mental health service delivery process consequent to escalated psychosocial stress and a shocking increase in mental health disorders in Kashmir. Over the years, SAWAB has been very silently striving to fight stigma, enhance awareness about mental health problems, provide access to counseling, and deliver expert psychiatric treatment and free medication to the needy at their doorstep. It has also been focusing on and facilitating the training of budding mental health professionals in the community over the years with very promising results (Kashmir Life Health interview, August 11, 2021).

Dr. Margoob is a member and an expert committee member of more than two-dozen organizations, including member of International Society of Traumatic Stress Studies. He has been a member of the national consultative committee for the National Mental Health program since 2006. He has received travel grants from the World Congress of Psychiatry for presenting his work on 'disaster' in Mexico City in 2018. He delivered an invited guest lecture in Montreal, Canada, on psychological interventions for communities affected by the disaster. Dr. Margoob has more than one hundred publications to his credit and is presently working on an innovative low-cost model of mental health services in rural Kashmir. Dr. Margoob is on the editorial board of many leading international and national journals.

Dr. Margoob has guided more than two-dozen postgraduates in his department and helped in the research work conducted by other departments related to psychiatry. Suicide, sexual problems, dermatological issues, psychiatric problems of terminally ill patients, behavioral disorders in Kashmir have been researched and written about threadbare . . .... (courtesy Dr. Margoob).

To sum up Dr. Mushtaq A. Margoob is an internationally recognized expert on humanitarian emergencies and disaster mental health. Dr. Margoob's innovative research work over more than four decades encompasses a wide range of topics ranging from seasonal mood disorders to drug use problems and stress. Besides behavioral neurosciences, the focus of his work has been on coping, resilience, and vulnerability following traumatic stress resulting from man-made and natural disasters in the developing world and its impact on the individuals as well as communities as a whole. His innovative self-reliant psychosocial/psychiatric intervention model for disaster survivors in impoverished regions of the world has been appreciated globally across all professional levels. In Kashmir, he is known for his professional leadership and outstanding contribution in transforming the most stigmatized and neglected sole psychiatric service setup to the present day advanced center. Dr. Margoob withstood the difficulties and turned the fate of mental health services in Kashmir. As a clinician, Dr. Margoob has provided more than half a million psychiatric consultations/counseling to suffering masses in the community, government hospital settings, and in his private center over past forty years. He continues to spend most of his time with different stakeholders in the community for promotion of mental health and prevention/treatment of mental health problems. He has ensured that whatever the degree of trauma and pain in Kashmir, mental health support is available.

Dr. Nazir Ahmed Wani

Dr. Nazir Ahmed was born in Downtown Srinagar on July 13, 1944, in a well-known and well-to-do business family. After early education in a local primary school, he studied at Central High School, Fateh Kadal. Dr. Wani was a meritorious student and qualified matriculation examination of Jammu and Kashmir University in 1960 with high merit. He studied PUC and first-year TDC classes at SP College Srinagar. Since early childhood, Dr. Wani felt the pain and agony of his people so always had the urge to help suffering people and thought that being a doctor was the best way to achieve his dream.

To pursue his dream, he joined Government Medical College Srinagar in 1963 for MBBS, which he completed in 1968. He secured first position in obstetrics and gynecology and overall second position in MBBS examination for which was awarded medals and Certificate of Honor. After his internship and house job, he joined general surgery at SMHS Hospital and was registered as a postgraduate student in surgery. Throughout his educational career, Dr. Wani remained a meritorious student. He completed his postgraduation in general surgery in May 1975.

Dr. Wani proceeded to the UK in 1976; for seeking further knowledge and to hone his skills in surgery, he worked in various UK hospitals. He qualified FRCS (Fellow Royal College of Surgeons of Edinburgh) in 1979. Dr. Wani had enough opportunities to stay and work in the UK, but he preferred to return to Kashmir and joined SKIMS in January 1983. Although mild and modest with down-to-earth nature, he was a man with many virtuous qualities.

To help the poor, suffering community at home brought him home. SKIMS had just started functioning in December 1982 and had a promising future as a center of excellence—so he joined it promptly and was one of the founding members of SKIMS.

Dr. Wani nourished the Department of General Surgery and worked towards its diversification. Dr. Wani was a surgeon with "golden hands" who performed all the surgical procedures with patience and perfection. He was a great academician who worked hard on inculcating knowledge and surgical wisdom to his colleagues. He was promoted to the post of professor in 1988 (August) and worked as professor and HOD of Surgery Department till his superannuation in July 2004. One of the major contributions of Dr. Wani was to start major and advanced surgical treatment for complicated GI diseases for which the people had to go to PGI Chandigarh and AIIMS Delhi. Procedures like pancreatic resection and major gastric and colonic procedures were started and perfected by Dr. Wani at SKIMS.

Apart from the surgical expertise, he was involved in starting postgraduate studies in surgery in 1986 and has been a guide to nearly thirty students and a teacher to nearly two hundred others. The postgraduate course was recognized by MCI, and skilled general surgeons and specialist surgeons were made available to the community where a deficiency of skilled surgeons existed. These well-trained surgeons are working in various health-care institutions of the state and other parts of India, the Middle East, USA, and the UK, where their efficient work is appreciated and acknowledged.

Dr. Wani was a great teacher and a surgeon who taught his skill to the juniors without bias. His interest in gastrointestinal surgeries kindled the interest of many surgeons in this field and ultimately led to the establishment of a separate Department of Surgical Gastroenterology at SKIMS. So Dr. Wani is the father of surgical gastroenterology in Kashmir. Dr. Wani has published various research papers in national and international journals. In all, nearly 160 articles are accredited to his name besides a chapter on the management of chronic pancreatitis. Three articles authored by him were included in the top ten papers of the year by the *Indian Journal of Surgery* in 2004–2006.

Dr. Wani served as the dean of Medical Faulty for two years from January 2002 to December 2003 during which many postgraduate courses were recognized by MCI and a few more courses were started in other disciplines. Dr. Wani attended regularly national and international conferences where he presented a number of papers, delivered lectures on various subjects, and chaired many sessions. Dr. Wani during his career was awarded a fellowship of the International College of Surgeons (ICS), membership of Collegium Internationale Chirgurvae Digestivae (CICD), New York Academy of Sciences (NYAS), and Fellow of the College of Laparoscopic Surgeons India (FCLS). Dr. Wani has been involved in organizing various medical events at the institute.

Dr. Wani was an external examiner for BDS, MBBS, and MS surgery to the Universities of Kashmir/ Jammu and Aligarh Muslim University. He was actively involved in the running of the SKIMS in way of being involved in various managements committee and managed the library as chairman library for nearly fifteen years. To sum up, Dr. Wani was the pioneering surgeon who shaped the Surgery Department in its initial years at SKIMS and introduced modern GI surgery in which he was an expert. He preferred to serve SKIMS rather than go in private where his skill would have fetched him a fortune.

Dr. Pirzada Abdul Rashid

Dr. Abdul Rashid was born on March 13, 1935, in Srinagar to Pirzada Ghulam Mohammad and Fatima Begum. He received his primary education in Srinagar and secondary school education from SP College, Srinagar. He did his MBBS from Gwalior Medical College in 1958 and, after serving in Kashmir, went for his postgraduate studies to London in 1965 and thereafter worked as a registrar at Leeds Medical School. Upon his return from London, he was appointed as an assistant professor in the Department of Surgery, SMHS Hospital, Srinagar, and worked under Prof. Mehmooda Khan. He was elevated to the level of associate professor and subsequently became professor and head of the Department of Surgery, GMC Srinagar. He also worked as an administrator at SMHS Hospital. He retired from GMC in 1993 and joined SKIMS Medical College, Bemina, and retired as its principal in 1999.

Dr. Pirzada was a strict disciplinarian who, with his powerful voice, could control the whole class. His students popularly called him "Peter." He has been a very jovial, full-of-life, and easygoing doctor who was caring and friendly too. He has been an excellent bedside teacher and a wonderful surgeon. As a surgeon he was competent and cool. He would teach his junior colleagues and give them ample opportunity to learn. He worked on the prevalence of thyroid-related diseases in Kashmir and was among the first surgeons to venture into performing thyroid surgeries in the valley. As an administrator of SMHS

Hospital, he modernized the Casualty Department in the SMHS Hospital.

He lives in Qamarwari, Srinagar, and spends winters with his children, who are based in the US, He enjoys listening to Kashmiri folk music and going out for long walks.

Dr. Rafiq Ahmad Pampori

GMC Srinagar has braved odds, borne crisis, and withstood with great resilience the tumultuous years of turmoil. It kept on rebuilding whatever the odds. The credit goes to the doctors, the paramedics, and the other staff for making it run when all else failed. When it started to blossom again after turmoil, floods tore it apart. Floods swept away materials and machinery, labs and classrooms, OPDs and wards, and half-a-century-old hospital became a mass of filth and dirt. But the hospital was restored, the college was rebuilt, and machinery was replaced in record time. Prof. Rafiq Ahmad led from the front, from mopping of hospital floors to spraying of disinfectants, from listing of instruments to the framing of specifications, from arguments with the secretaries to negotiations with the health ministry—he did all to not only restore what had been lost but also to acquire more and to rebuild the college and hospital, bigger and better. He was not required to do this all for a single hospital—floods had made five prime associated hospitals spineless. They were made functional in record time. The college that had suffered significant damage to labs, classrooms, auditorium, and library was made functional without students losing time. Crores were spent on reconstruction and rebuilding without any stale deals. Each penny was accounted for. We all heaved a sigh of relief!

And then when this all happend, Dr. Rafiq started with the difficult task of restoring the glory of GMC. He revolutionized radiology, biochemistry, pathology, gastroenterology, cardiology, and ENT. A 256-slice CT scan replaced 64-slice CT, 3 Tesla MRI replaced 1.5 Tesla MRI, Carl Zeiss microscopes replaced the conventional microscopes, and automated instruments were brought in pathology and pharmacology. His efficient and methodical approach helped GMC increase the allotted MBBS seats from 100 to 150. Under his stewardship, MD course in various specialities was recognized by MCI. MD was started in specialities of radiodiagnosis and microbiology. A number of conferences were held, mortality meets were started, and publications from GMC tripled. DBT and ICMR projects were allotted to GMC faculty. A state-of-the-art research lab was constructed in the lawns of GMC in record time. Like phoenix, GMC Srinagar rose from the ashes and reached a pinnacle. The flag of GMC Srinagar again fluttered high up in the skies of medicine.

This revivifier was born in Downtown Srinagar on February 13, 1956. He did his schooling from National School Karanagar. Bright and bold, he joined GMC Srinagar and completed his MBBS in 1979. As a student, he was actively involved in sports playing cricket and has been an active member of CASS Union GMC Srinagar. He was responsible for establishing "Fair Price Shop" at GMC Srinagar. He did his MS in otolaryngology from Government Medical College in 1983. He was appointed as a lecturer in ENT in 1990, promoted as assistant professor in 1996, and became a professor of ENT in 2006. He was an ICMR fellow in Neuro-otology at All India Institute of Medical Sciences, New Delhi, India. He is a member of the American Academy of Otolaryngology.

Dr. Rafiq has been a keen researcher and ventured into many challenging areas. He is an innovative ENT surgeon with expertise in skull base surgery and endoscopy. He has made impressive presentations at many international conferences, which include "The Role of FESS in Headache" at Riyadh, "Challenges of Skull Base Surgery to Otolaryngologists" at

Kuala Lumpur, and presented challenging cases in skull base surgery in a conference held at Dubai, UAE. He has sixty publications in various national and international journals. He has organized many conferences and workshops in GMC Srinagar—people from renowned institutions were invited to Srinagar on many occasions to deliver talks.

Dr. Rafiq has served GMC with commitment and has been one of its best teachers who has delivered in the worst of the times. He lives a life of a committed doctor who was never tempted by power or position. Dr. Rafiq is an exceptional human being who, besides his love for medicine, has a great hold on religion. He has authored more than two dozen books on Islam and translated many from Arabic and Urdu to English. He has guided, helped, and held the hands of many poor and downtrodden people. He has taken personal interest in his students' lives and would always counsel and guide all those who sought his advice and help. Known for his social activism and his austerity, he was instrumental in establishing Voluntary Medical Trust (VMT), which has alleviated the suffering of many patients with dialysis and helped poor people in need of medicine.

He started cochlear implants for the first time in the erstwhile state. This surgery is done on children and adults and has been a life-changing event for many children born with hearing impairment who otherwise had to live a life of isolation and disability. The implant costs in many instances are covered by various schemes, and these children are helped for free.

Dr. Rafiq spends his time teaching Quran, Hadith, and promoting peace, brotherhood, and morals in the society. He is a social reformer and a giver who distributes love, knowledge, and promotes charity. He lives with his wife and three children and grandchildren in Srinagar.

Dr. Sheikh Abdul Ahad

Dr. Sheikh Abdul Ahad was born in Seloo, Sopore, Kashmir, in a business family on the May 12, 1943. After completing his MBBS, MS (ENT), and senior residency from Maulana Azad Medical College, New Delhi, he joined GMC Srinagar and its Department of ENT in SMHS Hospital as an assistant professor in 1974.

He took over as professor and HOD of ENT and Head and Neck Surgery in September 1992 till his superannuation in May 2001. He contributed to the substantial development of the specialty equally in the areas of research, diagnosis, and treatment. Dr. Ahad's art of teaching earned him the name of a "great teacher." He trained twelve postgraduate scholars during his tenure as faculty spanning twenty-seven years. He always found time to keep himself abreast with all the advanced literature in otorhinolaryngology.

He has been a pioneer of modern otology in Kashmir and was among the earliest to start head and neck surgery in the department; in fact, a skillful and artistic surgeon, a treat to watch. He was a nature lover and was always eager to travel. He was so much special for me: he was my teacher and my friend.

He left this world with a smile on his face at SKIMS, Soura, on January 3, 2019.

(Penned down by Dr. Sajad Qazi)

Dr. Sushil Razdan

In 1990, as the Kashmiri Pandit community left the valley, Kashmir's most renowned neurologist, Dr. Sushil Razdan, left too and established his clinic in Jammu. But that did not stop his Kashmiri patients from visiting him. At his Jammu clinic, 80 percent of Dr. Razdan's patients are Muslims from Kashmir. He is no God-man, but his Kashmiri patients think their aches will go if he places his hand over their heads. "This has never made me feel that I have left my home in Srinagar," he says.

I read a news item from Rediff news dated July 25, 2003, about Dr. Sushil Razdan titled "Dr. Goodwill: Kashmir Loves This Pandit," which talks about the visit of Dr. Razdan to Kashmir and describes the love and affection showered on him by his patients and his admirers. This is how the news item describes his visit: "On a week's visit to Kashmir recently, Dr Razdan stayed at the house of a Muslim schoolmate, and was inundated with invitations from well-wishers across the valley. He spent considerable time meeting people over lunch/dinner or a refreshing cup of saffron-rich *kahwa*. During his stay in Kashmir, one point became abundantly clear—trust and amity between the two communities had in fact become firmer with distance. Even patients throng places where he goes. A two-day visit to the meadow of flowers, Gulmarg, was supposed to bring the busy practitioner some respite from his hectic schedule. But the news of his arrival spread like wildfire and hundreds of Kashmiris arrived there with MRI reports,

CAT scans and X-rays. 'The medical profession and anger are incompatible. You cannot treat patients if you suffer from intemperate behavior,' Dr Razdan said when asked whether such incursions into his privacy irritated him. His competence and compassion have made this Kashmiri doctor a celebrity and wherever he goes, his patients follow him. 'He is not just a highly competent doctor, he is essentially a nice human being. I have often intruded into his privacy at odd hours, but he has never shown a frown on his face,' said Ghulam Nabi, 62, whose son, who gets seizures, has been the doctor's patient for the last 20 years. Towards the end of his weeklong visit, during which Dr Razdan saw around a thousand patients without charging them anything, he went to see a journalist friend's family. The moment the doctor arrived at his friend's home, the entire place was converted into a makeshift clinic. Instead of entertaining their guest, the journalist and his family began regulating the flow of patients. When the doctor left for the airport, there were tears in the eyes of those he had attended to and also those who were waiting for his attention. The doctor was smiling, but tears were trickling down his face too."

This love for Dr. Razdan has not erupted in Kashmir all of a sudden. It is a result of faith in the "healing touch" of Dr. Razdan. He listens to his patients, counsels them, and guides them besides diagnosing and treating them. He knows what ails their psyche and what aches their heart. By just listening to them, he frees them from the miseries of their disease.

Dr. Sushil Razdan was born in Srinagar and is the son of a legendary teacher, Sat Lal Razdan, who is known in the valley as "*Masterji*"— who taught generations of Kashmiris-science. Dr. Sushil Razdan earned his medical degree from the University of Kashmir in 1973, where he was named Best Outgoing Medical Graduate and conferred the Gold Medal. He received his MD (general medicine) from the University of

Kashmir in 1978 and then went on to PGIMER, Chandigarh, to pursue his superspecialization (DM neurology) in 1980.

Dr. Razdan has held clinical and academic positions at prestigious institutions such as the SMHS Hospital in Kashmir, the Sher-i-Kashmir Institute of Medical Sciences, Srinagar, and ASCOMS in Jammu. He is a visiting faculty to Medanta, New Delhi. Dr. Razdan has conducted epidemiological research in South Kashmir on neurological disorders. He and his team have conducted research on deaf-mutism in Doda District (the highest concentration), as well as research on the cause of blindness in children in R. S. Pura's border areas.

Visit his clinic-cum-house at Bhagwati Nagar Jammu and you see crowds. One patient and four persons accompany to have a glimpse of Dr. Sushil Razdan. Patients keep coming to him from far-off places in the valley such as Tanghdar and Kupwara since 1990. Some patients bring *Haak* and some lotus stems (*Nadru*) for the doctor. "If he does not accept it, that shall break my heart. He saved my wife from death. He has never asked for a fee. We force him to accept it," say his patients outside his clinic. ("Sushil Razdan: a Doctor Loved by Everyone in our State," Chinar Shade by Autar Mota, February 3, 2010).

Besides being a celebrity doctor, his colleagues and friends hold tremendous respect for him. "No doctor has received so much love as he has received it. He is a darling not only of patients but of the general public also. He is a matchless doctor and a very pleasant human being. My all worries disappear when I am in his company. I really feel fresh and young when he talks to me. Long live Sushil!" says his friend and colleague at SKIMS, Dr. A. Wahid (Facebook post March 15, 2022). His world-famous fellow neurologist, Dr. Noor Ali, describes him the best: "A brilliant physician who introduced Neurology as a subspecialty to Kashmir. So much has been said about his popularity, his bedside manner and his integrity that I can't add any more. But this much I can say—he will always have a special place in my heart as a mentor, colleague and above all a wonderful and loyal friend. He transcends petty issues of religion, region etc and is loved by all." This in fact sums up Dr. Razdan.

Dr. T. S. Sethi

Dr. T. S. Sethi is a household name in Kashmir. He has spent a greater part of his career managing orthopedic trauma that came in epidemic proportions to Kashmir in the '90s. He pioneered the management of open fractures in gunshot injuries and blast injuries. Dr. Sethi was born in August 1944 at Maisuma Bazar Srinagar, Kashmir. He did his matriculation from CMS Biscoe School, Srinagar, in 1959 and thereafter FSc from SP College, Srinagar, in 1962. Dr. Sethi did his MBBS and MS in orthopedics from Prince of Wales Medical College, Patna, Bihar, in 1970.

Dr. Sethi joined the Government Medical College, Srinagar, as registrar in December 1970 in the Department of General Surgery as there was no Department of Orthopedics in Government Medical College, Srinagar, at that time. As the department of orthopedics started expanding need for a separate hospital for orthopedic diseases was felt and Dr. Sethi was at the forefront during the founding years of the hospital and working tirelessly for its success. Subsequently, he was promoted as an assistant professor in the Department of Orthopedics of Government Medical College, Srinagar, in 1976. He then became associate professor in 1982 and professor in 1986. Dr. Sethi retired in 2002 but continued to serve his people while working in his private clinic.

Dr. Sethi was trained in orthopedic surgery under the expertise of Professor Mukhapadya from Patna, Prof. Karan

Singh of Grewal Amritsar, and Prof. Farooq Ashai of Kashmir. He introduced the system of internal fixation of fractures in Kashmir. Thus, he worked with the masters of orthopedics honing his skills and innovating.

During the peak years of turmoil, the proportion of orthopedic trauma increased substantially. Catering to the inflow of mass casualties in Kashmir during the '90s was a tough task. Dr. Sethi and his colleagues in the Bone and Joint Hospital managed the trauma very well and no wonder received a letter of appreciation from WHO regarding the management of "gunshot and blast injuries" and compared the management of these cases to those who suffered in the Afghanistan war. Dr. Sethi received President of India's Award in 2000 for the management of physically disabled persons. He has the honor of heading the surgical team for the management of the largest series of prolapsed lumbar intervertebral discs.

Dr. Sethi was elected president of the North Zone Association of Orthopedic Surgeons, Srinagar, in 1998. He has been an excellent teacher and trained almost fifty postgraduate students, and a few of them headed the Department of Orthopedics of the institutions of repute.

Dr. Sethi is a skilled surgeon, an excellent teacher, and works still in his private clinic to help his patients. He is in love with his motherland and his people and in spite of difficulties never left Kashmir.

Prof. Taffazull Hussain

A teacher par excellence

Biochemistry for a beginner in a medical School is perhaps the most difficult subject that needs ample hard work, great memory, and a great teacher. The students at GMC Srinagar for many decades were lucky to have an extremely dedicated teacher in biochemistry who is a master of his subject. His behavior, attitude toward his students, and ability to make his students understand the most difficult reactions and mechanisms taking place within and outside the cell made him a lovable teacher of his times. Though himself not a medico, he inspired generations of medicos in Kashmir and abroad with his stimulating mind and exceptional teaching skills. There cannot be a better story than the one that is told by one of his bright students who credits his success as an oncologist at Harvard to Mr. Tafazul Hussain. I did not dare to edit what he wrote; please read on.

"By way of my introduction, I am an Associate professor of medicine at Harvard Medical School, and I lead NK cell immunotherapy program at Dana Farber Cancer Institute, Boston. I am an Oncologist who treats patients with leukemia and those undergoing stem cell transplantation. I graduated from GMC Srinagar in 2003 and was blessed to have Prof. Taffazull Hussain as one of my teachers in the Biochemistry department.

"I vividly remember my first interaction with Taffazull Sir, it was during one of my biochemistry classes in the first year of my medical school. During this class, he taught us about signaling mechanisms of the G-protein linked receptors. I was highly impressed by his hold on the subject and his passion for teaching. I met him right after that class and our mutual love for molecular biology led to a lifelong mentor-mentee relationship. His depth of knowledge from the basic enzymatic reactions in the Krebs cycle to the antibody generation in plasma cells is quite amazing. Our discussions regarding intricate mechanisms of the gene segment rearrangements in the B and T cells and how this helps generate immense immune receptor diversity, made me fall in love with immunology. During the 2nd year of my medical school, Taffazull Sir lent me an immunology textbook (*Basic Immunology* by Abass). By the time I graduated from medical school, I had read many of contemporary immunology textbooks, all thanks to Taffazull Sir for having introduced me to this field. During the final year of my medical school, I became obsessed with learning about alternative stem cell donors including cord blood. Taffazull Sir again helped me find the relevant literature and, we tried to see what it would take logistically to start a cord blood-banking program in the valley. Unfortunately, we failed in this endeavor, however, I learned a great deal about stem cell transplantation, which deepened my desire to pursue further training in the field of hematology and oncology.

"During my intern year when I was trying to figure out my career path, he advised me to follow my passion and pursue higher studies in the US, and this advice changed my career trajectory forever.

"In my opinion, mentorship is the single most important factor that ensures success in academia and I cannot think of anyone who has done a better job than Taffazull Sir in mentoring so many GMC students including myself.

"Over the years I have worked at several major universities in the USA and Taffazull Sir stands out as one of the most dedicated teachers and mentors. Taffazull Sir is held in high regard by all of his students as he always went above and beyond to ensure that his students understood the major concepts in biochemistry in detail. There is absolutely no dearth of great talent in the valley, however, talent needs the right academic environment to thrive, and teachers like Taffazull Sir exactly serve this role by providing support and mentorship to the students. There is hardly ever a Kashmiri gathering in the USA where GMC graduates don't talk highly about him. It is amazing how every single GMC graduate remembers him as one of his or her favorite teachers.

"During his tenure at GMC Srinagar, Taffazull Sir also ran the clinical biochemistry laboratory at SMHS Hospital. I routinely visited him there and was always amused and impressed by the fact that he would try very hard to fix errors/ minor glitches in the machines on his own. He always tried to maintain the latest high-tech equipment in the lab so it could be at par with the best labs in the country.

"While most of us know Taffazull Sir as one of our beloved biochemistry teachers from GMC Srinagar, however, his talent extends beyond biochemistry and molecular biology. He is a well-established writer, having published several books in Urdu and the English language. In 2015 when I visited SKIMS, he gifted me one of his signed books which I enjoyed reading; it also made me realize and appreciate a completely different side of Taffazull Sir. I have kept in touch with him over the years though wish I could visit him in person frequently and be blessed with his sage advice for my academic and non-academic life.

"Teachers like Taffazull Sir are a true treasure for our nation and therefore deserve all the respect and appreciation. He is a perfect role model as a teacher and a mentor, and it is my deep desire to try to fit into his shoes for my own students and mentees.

"Taffazull Hussain, a teacher par excellence has inspired multiple generations of students at GMC Srinagar" (Dr. Rizwan Romee, MD).

While I struggled to know more about Professor Taffazull, trying to contact him through email and personal contacts, I could not get any other information about him, and while I was convinced a teacher lives best in the mind and heart of a student . . . the write-up by Dr. Rizwan did not end up my queries about Professor Taffazull, and the Golden Jubilee issue of *KASHMED* provided more information about him.

While summing up his life at GMC, precisely thirty years, in an essay titled "Vignettes of GMC," Taffazull Hussain talks about various aspects of his life. In a column on GMC students, he says, "The students of this institution are real uncut diamonds. It is my eternal regret that I and many of my colleagues have miserably failed to cut and polish them, as they deserve. Biochemistry is taught in the very first year of a student joining this institution. The newcomer has his sights fixed on the stars. Unfortunately by the time, he leaves the institution much of this heavenly manna has evaporated away. I often feel that for this disillusionment we the teachers cannot but share at least a part of the blame." About his experience before joining GMC, he says, "I had spent many years as a research fellow at the Central Drug Institute, Lucknow. I had worked with scientists who had been persuaded to come back to India and had worked in the best institutions of the world. When I came to GMC, I was a little disoriented. Things did not come easy." He quotes an example of requesting for an auto-analyzer annually for many years till it was finally installed twenty-five years after the first request. Such are the hiccups of working in an underdeveloped country. Prof. Taffazull believes that each technician should be trained in a particular specialty to render the best services possible. Despite being a loved teacher and nourishing a big department in GMC, Mr. Taffazull would not like to serve again as a public servant. Public service per him is a thankless job. This is an honest opinion and an honest review by one of the tallest teachers of GMC Srinagar.

Dr. Zubaida Jeelani

Dr. Zubaida Jeelani was born in Askardu in 1943 to a pious and educated family. Her father, Khwaja Noorudin, was a great academician and the first Kashmiri vice chancellor of Kashmir University. Dr. Zubaida, a green-eyed girl, showed brilliance in studies and leadership qualities from early childhood. She lived up to her rich heritage when she stood first in the matriculation examination in Kashmir Province in 1959 and showed great prowess as a debator in the Mallinson School, where she was exposed to a blend of sports and studies.

During her studies for MBBS in the Government Medical College Srinagar, she was awarded Certificate of Proficiency in the prefinal Eye and ENT examination. After completing residency in obstetrics and gynecology in SMHS Hospital, she opted to do MD in pharmacology, a nonclinical subject, so as to pursue teaching profession like her father. She devoted her time and energy to shaping the department, and scores of doctors were being trained in this vital branch of medicine at Government Medical College, Srinagar.

After serving as an assistant professor in the Department of Pharmacology as a very popular teacher for a decade, she was deputed to PGI Chandigarh for DM in the recently introduced subject of clinical pharmacology to establish a similar department in the newly created SKIMS Soura. Being highly motivated, she was one of the first DM candidates in this superspeciality in India and was exposed to this novel course under the guidance of teachers like Prof. R. R. Chowdhury, the then head and dean at PGI, visiting professor T. C. Dollery, Prof. Paul Turner, and Prof. Alasdair Breckenridge of international repute, who constantly encouraged her and were impressed by her dedication and leadership qualities. She was also good at research work. She was extremely friendly and sociable and had a very cordial and healthy relationship with both junior and senior colleagues.

Under her chairmanship of the Pharmacology Department at SKIMS, drug-level estimation of drugs like lithium, carbamazepine, etc and trace elements,. was started by using HPLC for the first time in the state. The department started "lung function tests" also for the first time in the state. Many papers on drug estimation were published by the department in national journals.

Recognizing the administrative and leadership qualities of Dr. Zubaida, the first project director of SKIMS, the dynamic and charismatic Dr. Nagpal would closely involve her in day-to-day administrative decisions; as such, she used to deputize for him a number of times as she was the first senior faculty member to join the SKIMS in 1981. She also had training in clinical pharmacology in West Germany at Hoechst Lab, training in UK at Hammersmith and Milton Keynes, which gave her a broad insight into clinical pharmacology. During her chairmanship of the department, she organized the 19th Annual Conference of IPS in 1985, which was a great success, widely attended by delegates all over.

She was an MD examiner at Kashmir University, Delhi University, Aligarh Muslim University and was a member of the national board of examinations for Diplomats of National Board (DNB). She was a member of the editorial board of the *Indian Journal of Pharmacology* and member of Indian Academy of Neurosciences and chief editor and convener of Annual Report, SKIMS.

After the retirement of General Thirumulai, she was appointed as the subdean of the faculty by the governing body

SKIMS and later the dean, a post she held for longest five years after the SKIMS was declared a university by an act of JK Assembly under the then director, Prof. B. K. Anand. She also was a member of the university syndicate to advise regarding the establishment of private hospitals and institutions like Imam Hussain Hospital and SKIMS Medical College for MBBS.

During her deanship, she was instrumental in pushing for a common entrance test for MD examinations against all odds and to give a fair chance to all good students rather than leaving it for the faculty and Heads of departments to choose blue-eyed boys for such courses during the political turmoil of the '90s. She would listen and help common but brilliant students and the staff of the institute and conduct various examinations without bias and favoritism.

She also encouraged a lot of Muslim girls to join the noble profession of nursing, which was still a taboo in Kashmir in those days. She would fight for the rights of the staff and doctors at the highest level fearlessly with persistence and dedication. Like her father, she hated illiteracy and left to herself would have loved to make illiteracy a crime. At a socioeconomic level, she helped financially weaker people and helped many girls, some of them orphans, to pursue nursing and the teaching profession; some of these girls were accommodated by her in her own home for a long time, where they took shelter and studied also.

As the director of the prestigious SKIMS for a short period during the toughest phase of turmoil, where on an occasion there was a question mark on her personal safety, this highly sensitive lady faced the challenge like a fighter and proved to be an able administrator. As the first female director of SKIMS, she inspired many female doctors who wanted to emulate her. Even when many stalwarts of SKIMS, including her husband, Dr. Wani, found the conditions unbearable and chose to work abroad, she stayed back to take care of SKIMS.

In 2002, she took voluntary retirement to join her husband, who was working as a cardiologist in the Middle East. They are blessed with two daughters, both doctors working in the West with their families.

On a personal level, Dr. Jeelani had more than her profession to tend to. Her father lost his life to a creeping malignant disease at the young age of fifty-nine while he was the VC. She had younger brothers and sisters, some still in their formative years. She threw her protective wing over them and helped them grow into responsible human beings, motivating them to lead meaningful lives. Three of her younger siblings became highly qualified doctors; two became engineers, who held positions of importance in the JK State. Her two sisters also made a mark in the education department. She served her mother for many years during her illness.

She passed away quietly in Saudi Arabia in 2009 and was buried in Riyadh as per her last wishes. So, Kashmir lost a bright doctor who, with her dignified appearance, her sea-green eyes, her graceful demeanour, sparkled in a crowd. A loving wife, a dedicated mother, a noble soul, and one of the pioneers of medical education in Kashmir was no more.

Her charismatic personality and leadership qualities will always be remembered. Dr. Nagpal, ex-director, called her an intelligent, hardworking, methodical, and conscientious worker who always maintained a high standard of work. Her senior colleagues remembered her as an upright lady with uncompromising principles and an equally warm and affectionate personality. Her contribution towards medical education, her work as one of the first consultants at SKIMS, the first Kashmiri woman to do DM in pharmacology and hold the post of dean and director SKIMS are enough reasons for us to include her in this list of one hundred Kashmiri doctors.

(Inputs from Dr. Bashir Wani and Dr. Javid Iqbal, from his article on Dr. Zubaida Jeelni July 4, 2009, in Greater Kashmir)

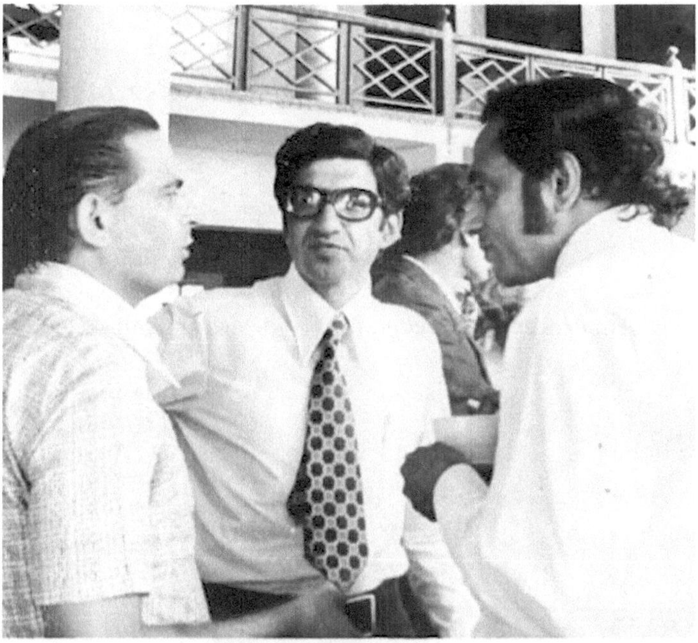

Prominent teachers of GMC Srinagar (L to R): Dr. Sayeed, Dr. A. H. Fazili (middle), Dr. H. A. Durrani

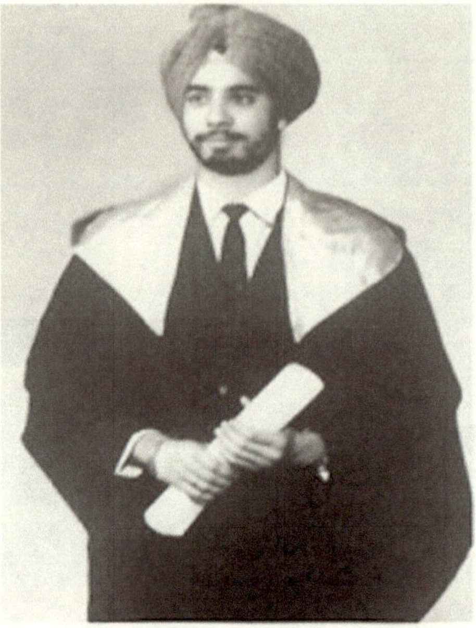

Dr. Amarjeet Singh (receiving Gold Medal from AIIMS)

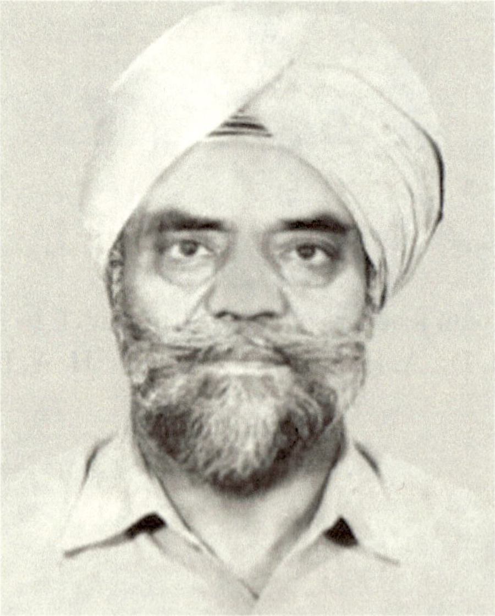

Dr. Jagdish Singh (popularly called J. Singh)-
the famed anatomy professor at GMC.

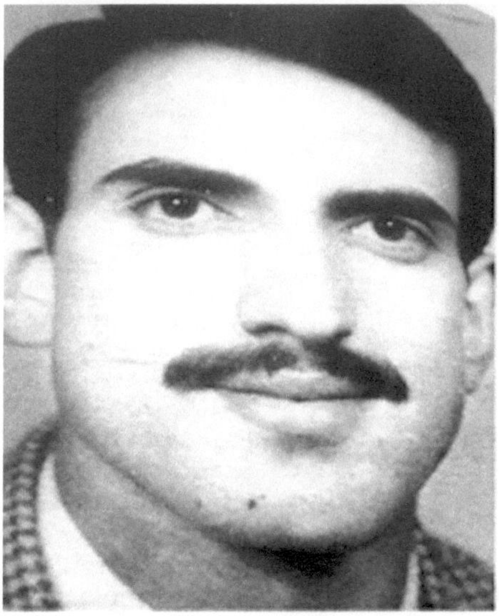

Dr. A. R. Khan—a dedicated pathologist who has rendered an incredible service to Kashmir for more than four decades.

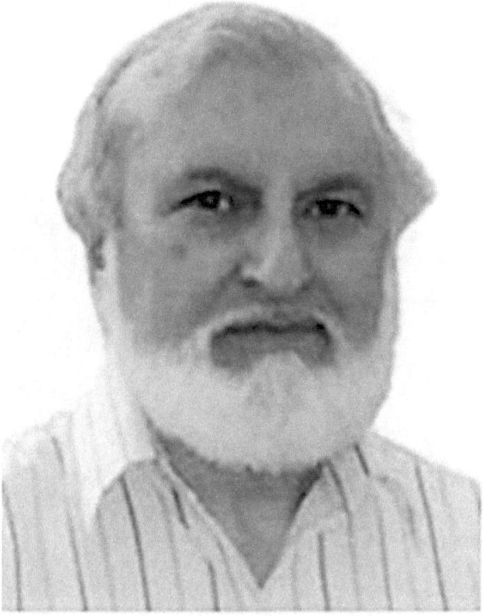

Dr. G. M. Dhaar—contributed to the Departments of Preventive and Social Medicine at GMC Srinagar and SKIMS.

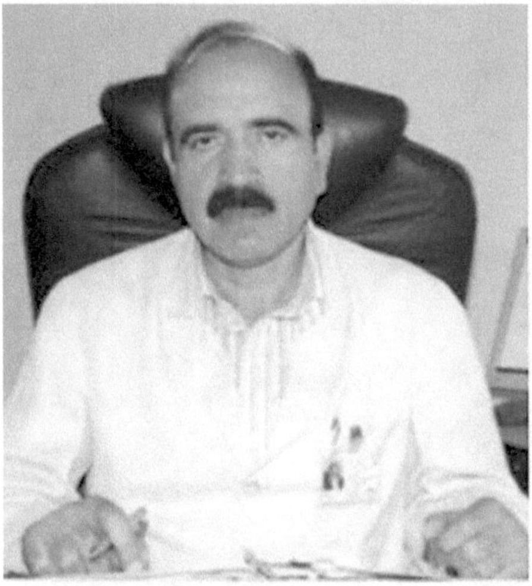

Dr. Abdul Hamid Zargar—the endocrinologist researcher at SKIMS whose research on diabetes, thyroid, and pituitary helped to douse the flames of an imminent disaster by introducing lifestyle modifications and policy changes by the government.

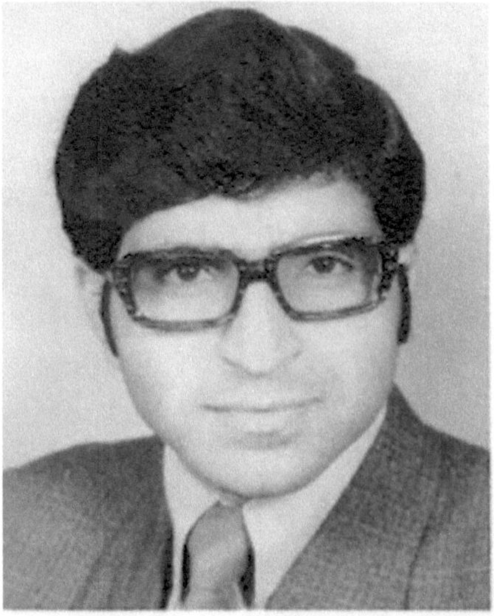

Dr. A. A. Beig—the soft-spoken psychiatrist who helped to remove the "stigma" around psychiatry.

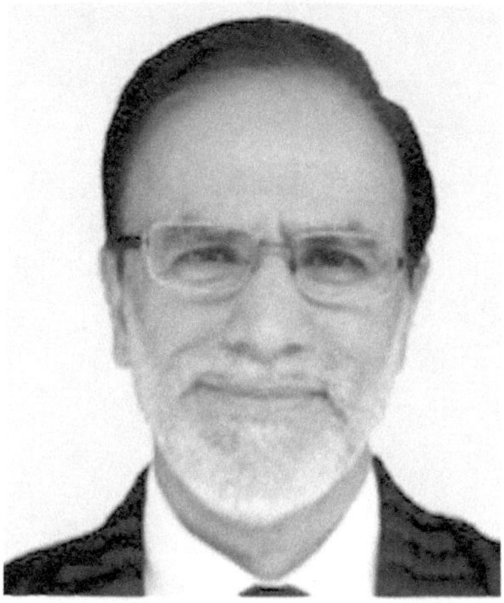

Dr. Mushtaq A. Margoob—amid an explosive increase in psychiatric diseases helped to convert a mental asylum into IMHANS.

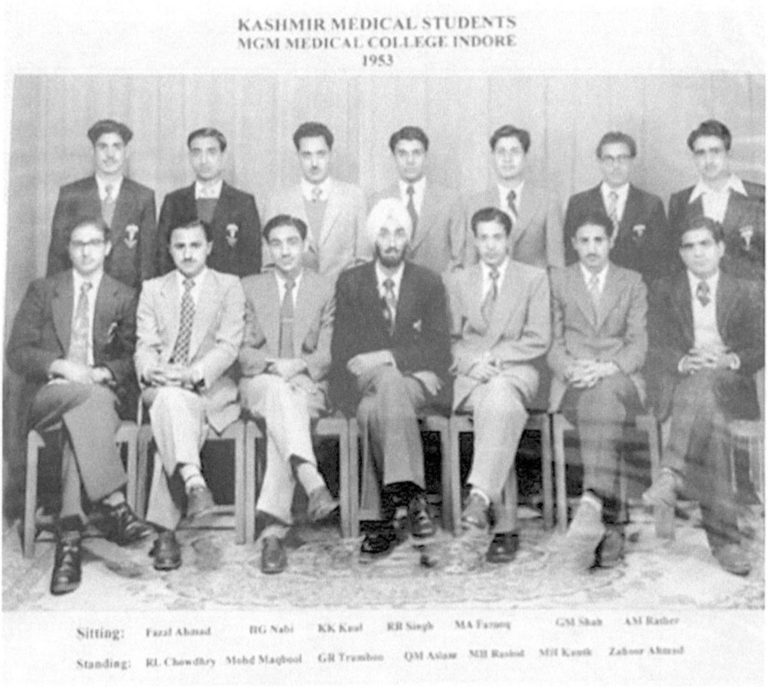

Photo courtesy of Dr. K. K. Kaul

The Flag Bearers

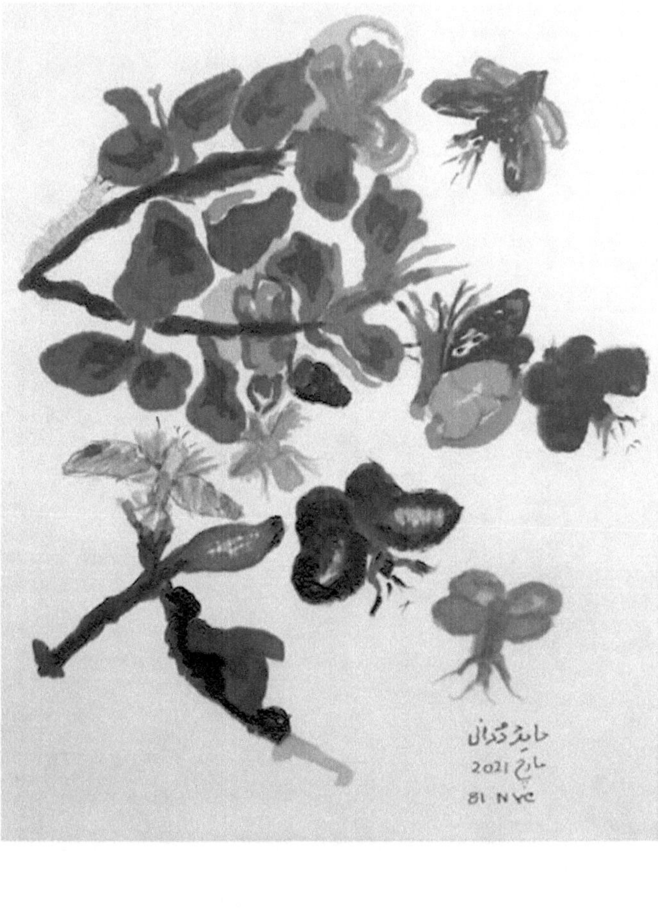

1. **Dr. Anil Bhan**
2. **Dr. Azra Shah**
3. **Dr. Farhat Jabeen**
4. **Dr. Feroze Shaheen**
5. **Dr. Ghulam Hassan Malik**
6. **Dr. Ghulam Jeelani Qadiri**
7. **Dr. Ghulam Mohammad Malik**
8. **Dr. Khursheed Aslam Khan**
9. **Dr. Khurshid Iqbal**
10. **Dr. Mehraj-ud-din**
11. **Dr. Mohammad Maqbool Lone**
12. **Dr. Mohammad Saleem Wani**
13. **Dr. Muneer Khan**
14. **Dr. Murtaza Chishti**
15. **Dr. Muzaffar Ahmad**
16. **Dr. Nisar Ahmad Chowdri**
17. **Dr. Nisar Ahmad Tramboo**
18. **Dr. Omar Javed Shah**
19. **Dr. Parvaiz Ahmad Koul**
20. **Dr. Shabir Iqbal**
21. **Dr. Shahida Mir**
22. **Dr. Shariq Rashid Masoodi**
23. **Dr. Shiekh Aejaz Aziz**
24. **Dr. Showkat Ali Zargar**
25. **Dr. Upendra Kaul**

Dr. Anil Bhan

Dr. Anil Bhan is an impressive cardiac surgeon born in Srinagar and had his initial education from Tyndale Biscoe School, Srinagar. Right from his school days, he excelled both in sports and studies. He was awarded the Certificate of Honor as the Best All-Round Boy in school. He was also awarded the Certificate of Honor for his performance in matriculation, as he stood first in matriculation in Kashmir Province. He is the recipient of a Certificate of Distinction for first rank in premedical examination at the University of Kashmir. He graduated from Medical College, Srinagar, with a distinction in pharmacology, pathology, forensic medicine, internal medicine, surgery, and gyne/obst. He received a Certificate of Distinction for securing the first position in order of merit in the MBBS examination of the University of Kashmir. His friends and class fellows remember him as a brilliant student who excelled at everything.

Dr. Anil did his internship at Christian Medical College Vellore. Being the son of a pioneer in surgery who was instrumental in laying the foundations of surgery in Kashmir (Dr. B. M. Bhan), the art of surgery came naturally to him. He competed at the national level and did his MS in general surgery from the prestigious PGI Chandigarh and was awarded the Silver Medal at PGI for his performance in the MS general surgery examination. He worked as a "pool officer" in cardiothoracic and vascular surgery at All India Institute of Medical Sciences and completed his MCh in cardiothoracic and vascular surgery from All India Institute of Medical Sciences New Delhi. He was inducted as a faculty member in All India Institute of Medical Sciences (AIIMS) and was involved in academics and patient care and stood at the gateway for the revolution in cardiac surgery that was happening in the world as well as at the institution where he was working. He was part of the iconic and celebrated team that conducted the first successful heart transplantation in India under Dr. Panangipalli Venugopal on August 3, 1994. At AIIMS, New Delhi, Dr. Anil supervised the thesis of twelve postgraduates at AIIMS and was involved in academic activities that resulted in getting more than two hundred papers published in high-impact journals.

Dr. Anil Bhan worked at AIIMS New Delhi till 2004 and resigned as the additional professor in cardiothoracic and vascular surgery. Dr. Anil Bhan left AIIMS and opted to work in private and is the cofounder of Max Heart Institute Saket, New Delhi, where he worked as the director and chief coordinator of Cardiothoracic and Vascular Surgery from 2004 to 2008. He was awarded the Lifetime Achievement Award at the World Congress of Clinical and Preventive Cardiology in 2006 conferred by former president of India Dr. A. P. J. Abdul Kalam in Rashtrapati Bhawan. The Indian Association of Cardiovascular Surgery conferred him with K. N. Dastur Oration and the PK Sen Oration in 2009 and 2013, respectively. Dr. Anil published stellar data on "adenosine preconditioning of the myocardium in patients with ventricular dysfunction undergoing myocardial revascularization," which was published in the *European Journal of Thoracic and Cardiovascular Surgery*.

Dr. Anil Bhan is one of the best pediatric cardiac surgeons in India and conducted the coronary artery bypass surgery for the youngest—a patient aged twenty months. He developed one of the largest pediatric surgical programs in the country. When at AIIMS, he was instrumental in shaping the neonatal cardiac surgical program, and even now his team performs all kinds of complex pediatric cardiac procedures. He described a new operative technique for the repair of supracardiac total anomalous pulmonary venous drainage (published in *Annals of Thoracic Surgery*, USA).

He modified the circuit for retrograde central perfusion published in *Asian Cardiovascular Thoracic Annals*, 2003 (aortic surgery program). Dr. Anil is a passionate aortic aneurysm surgeon who has developed one of the largest aortic aneurysm programs in India. His team operates all cases of complex dissecting and nondissecting aneurysms. He is a pioneer in myocardial revascularization technique and has mastered both on- and off-pump myocardial revascularization techniques. He has developed special techniques and instruments for the safe conduct of off-pump myocardial revascularization procedure. Dr. Anil Bhan is an innovative surgeon who has designed and developed more than fifty instruments for minimally invasive cardiac surgery, thoracic and thoracoabdominal aortic aneurysms, mitral valve surgery, and the beating heart coronary artery bypass surgery. Dr. Anil has designed an OPCAB sternal retractor for the safe conduct of beating heart surgery.

Dr. Anil Bhan is credited with developing the first minimally invasive cardiac surgical programs in India. He developed various new instruments to perform these minimally invasive procedures. He and his team have extensive experience in valvular heart surgery—both replacement and repair procedures. He holds a special interest in the Ross procedure for native aortic valve disease, which is done by very few cardiac surgeons.

Dr. Anil Bhan is working toward the role of stem cells in cardiac diseases and also the use of robotics in cardiac surgery. Dr. Anil Bhan, for his meritorious service in the field of CTVS, has received more than twenty awards from various associations and NGOs, which include awards from the Rotary Clubs of

Faridabad (2005); IMA Academy of Medical Specialties, New Delhi Branch (2007); Felicitation by the Kashmir Medicos—Old Students Forum (2007); Lifetime Achievement Award by the Human Care Charitable Trust (2014); DMA Chikitsa Ratan Award by Delhi Medical Association (2014); Lifetime Achievement award by KECESS (Kashmir Education, Cultural and Science Society) in view of his outstanding contribution in the field of medical sciences (2015); and Felicitation by the Society of Heart Failure and Transplantation in Kochi (2016) in recognition of the contribution in the thoracic organ transplantation in India.

Dr. Anil Bhan is happy as well as sad when he sees Kashmiris outside his chamber not only looking for treatment but also wanting to talk to him. They come to him for the trust they have in him and out of their love for him. He is keen that cardiac surgery facilities are improved in Kashmir and would consider himself lucky if he could be of some help in this regard. Dr. Anil Bhan is a messiah for so many . . . more so for the Kashmiris who come flocking to his clinic with their diseased hearts . . . some he mends and some he holds for a lifetime with his tender touch and soft words. A humble gentleman with a mission to lead and many goals to accomplish, he has rendered the ultimate service in his chosen field. He makes us all proud!

Dr. Azra Shah

It was the early '90s, and there was turmoil everywhere in Kashmir. Many faculty members left SKIMS, and many departments literally faced closure. Post-turmoil, the Department of Microbiology at SKIMS owes its existence to a lady who accepted the responsibility of heading the Department of Microbiology after all the faculty members had migrated and the department had no one to lead it. The postgraduates had no guide. She accepted the leadership in a difficult time at a difficult place. Under her leadership, the Department of Microbiology continued to provide diagnostic services, and postgraduate course continued. This responsibility was shouldered by her till the department had its own faculty. This graceful woman stood by SKIMS in its most difficult time and quietly complied with whatever she was asked to do. This woman named Dr. Azra Shah came as savior of a department and its postgraduates.

Dr. Azra was born in Srinagar in 1947 to Mr. Syed Ahmad Shah and Salma Shah. She belonged to a highly educated and influential family and received her schooling from Presentation Convent School, Rajbagh, Srinagar. She was a meritorious student who secured a position in her matriculation examination and pre-university boards. She did her MBBS from Government Medical College (GMC), Srinagar, in 1969 and passed all professional examinations with distinction. She had an opportunity to do her postgraduation from PGI Chandigarh and worked as a junior resident and postgraduate student in the

Department of Pathology, PGI, Chandigarh, from 1976 to 1977. After studying at PGI, she worked as a tutor/demonstrator in the Department of Pathology, GMC, Srinagar, from 1978 to 1980. She was inducted as a lecturer in the Department of Pathology, GMC, Srinagar, from 1980 to 1981.

When the SKIMS was in its initial years, Dr. Azra chose to work there as an assistant professor in the Department of Pathology and was instrumental in shaping up a highly specialized department with state-of-the-art services that were not available anywhere in North India. She joined the department in 1981 and rose to the rank of professor and head of the department. She received the WHO fellowship in gastrointestinal pathology at St. Mark's Hospital, London, in 1984 and was trained by a world-renowned gastrointestinal pathologist, Prof. B. C. Morson. She also received WHO fellowship in advanced histopathology at Royal Postgraduate Medical School, Hammersmith Hospital, London, in 1984 and worked with Prof. Nicholas Wright. Dr. Azra was awarded a Fellowship of the Indian College of Pathologists. She took over as head of the department when most of the faculty had left SKIMS because of turmoil. She ran the department efficiently and put it back on the rails.

Dr. Azra worked as controller of examinations at SKIMS and as dean at SKIMS. She was instrumental in starting the postgraduate program (MD) in pathology and getting it recognized by MCI. She was a member/chairperson of various important committees of SKIMS. She has been a founder member/executive member of the Indian Leptospirosis Society and held the important position of treasurer. Dr. Azra has been a life member of many associations, including life member of the Indian Association of Pathologists and Microbiologists (1976) and life member of Indian Association of Cytologists (1989). She has received many awards, including the Award of Excellence in recognition of outstanding contribution towards medical education by SKIMS in 2009 and the Distinguished Leadership Award by the American Biographical Institute in 1998.

Dr. Azra has authored more than a hundred papers in various national and international journals and authored two books—namely, *MCQs in Pathology with Explanations and Text* and *A Dictionary of Medical Syndromes.* Dr. Azra has been on the editorial board of various journals, including the prestigious *Indian Journal of Pathology and Microbiology.* She has been an examiner for MBBS, BDS, and MD in pathology. Dr. Azra has been an expert for the selection of faculty of Aligarh Muslim University and an advisor for the selection of faculty by the Union Public Service Commission (UPSC) and J&K Public Service Commission. She has been on the task force advisory committee of ICMR and the task force advisory committee of the Directorate of Science and Technology, Government of India.

Dr. Azra has been a highly respected faculty member of SKIMS who has helped the institution tide over very difficult times. She is a sober human and a highly professional pathologist who is respected all over India for her professional competence. She is the devoted wife of Prof. Abdul Rauf, ex-principal at GMC Srinagar, and has two children who work abroad. She lives a happy postretirement life with her children and grandchildren.

Dr. Farhat Jabeen

Amid the stress of work that is so prominent in our overburdened and overcrowded hospital of gynecology and obstetrics—namely, Lal Ded Hospital—is a vibrant woman with a charming and ever-smiling face. A hardworking and dedicated doctor she is, and her calm temperament makes her a darling teacher too. Report if you watch her in anger, panic, or rage! This woman has been one of the biggest pillars of one of our biggest hospitals for the last many challenging decades of turmoil and unrest. That's how we the students fondly remember Dr. Farhat Jabeen, who, without doubt, maintained her calmness, cool temperament, and competence through tough years of turmoil and extreme pressure of work. Dr. Farhat recently retired from her position as the head of the Department of Gynecology and Obstetrics at Lal Ded (LD) Hospital and is at present rendering her services in the private sector.

Dr. Farhat Jabeen was born in Sopore, Kashmir, in a renowned family. The family is known for the public service that the family has rendered to the people of Sopore for many generations. She inherited this spirit from her father, Dr. Hakim Atiquallah, and Mrs. Haneefa Begum, her mother. Her father has been a renowned physician of Northern Kashmir and has served every nook and corner of that area for many decades. Dr. Farhat did her early schooling from Janatul Islamia School and went to Women's College Sopore after that. She was highly impressed by the teachers of her school who inspired her to do good in life and supported her. She was a bright student who had a passion for medicine, and her father greatly stimulated her to join medicine. She was always impressed by the hard work, dedication, and commitment her father displayed toward his patients, his service to his fellow beings, and his love for medicine. Her brothers—namely, Dr. Shad Salim Akthar (who was the first medical oncologist of Jammu and Kashmir and a pioneer in his field) and Dr. Mushtaq Hakim (who was the first orthodontist of Jammu and Kashmir)—further added to her desire to pursue medicine. She was selected for MBBS at GMC Srinagar in 1977 and completed it in 1982. After working as an assistant surgeon and a junior resident, she was enrolled as a postgraduate in gynecology and obstetrics in 1987. She completed her MD in 1989 under the guidance of her mentor and guide, Prof. Wazira Khanam.

Dr. Farhat worked as a registrar in the Department of Gynecology and Obstetrics, Lal Ded Hospital, Srinagar, for a long turbulent decade from 1989 to 1999. This was a time of extreme pressure on LD Hospital as most of the staff had migrated because of turmoil and the peripheral setups for obstetric care had almost collapsed. Dr. Farhat, along with her few colleagues, was in a responsible position managing the hospital amid curfews, hartals, and bomb blasts. Whatever the situation outside and whatever the conditions inside, Dr. Farhat would be available 24-7 for any eventuality, any emergency, or any exigency. I remember Dr. Farhat as an omnipresent face at LD Hospital during my years of training. The kindness and ethics, which are the first casualty in any kind of stress, could not overpower the will of this dynamic surgeon and teacher. Her soft touch and smile are the greatest virtues she has, and I believe she persistently preserved these traits for all her patients and students.

Dr. Farhat was inducted into the faculty at GMC Srinagar in 1999 as a lecturer. She was promoted as an assistant professor in 2003 and became an associate professor in 2009. She became the professor in 2014 and retired from her services in 2021. Dr. Farhat has authored many papers published in national and international journals, attended many international conferences, and presented her papers. She is the vice president of the Srinagar branch of Obstetrics and Gynecology Society of India. She is holding this prestigious position since 2013. She has been a counselor for PGDMCH courses of IGNOU. She has organized many conferences and workshops, notable being a conference on operative endoscopy in gynecology at GMC Srinagar.

Dr. Farhat conducted the FORCE program for postgraduate scholars in collaboration with FOGSI in 2013. She is a coinvestigator in many ICMR projects and has been a guide and coguide for many postgraduates. She has collaborated with scientists from other institutions for many research projects.

Dr. Farhat is a capable surgeon who has tried her best to pass on her skill to the younger colleagues. Her juniors would see her as a caring boss who would love to work in a team and never exploit them. She would share the responsibility wholeheartedly. She is thankful to her mentor, Professor Wazira, and her other senior colleagues and teachers.

Dr. Farhat is a mother to three wonderful daughters, who are doctors too. She is married to Dr. Kaiser, a busy pediatrician. She and her family of competent and humble doctors make a perfect family!

Dr. Feroze Shaheen

Dr. Feroze Shaheen holds the distinction of being one of the brightest radiologists who started intervention in cardiac and neuroradiology at SKIMS. He is academically oriented and has been trained extensively in all the major institutions of the country in cardiac and neuroradiology. Dr. Feroze Shaheen is a gentleman who put his efforts together to bring the Department of Radiodiagnosis at SKIMS at par with the best institutions of the country.

Dr. Feroze Shaheen was born on November 11, 1964, to Mr. Ghulam Mohammad Wani and Maryam Bano. He received his initial education from Government Higher Secondary School Nagam. He did his MBBS from GMC Srinagar. During his college days, Dr. Girja Dhar, whom he admired for her impeccable integrity, discipline, impressive personality, and poise, inspired him. Dr. Muneer Khan from Surgery also inspired him. When clinical branches were considered to be attractive and appetizing, Dr. Feroze Shaheen chose to follow his passion to pursue the challenging field of radiodiagnosis and imaging. Dr. Feroze did his MD in radiodiagnosis and imaging from GMC Jammu in 1996.

Dr. Feroze chose not to practice radiology in private, where it would be attractive monetarily, but opted for an academic institution like SKIMS. There was an expansion and tremendous advancement in radiodiagnosis, much of which was unexplored in Kashmir, SKIMS was at crossroads, and a robust radiodiagnosis department was the need of the hour. Dr. Feroze joined the department at SKIMS as an assistant professor in 2001. As a faculty member, he was instrumental in upgrading the department and doing challenging interventions. He was also instrumental in starting the postgraduation in radiodiagnosis along with his other colleagues.

Dr. Feroze received special training in cardiac CT from Madras Medical Mission, Chennai, and training in color Doppler from AIIMS, New Delhi. He was trained in neuro and cardiac radiology from Bombay Hospital and Research Center and from Sayadhari Super Specialty Hospital, Pune, India. He also received training in USG and CT-guided interventions from Bombay Hospital and Research Center. He went for training in interventional and diagnostic neuroradiology at the National Institute of Mental Health and Sciences, Bengaluru. This training gave him an exposure to multiple institutions with advanced radiological services. He tried his best to use this expertise for the benefit of patients at SKIMS. Presently, he is the professor and head of the Radiodiagnosis Department at SKIMS.

Dr. Feroze is a "know-all" radiologist who excels in all radiological subspecialties with a special interest in cardiac and neuroradiology. Dr. Feroz has supervised the execution and reporting of all imaging modalities, especially the superspeciality modalities like cardiac CT, cardiac MRI, and interventional procedures of a high-risk nature like CT fluoroscopic guided mediastinal biopsies. He is an excellent teacher involved in teaching of postgraduates, senior residents and postdoctoral students from cardiology, CVTS, neurosurgery, gastroenterology, plastic surgery, etc. He has published his research work in high-impact journals like *American Journal of Radiology*, *Applied Radiology*, *European Journal of Radiology*, and *Journal of Gastrointestinal Surgery*.

According to Dr. Feroze we should embrace the technological boom that has revolutionized radiodiagnosis. He says, "In this era of knowledge boom, one has not only to continuously update the knowledge and skills but also to unlearn redundant practices and work habits. We are witnessing an exponential growth of cross-sectional imaging that is increasingly being AI-enabled. Knowledge of radiological sciences and image interpretation skills accumulated over decades of work is the greatest asset with the radiologist that can be of immense use in deciding the treatment of patients from all domains of disease profiles. It can also be leveraged to produce robust AI protocols in diagnosis and interpretation."

Dr. Feroze has inspired some of the brightest minds in Kashmir to pursue radiology and excel in it. According to Dr. Feroze, "My dream has always been to crave for professional excellence, to be in love with your roots and to be humble in any circumstance. My ultimate dream is imparting the skills and knowledge acquired to the next generation." Talking about his dream further, Dr. Feroze says, "I aspire to be an enthusiastic contributor to the incoming paradigm shift in imaging technology driven by AI and 6G communication. I hope Kashmir with its immense talent has this window of opportunity to leapfrog into a knowledge economy by leveraging this talent and high standards of medical education. We could become the next hub in the Tele-radiology, the Tele-diagnosis and Tele-medicine for most of Asia and Europe." I hope his dream is realized and we live to see things happen for the benefit of our community.

Dr. Feroze is married to Hina Rehman, who is also a doctor, and lives with his wife and children in Srinagar.

Dr. Ghulam Hassan Malik

A zealous young researcher presented his work titled "Chronic End-Stage Renal Disease at Chandigarh—Prevalence and Management by Dialysis and Transplantation" at the First Asian Pacific Congress of Nephrology in Tokyo, Japan, on October 1979. The youngster made his presentation in front of an impressive international audience, which included stalwarts in nephrology. The audience was highly appreciative of the work he presented. This was the work of a DM scholar pursuing superspecialization in nephrology at PGI Chandigarh. This youngster named Dr. Ghulam Hassan Malik went on to become the first qualified nephrologist from Jammu and Kashmir. His research included bold and outstanding work on renal failure secondary to torture, discussed on academic forums throughout the world.

Dr. Ghulam Hassan Malik was born on March 11, 1946, in Aloosa, Bandipora, to Mr. Mohammad Rajab Malik and Zeba Malik. He received his early education from Aloosa and later on went to Government Degree College, Sopore. Dr. Malik was selected for MBBS at GMC Srinagar in 1964 and completed it in 1970. He did MD in general medicine from GMC Srinagar in 1975. He was deputed to PGI Chandigarh for a six-month training in nephrology, and, after he came back, he started both peritoneal and hemodialysis at SMHS Hospital. This training kindled his interest in nephrology, and he eventually did his DM (nephrology) at the Postgraduate Institute of Medical Education and Research, Chandigarh (India), in 1980.

Dr. G. H. Malik was appointed as lecturer, Department of Medicine, Government Medical College, Srinagar, Kashmir, in 1980 and worked there from 1980 to 1985. He was one of the founding members of the Nephrology Department of SKIMS Srinagar. He worked as an associate professor in the Department of Nephrology, Sher-i-Kashmir, Institute of Medical Sciences, Srinagar, from 1985 to 1987. He was promoted as an additional professor and worked in this capacity from 1987 to 1993. At SKIMS, he was a postgraduate teacher and MD examiner, and many candidates had their theses and degrees in medicine completed under his guidance.

Dr. Malik has an excellent research record. He has authored some of the classic papers in nephrology. His remarkable research work on acute renal failure following physical torture, published in *Nephron* (Malik, GH, Sirwal IA, Reshi AR, et al. "Acute Renal Failure following Physical Torture." *Nephron*, 1993; 63: 434–437), was considered to be a bold and a daring paper that brought to fore different nephrological aspects of physical torture in a conflict zone. His other paper (Malik GH, Reshi AR, Najar MS, Ahmad A, Masood T., "Further Observations on Acute Renal Failure following Physical Torture," *Nephrology Dialysis Transplantation*, 1995, 10; 2: 198–202) became a talk of various editorials and was widely discussed paper very relevant to a conflict zone. Commenting on the "Nephrological and Moral Aspects of Physical Torture," N. Lameire and E. Vermeersch, the editors of the prestigious journal in which it was published, had all praise for the paper Dr. Malik published. Appreciating the efforts of the authors, they said, "We feel they (authors) should be congratulated for the courage to publish this and a previous paper on this subject," And they further note, "This paper encourages the discussion of a number of important issues related to physical torture."

In a concluding remark, they write, "It should be said for the authors of the article by Malik et al. that most probably in difficult circumstances, they have been faithful to the duties inherent to their profession" ("Nephrological and Moral Aspects of Physical Torture," *Nephrol Dial Transplant*, 1995: editorial). His work on rhabdomyolysis and torture is a work of class and courage, which no one from Kashmir or India has been able to replicate. His work forms an essential reference in all books related to nephrological manifestations of torture. These avant-garde papers in nephrology were presented by him in a number of national and international conferences. He has authored two book chapters on pregnancy-related kidney diseases published by Elsevier.

Dr. Malik worked as a consultant nephrologist at Security Forces Hospital, Riyadh, Saudi Arabia, from 1993 to 2004. Security Forces Hospital is a five-hundred-bedded Tertiary Referral Center recognized by the Saudi Medical Council for Postgraduate Medical degrees. Dr. Malik was committed to research and teaching in Saudi Arabia too and has published more than thirty papers from there in high-impact medical journals.

Dr. Malik has been the president of North Zone Indian Society of Nephrology. He is a life member of more than six nephrology associations, including life member, the Indian Society of Nephrology and the International Society of Nephrology. He received the Dronachary Award in 2016 and an award by the Delhi Nephrology Society in 2016 at New Delhi. He also received the Lifetime Achievement Award conferred by the North Zone Indian Society of Nephrology on February 16, 2018, at Jaipur. He has been awarded Foundation Award from TANKER (Tamil Nadu Kidney Research) on January 25, 2019, in Chennai. He is a reviewer for the *Saudi Journal of Kidney Diseases and Transplantation* and the *Indian Journal of*

Nephrology. He is a member of the editorial board of the *Saudi Journal of Kidney Diseases Transplantation*.

The space of a profile is limited, I cannot quote all the publications that Dr. Malik has authored, but while going through his CV, a paper by three legends of SKIMS could not escape my attention (Khuroo, MS, Guru AA, Garyali RK, Malik GH, "Ascites of Undetermined Origin in Patients with Pneumatosis Cystoides Intestinalis," *J. Ass. Phy. India* 24, 5, 1976). This paper does depict how the legends at SKIMS coordinated interdepartmentally for patient care and research. Dr. Malik has done extensive work on pregnancy with underlying renal diseases and lupus.

Dr. Malik has pioneered nephrology in Kashmir and has authored excellent research papers, which are read with interest not only by medical researchers but also by all those interested in the studies related to a conflict zone. He has established and runs a dialysis center since 2004 at Soura Srinagar. Presently; he is the director/senior consultant nephrologist at Well Care Medical Center, Soura, Srinagar, Kashmir. He manages to provide nephrology and dialysis services to his patients.

Dr. Ghulam Jeelani Qadiri

Dr. Ghulam Jeelani Qadiri was born on April 1, 1949, in the Downtown Srinagar in a well-to-do family. His father, Peerzada Ghulam Mohammed Qadiri, and mother, Maimouna Begum, were keen to see their children receive good education. He had his early schooling from Srinagar and Jammu. He went to MPML Higher Secondary School and SP College Srinagar. He was selected for MBBS course at GMC Srinagar in 1966. In GMC Srinagar, he was greatly influenced by Prof. Naseer Ahmad Shah and Prof. R. S. Manhas. Dr. Jeelani, rates them as the best teachers in the medical college.

After his MBBS from GMC Srinagar, he worked as a postgraduate resident, Department of Hospital Administration and Medical Care, National Institute of Health and Family Welfare, New Delhi (April 1977 to March 1979), and did MD in hospital administration from the University of Delhi. After MD in hospital administration from Delhi, he returned to Srinagar and worked as the deputy medical superintendent, Government Medical College Hospital, Srinagar (April 1979 to May 1981). He became a consultant (assistant professor), Department of Hospital Administration, and deputy medical superintendent at SK Institute of Medical Sciences, Srinagar, Kashmir (June 1981 to June 1985). He was promoted as an associate professor, Department of Hospital Administration, and medical superintendent at SKIMS and worked in this capacity from 1985 to 1989. He became the professor and head of Department of Hospital Administration (July 1989 to 1996). He also served SKIMS as the chief of Materials Management (1997 to March 1999).

Dr. Jeelani has done a commendable job as the professor and head of Postgraduate Department of Hospital Administration SKIMS and as the medical superintendent of SKIMS in the most difficult years of turmoil surrounding the valley and SKIMS during 90's. He had to face the situation on the ground, which was in no way healthy. To run a hospital during those times was a herculean task that was done to perfection by Dr. Jeelani. The times were so hard that to keep the hospital working against the odds meant compromising one's safety and security. Dr. Jeelani looked after SKIMS in those times and held together the institution and his own department very skilfully.

Dr. Jeelani worked as a specialist in public health, directorate general of hospital administration, Ministry of Health, Kingdom of Saudi Arabia (March 1999 to November 2000). He was appointed as the principal, Government SKIMS Medical College, Srinagar (October 2005 till March 31, 2009), and was the dean of medical faculty, S. K. Institute of Medical Sciences (Deemed University), Srinagar (October 2007 to March 31, 2009). Dr. Jeelani took up the assignment of the professor and head of Postgraduate Department of Hospital Administration and principal dean, Yenapoya Medical College, Mangalore, Karnataka (June 2009 to July 2018). This was a very challenging role for Dr. Jeelani. He transformed Yenapoya Medical College and helped it to fulfill all the NMC requirements, and thereby become an excellent medical college in the private sector where quality education was provided and youngsters were stimulated to excel.. After his retirement, he continues to work as the professor emeritus, Postgraduate Department of Hospital Administration, Yenapoya Medical College, till date.

Dr. Jeelani has many awards to his credit. He has received Eminent Educationist Award by the International Institute of

Education and Management, New Delhi, in 2012, Lifetime Achievement Award by International Institute of Education and Management, India, in 2016, Outstanding Achievements Award in Health Care by the Global Achievers Foundation of India in 2016, American Order of Merit by American Bibliography Institute USA in 2010 and was awarded Shiksha Rattan Puroskar (Certificate of Excellence for Meritorious Services, Outstanding Performance and Remarkable Role) by the Indian International Friendship Society at New Delhi in 2010.

Dr. Jeelani has authored seventy-eight scientific papers chaired many scientific sessions and delivered talks in various scientific conferences and training programs in India and abroad. He has authored books, book chapters, and manuals for hospitals. This includes

- *Hand Book of Patient Care and Hospital Medicine* (1997)
- *Nursing Operational Manual* (1999)
- Chapter on "Materials and Equipment Management in Hospitals and Organization of Dietary Services in Hospitals" (for Course Material for One-Year Distance Learning Program in Hospital and Health Management conducted by National Institute of Health and Family Welfare, New Delhi)
- *Residents and Nurses Manual*, Medical College Hospital, Yenepoya University (2013)
- Chapter "Manual on Safety in Hospital Laboratories," Yenepoya University (2014).

Dr. Jeelani received PhD from the Gatesville University, California, USA, in 2016. He is a life member of many national and international bodies and associations. He is the examiner MHA, awarded by the SKIMS Soura, AIIMS New Delhi, NIMS Hyderabad, RGUHS Karnataka, and MAHE Manipal Karnataka.

He is also the examiner of the DNB, awarded by National Board of Examinations. He has been the chairman/member of various expert committees, selection committees, planning and advisory committees at SKIMS, SKIMS Medical College, Srinagar, and Yenepoya (deemed to be university) Karnataka. He has been a member of Core Group MHHM/PGDHHM, Indira Gandhi National Open University, New Delhi; member of Working Group MCI at New Delhi for the specialty of Health Service Management; expert, Faculty Selection Committee, Indira Gandhi National Open University, New Delhi, MAHE Manipal, Karnataka; and expert, Faculty Selection Committee, National Institute of Health and Family Welfare, New Delhi. He has also held various honorary offices, including regional director, Academy of Hospital Administration, Mangalore—Manipal Chapter, 2010–July 2018. He has been member of Working Group MCI at New Delhi for the Specialty Board of Health Administration and the secretary, Academy of Hospital Administration, Kashmir Chapter, 1994–2008.

Dr. Jeelani has thirty-two years of administrative and teaching experience in the specialty of health and hospital administration. He has practiced and taught various concepts of hospital and health management in different medical colleges and health-care institutions. The study tours to various hospitals and health-care institutions in India and outside India (UK, USA, Malaysia, KSA, and Nepal) provided him with opportunities to learn and assess various systems of medical care and understand planning, operations, evaluation, and quality management aspects of health care administration.

He has taken up many challenging assignments in Kashmir and outside Kashmir. The most challenging of all the assignments has been the job of the medical superintendent and head of the Department of Hospital Management at SKIMS in the tough years of turmoil. As the principal of SKIMS Medical College, Srinagar, and Yenepoya Medical College, Mangalore,

Karnataka, he was involved in tackling the challenges facing these institutions and known for his student-friendly and faculty-friendly behavior. He is one of the few administrators who worked beyond Kashmir after his retirement and continued to contribute towards health-care and medical education.

Dr. Ghulam Mohammad Malik

When health care in Kashmir was in total chaos because of the turmoil, who would think of writing a scientific paper and getting it published? The process was tedious, the postal services were dismal, and the Internet was nonexistent—those passionate to write hardly had avenues. All did not have the stamina or the passion to cross the hurdles and bulk of work from Kashmir would remain unpublished. The thought of getting Kashmir onto the medical publishing platform came to Dr. G. M. Malik, who launched *JK Practitioner*, the first medical journal from Jammu and Kashmir, in 1994. *JK Practitioner* not only served as a launch pad for budding researchers and writers but also removed the fears that having a medical journal in Kashmir was an achievable task. *JK Practitioner* introduced Kashmir and its diseases to the world and gave recognition to the hardworking and dedicated community of doctors at the national and international stage. Incidentally, I and many of my friends and colleagues had *JK Practitioner* as the journal for our first publication. Dr. Malik put together a great team of professionals, under talented Dr. Zaffar Abass, to do the job, who, in spite of the difficulties, has managed the show well.

Dr. G. M. Malik was born in Galoora, Handwara, Kashmir, in 1948 to Mr. Khazir Mohammad Malik. He was bright and innovative from his childhood and made his way into the GMC Srinagar and completed his MBBS in 1973. He did his MD in internal medicine in 1977. He was one of the toppers of his class and was awarded ten medals and certificates for his academic excellence. He worked as a fellow in Queens LUH, Prince George Hospital, Maryland; Long Island Jewish Hospital, New York; and Thomas Jefferson University, Philadelphia, USA. He has received fellowship from the American College of Gastroenterology (FACG) in 1994 and the Indian College of Ultrasound in 1995. He served as a faculty member in internal medicine and became the professor and the head of the Department of internal medicine at GMC Srinagar. He worked to establish gastroenterology services in GMC Srinagar in close collaboration with Dr. Hamid Durrani.

At GMC Srinagar, students' interests were very dear to Dr. Malik, and he was an active member of the CASS union. He organized many national and international conferences and was instrumental in getting computers for the GMC library. Dr. G. M. Malik has been an exceptional teacher and has guided nearly fifty postgraduate students in medicine. He has been an internal and external MBBS and MD examiner for more than a dozen universities in India. Dr. Malik served as a link between nonresident Kashmiri doctors and the medical faculty of Kashmir. It was through him that the medical fraternity of Kashmir would collaborate for various projects, conferences, and fellowships with nonresident Kashmiri doctors who wished to help their brethren back home. It was through him as a resource person that essay competitions supported by Dr. Faroque Khan were organized at GMC Srinagar and the topics mostly related to health-care issues confronting Kashmir.

Dr. G. M. Malik has served in Riyadh Central Hospital, Saudi Arabia, and has been lauded for his services there too. After retirement from government services, he worked at ASCOMS Jammu and SKIMS Medical College, Srinagar, as the professor of internal medicine.

Dr. Malik has been the state president of the IMA (Indian Medical Association) and has worked towards the creation of an

IMA house in Srinagar. He is the state president of IDPD (Indian Doctors for Peace and Development). He has been awarded by DAK (Doctors Association of Kashmir) for his exceptional work in launching a medical journal in Kashmir. Dr. G. M. Malik is also the chairman of JK State Medical Council. He has received IMA Professorship and Academic Excellence Award, which was conferred to him at New Delhi in September 2021. Dr. G. M. Malik has collaborated for the award of international fellowships to the UK and Australia, including MRCP and fellowships in emergency medicine and family medicine.

Dr. G. M. Malik has published his work in many international journals, including *NEJM*, *Lancet*, *American Journal of Gastroenterology*, *Endoscopic Journal of Japan*, etc. His dauntless letter published in *Lancet* about stopping the use of landmines in conflict-ridden Kashmir helped to create awareness about land mines in rural Kashmir that had created havoc in the villages living close to the border areas (Malik, G. M. and J. A. Basu, "Landmines—Time for a Ban" (letter), *Lancet*, September 20, 1997, 350 (9081); 891).

Dr. G. M. Malik is active and readily participates in all academic events held in Jammu and Kashmir. He works in his private clinic and endoscopy lab and sees patients regularly. He lives with his wife, his son, and his grandson in Srinagar and keenly follows the construction of a Government Medical College in his hometown, Handwara, where he wants to contribute.

Dr. Khursheed Aslam Khan

Kashmir is a place where we do not usually celebrate "doctors and their accomplishments." To my great surprise, I saw a photo of a familiar face in one of the leading local newspapers with a note of thanks from SKIMS employees summing up the qualities of the doctor in a brief note on his retirement. The same photo was part of many Facebook posts, and thousands of comments followed these posts—the comments came from hundreds of thankful patients, employees, colleagues, friends, and coworkers. I was amused by the popularity of the doctor and the respect that people had for him. This most popular and gentle doctor named Dr. Khursheed Aslam Khan has served as a cardiologist at SKIMS and is admired by one and all for his exceptional qualities. Dr. Khursheed Aslam Khan is regarded as one of the most decent, soft-spoken, and down-to-earth doctors of Kashmir who, in spite of his busy schedule as a cardiologist, did not let go of his mannerisms and his humility. He served the community and SKIMS all along with commitment and dedication. He along with the other stalwarts of SKIMS cardiology worked hard towards making SKIMS cardiology what it is is today—a seat of excellence.

Dr. Khursheed was born in Srinagar in 1958. He received his initial education from CMS Tyndale Biscoe School. He did his MBBS from Government Medical College, Srinagar, in 1981 and his MD in internal medicine from Government Medical College, Srinagar, in 1987. He did DM in cardiology from Sher-i-Kashmir Institute of Medical Sciences, Srinagar, in 1998. He did his fellowship in interventional cardiology from the University of Buffalo, New York, USA, in 2006. He is a life member of reputed cardiology societies, including the Cardiology Society of India and the Indian College of Cardiology (FICC). He is a fellow of the American College of Physicians (FACP) and a recipient of the International Overseas Fellowship Award from the American College of Physicians. He is a fellow of the American College of Cardiology (FACC) and a fellow of the European Society of Cardiology (FESC).

Dr. Khursheed has more than sixty publications in national and international journals. He has presented complex and challenging cases at national interventional cardiology conferences (India Live, National Interventional Council, CAD India). He has presented interventional cases at C3 International Cardiology Conference in Orlando, Florida, USA. He has chaired and moderated scientific sessions at various national cardiology conferences and workshops. He has been the coordinator for the India Heart Study (the largest Indian study on hypertension). Dr. Khursheed has been conferred many awards by the SKIMS administration, including the Lifetime Achievement Award. Dr. Khursheed has been a popular teacher who would make it a point to teach his younger collegues the skills that he excelled in. One of his students told me this, "I wish I would become like Dr. Khursheed. He is calm and competent, graceful and cheerful, firm and generous. He has the qualities that most of us lack-he listenes, he smiles, he cares and he is accessible. He is smart and he is so well dressed".

After his retirement from SKIMS Dr. Khursheed works in private and he displays the same courtesy in his private clinic as he displayed at SKIMS. My mother is Dr. Khursheed's regular patient, and as I stand next to her in Dr. Khursheed's chamber, I am wonderstruck by the mannerism and ethics displayed by Dr. Khursheed. We need many more teachers like Dr. Khursheed to teach us what we are lacking.

Dr. Khurshid Iqbal

I have not heard a better story than this one about time management. It was early '70s; the city of Srinagar was lit and excited to host a "show" in the backyard of Kohimaran. All kids would come to watch the "show," which was focused on Kashmir history. The program would extend for a few hours well into the night. While the rest spent hours at the show, a boy knew how to manage his time. He, too, watched the show, but every day for half an hour so as not to tire himself and to manage his time and his daily engagements. If, for instance, he would watch the show from 4:30 p.m. to 5:00 p.m. one day, next day he would watch it from 5:00 p.m. to 5:30 p.m. This meant the routine was not disturbed and the "informative show" was not missed. This youngster named Khurshid Iqbal went on to be an Iqbal—a genius of hearts and a Khurshid, an illuminating sun, too! This boy raced on excelling, scoring honors in his school, ultimately topping the twelfth class examination from Islamia College, Srinagar, in 1971.

Once Dr. Khurshid went into the premier medical college of the state—namely, Government Medical College, Srinagar—he excelled there too. His teachers at GMC had the treat of their times; a bright student who excelled in every aspect of medicine—mannerism and gentleness included—was their student! He completed his MBBS in 1977. He did his MD in internal medicine in 1983 from GMC Srinagar (University of Kashmir). Destiny chose this gifted doctor to be a cardiologist, and he was trained in cardiology at PGI Chandigarh. He did his DM in cardiology from PGI Chandigarh in 1988.

Born into a family of Unani and allopathic physicians (Kozgars) from Khanquahi Moulla, Srinagar, his father, Dr. Ghulam Nabi, was an eye and ENT specialist and a faculty at SMHS Hospital/GMC Srinagar. His mother, Mrs. Hajra Begum, was an educationist having a master's in Urdu and English and served the School Education Department, Government of Jammu and Kashmir.

The birth of Sheri-Kashmir Institute of Medical Sciences (SKIMS) as a superspecialist hospital saw Dr. Khurshid being inducted as a lecturer in the Department of Cardiology at SKIMS.

From a founding member, he continued as a pillar getting stronger and sturdier with each challenge. He rose to the position of a professor of cardiology in 2001 and became head of the Department of Cardiology SKIMS thereafter. Times changed, turmoil came up, good ones and "would-be great ones" left SKIMS in search of better opportunities—but he stayed back fighting and managing the disasters and their consequences and moving on . . . The difficult times we faced gave us personality disorders, but this gentleman continued to be human, humble, and dedicated.

I remember a day at SKIMS in the early '90s when, as a student, I went to the library there and saw a gloomy, deserted hall with a few whispers coming from one of the rooms at the extreme end of the library. Curious to know what was going on, I saw Dr. Khurshid Iqbal with a few postgraduates on a computer (which was a rare sight those days) teaching students how to operate it and how to take out medical references. In a disorder that rendered us selfish, scary, and wrapped us up in a laid-back attitude, Dr. Khurshid was doing much more than his job demanded him to do. True to his name, *Khurshid* . . .

Dr. Khurshid nourished and nurtured his department, transforming SKIMS Cardiology from ordinary to a department excelling in interventional cardiology. He took care of the heart and its beats, restoring pulse to pulseless, synchrony to the asynchronous, and hope to the hopeless. Taking charge of a department ravaged and looted by turmoil, he restored order and pulled it out carefully from nothingness to hope . . . I remember how we had to refer hundreds of our patients to Delhi and other cardiac centers of India for cardiac interventions. Dr. Khurshid and his team came up as a blessing to thousands of poor patients of Kashmir Valley who could not afford expensive treatment outside. Also, a lot of state exchequer was saved as referrals to outside minimized.

While Dr. Khurshid is the unchallenged master of cardiology in Kashmir, his contribution in academics and research is unparalleled. As a dean of medical faculty from 2012 to 2014, he streamlined academics at SKIMS. During his tenure as the dean, a number of departments at SKIMS got MCI recognition. He was instrumental in introducing new courses and upgrading the existing ones. He broke the tradition and replaced the conventional methodologies with simple and modern technology to upgrade the Deemed University of SKIMS. His expertise in computers and information technology ensured that under his chairmanship, computers became an essential part of SKIMS working. He worked toward making SKIMS a paperless institution.

A genius is not limited by time and age, but opportunities bring out the best in him. I wish Dr. Khurshid had more opportunities, better infrastructure to work with, and a better appreciation for the work he did for many decades. He has been an achiever, a savior who has led at the forefront with his bare hands and whatever available little he had at hand. He saved lives and cared for the sick and suffering. His peers who left the valley are leaders of their profession elsewhere, but Dr.

Khurshid has helped build a department and helped shape an institution. He may not have invented a novel technique, but he has lived an exemplary life and kept the tradition of excellence, care, and compassion alive. His taught spread in all corners of the world practicing cardiology to perfection is an indication that great skills have been taught to them by wise minds in one of the remotest areas of the world.

A lot needs to be said about Dr. Khurshid; I feel short of words to describe him, but a farewell note to Dr. Khurshid on his retirement day by Dr. Parvaiz Koul, another genius and present director SKIMS, described Dr. Khurshid Iqbal to a great extent. This is what Dr. Pavaiz Koul said: "Dr. Khurshid transformed areas in SKIMS, especially the academics department. He revamped the examination system in SKIMS and added the modern-day technological advances into routine practice. His genius as a cardiologist was acknowledged by none other than his very successor in the department, Dr. Nissar. Dr Nissar in plain non-sugar-coated words described Dr Khurshid's contribution for every 'first' in cardiology in the state. His taking pride in serving as Dr Khurshid's first Assistant speaks volumes about the man and the systems that he inculcated into the routines of cardiology. What more does a person need to look back with pride and satisfaction? When Dr Khurshid mentioned, 'We are all because of SKIMS and SKIMS is not because of us,' he just spoke about a fact that many of us conveniently lose sight of. On its part, however, SKIMS owes a lot of gratitude to this man for whom greener pastures were always on the platter but he stayed stuck and 'made the difference.' He remained a distinct leading light for so many, including me. Dr. Khurshid remains an institution unto himself. SKIMS will take a long time to recover from his absence. People in SKIMS will have to come to terms with the fact that 'voids' have to be recognized and tolerated as 'voids,' even as life moves on. I will miss his ever-smiling face in the institute. He was always available for seeing my patient, unlock my 'hung phone' or provide advice on the new iPad software. For many of us, the lunch hour will never be the same. He will be missed by all but most by a select few of us with whom he shared his moments most. I salute this man from the core of my heart and wish him great success in his new chapter of life."

After his retirement, Dr. Khurshid chose to work at Florence Hospital, Srinagar, and works there as a consultant cardiologist. Dr. Khurshid is a great clinician, a composed human being—his dignity, behavior, and mannerism are something all of us should try to follow. His genius is something beyond us! He is truly called the "master of hearts"!

Dr. Mehraj-ud-din

Dr. Mehraj-ud-din was born in Srinagar and did his MBBS from Government Medical College, Srinagar, in 1967. Thereafter, he went to London, where he completed his DA (Diploma in Anesthesia) from the Royal College of Surgeons and Anesthetics, London, in 1974. He did his primary FFARCS at Royal College of Surgeons and Anesthetics, London, in 1975 and his Final FFARCS in 1977. He served as a locum consultant at General Hospital, Yarmouth, England, and as registrar of anesthesiology at Victoria Hospital, Blackpool, England. He returned to Kashmir and was appointed as lecturer, Anesthesiology, Government Medical College, Srinagar, in 1978. After a brief stint again in England in 1981, he was inducted into the faculty at Sher-i-Kashmir Institute of Medical Sciences (SKIMS), Srinagar, as an assistant professor in 1981. He was promoted as associate professor in 1984 and became a professor in the same year.

While in England, Dr. Mehraj-ud-din worked in different hospitals to gain experience in administering anesthesia to patients requiring surgical intervention in all the general specialities. He also was trained to administer anesthesia to patients requiring open-heart surgeries and neurosurgical procedures. He had been trained to manage patients in critical care and ICU settings as well.

After Dr. Mehraj-ud-din returned to Kashmir and got inducted into the faculty at Government Medical College, Srinagar, his job was to administer anesthesia to patients of general surgical specialities and for teaching assignments of undergraduates and postgraduates in anesthesia. He established, the Department of Anesthesiology at SKIMS which was a very advanced and sophisticated department. He joined the Department of anesthesiology in 1981 well before the hospital was commissioned in December 1982. He established the most modern operation theater with seven-bedded intensive care unit at SKIMS. In SKIMS, he was instrumental in administering anesthesia for open cardiac surgeries, for neurosurgical patients, and for the care of patients in intensive care units. Dr. Mehraj-ud-din has done exemplary work in tackling emergency cases during peak years of turmoil in Kashmir. He has spent sleepless nights and hectic days attending to critically ill patients during turmoil. When the entire valley was under curfew, at the risk of his own life, he would attend to his patients at odd hours. The health-care experts would say that the difference between SKIMS and other hospitals of the state during the peak years of turmoil has been Dr. Mehraj-ud-din. Dr. Mehraj-ud-din was the first anesthesiologist of Jammu and Kashmir State with a foreign fellowship who returned to serve his native place. With the start of postgraduation in anesthesia at SKIMS, the department developed a dynamic workforce to provide anesthesia services to not only the major hospitals of the state but also the peripheries and remotest areas of the state. Many trained anesthetists found good openings in reputed institutions in the country and abroad. Dr. Mehraj-ud-din has been a guide to many postgraduate students and an examiner at prestigious institutions of the country, including PGI Chandigarh, Lady Harding Medical College, Aligarh Muslim University, and Banaras Hindu University (BHU).

Dr. Mehraj-ud-din received a major assignment as director of SKIMS in 1995 and continued as the director SKIMS till 2003. As the director of SKIMS, he took charge of the SKIMS in very testing and difficult times. Dr. Mehraj-ud-din was one of the longest-serving directors of SKIMS and contributed toward subspecialization and superspecialization of the Department of Anesthesiology at SKIMS. New courses were started in many departments, and many departments like Cardiology and Radiotherapy were upgraded. Kidney transplantation was started at SKIMS under his leadership. He ensured that MD/MS/DM/MCh in many departments was recognized by the Medical Council of India even in times of troubling turmoil. One of the major achievements of Dr. Mehraj-ud-din was the takeover of Jehlum Valley Medical College (now SKIMS Medical College) and streamlining its functioning and seeking the recognition of the degree granted by it by the Medical Council of India. It was a frustrating scenario in which the fate of more than five hundred students was at stake. This decision led to the creation of another medical college in the state—adding up to fifty seats per year. The college now has an intake capacity of 125 students per year.

Dr. Mehraj-ud-din is a jovial human, an excellent teacher, and a skilled anesthetist. He is known for his ethics, punctuality, and standing up against the odds.

Dr. Mohammad Maqbool Lone

Cancer is one of the prime concerns of Kashmir's health-care system. All cancers are on the rise, and the existing facilities seem to be inadequate. There is a man in Radiation Oncology who spent sleepless nights to give to Kashmir its dedicated cancer centre in the premises of SKIMS. This committed gentleman named Dr. Mohammad Maqbool Lone, who served the Department of Radiation Oncology SKIMS as the professor and head of the department (July 2008 to 2020) was instrumental in doing this task and trying his best to help SKIMS tackle the huge burden of cancer cases. He worked to provide facilities for advanced diagnostics and management of cancer patients. Indeed a great accomplishment!

Dr. Mohammad Maqbool Lone was born in Krusan, the beautiful valley of Lolab, Kupwara, in 1958 to Mr. Abdul Khaliq Lone and Zeba Begum. He lost his greatest support, his father, when he was in primary school only. His mother worked hard on him to make him a responsible human being. Despite being illiterate, she guided him well and provided all the support to him. No wonder his mother has been his biggest inspiration in life. It was she who inculcated in him ethical and moral values to which he clung throughout his life. Dr. Maqbool received his initial education from Government Primary School, Krusan, Lolab, and Government High School, Maidanpora, Lolab. At the school, he was inspired greatly by Mr. Jawahar Lal (from Sogam), who was an exceptional teacher.

He inspired Dr. Maqbool to work hard and pursue medicine. Dr. Maqbool studied later at SP College, Srinagar. He was brilliant in academics and always topped the class from primary to matriculation. He did his MBBS from GMC Srinagar in 1983 and MD (radiotherapy) from SKIMS in 1991. He pursued a fellowship in radiation oncology from the Methodist Hospital, Houston, Texas, USA.

Dr. Maqbool was inducted into faculty at SKIMS in 1991 and all along served SKIMS, retiring as the professor and the head of Radiation Oncology in 2020. He worked in various responsible positions at SKIMS and has been a committed professional known for his honesty and upright character. He has been the chief warden of hostels at SKIMS and submitted a proposal to the then director of SKIMS for the construction of a hostel and a *Sarai* for the attendants from far-flung areas. This proposal was pursued by the administration at SKIMS, and the *Sarai* has been in operation for many years now and has greatly helped patients especially those from far-flung areas needing chemotherapy or radiotherapy. Dr. Maqbool has been the chairman of various committees including various inquiry committees at SKIMS. He did his work honestly and maintained decorum and ethical standards to the highest level while not compromising on truth and facts without favor or influence. He has contributed to academics by being the controller of examinations and subdean of academics. Dr. Maqbool has been a guide and a coguide to scores of PGs and postdoctoral fellows. He has published more than seventy-eight papers. He has been examiner (MD radiotherapy) at various universities in India. He organized a successful conference at Srinagar in 2009. To address the rising cases of cancer in Kashmir, he has conducted various awareness programs on TV, radio, in schools, and in public places in collaboration with the Cancer Society of Kashmir.

Dr. Maqbool's most notable contribution has been as regards the diagnosis and management of cancer, which is assuming the dimensions of an epidemic in Kashmir. As the nodal officer, Regional Cancer Centre (RCC), the already existing "Cancer Registry" maintained at the Department of Radiotherapy was reorganized to include all cancer patients managed by various other departments of SKIMS. The data analyzed has been an important source for various studies done by PGs, faculty, and other researchers, not only from SKIMS but from other universities as well. This data was submitted to the central government, and money was released for improving the infrastructure of the Cancer Center at SKIMS. This made procurement of some important equipment for the institute possible—for example, high-dose brachytherapy (for which patients had to go out of state for treatment) was procured. The efforts in RCC paved the way for establishing an important center at SKIMS . . . the State Cancer Institute. The establishment of the State Cancer Institute (SCI) was a marathon effort on part of Dr. Maqbool—something of which he is proud. He had to put in a lot of hard work and virtually had to beg people at SKIMS and had to convince the authorities at Health Ministry in Delhi to sanction this center for SKIMS. Thus, the erstwhile RCC was upgraded to SCI, and 120 crore rupees sanctioned for its construction and equipment. Major equipment proposed was high-end linear accelerator, 4D CT simulator, MRI, digital mammography, bone marrow transplant unit, theater equipment for surgical oncology, and Digital Radiography System (DRS).

The proposal for Hospital-Based Registry (HBCR) was submitted to NCDIR, and it was approved with Dr. Maqbool as the principal investigator. This helped SKIMS to further organize the cancer data because scientists, data entry operators, statisticians, and social workers were hired for the job. This project is still functional at SKIMS. The Population-Based Cancer Registry (PBCR) came up as an important project at

SKIMS as it was for the first time that the data from Kashmir was published and referred by the NCDIR subsidiary of the ICMR. This has given further recognition to SKIMS as an effective high-volume cancer center of North India. Twenty-three professionals including research scientists (doctors), statisticians, social workers, and data entry operators are currently working (against handsome salaries) in HBCR and PBCR producing authentic data on cancer burden in Kashmir. High-end equipment procured included Babhatron, a teletherapy machine linear accelerator, CT simulator, and HDR brachytherapy unit.

After his retirement from SKIMS, Dr. Maqbool was appointed as the professor of radiotherapy at GMC Baramulla, an upcoming medical college and hospital in North Kashmir. He is in the process of establishing a Comprehensive Cancer Center at GMC Baramulla. He has submitted a detailed proposal to the government for starting OPD services for patients suffering from various cancers. He has started Daycare Chemotherapy Services helping cancer patients of Baramulla, Kupwara, and Bandipora. Thus, patients do not have to move to Srinagar for cancer treatment. Dr. Maqbool is in the process of applying for an HBCR at GMC Baramulla. He is actively involved in cancer awareness and organized a breast cancer awareness event for the public at GMC Baramulla in 2021. He also conducted a successful webinar in collaboration with the British Kashmiri Medical association in 2022.

Dr. Maqbool is a champion of cancer awareness and a part of various groups working to help patients suffering from cancer. He is the vice chairman of the Cancer Society of Kashmir and the founder member and vice chairman of Kashmir Oncology Forum (KOF). He is a life member of many associations, including life member of Association of Radiation Oncologists of India (AROI), member of the Indian Cooperative Oncology Network (ICON), member of National Cancer Grid

(NCG), and member of Institute Ethical Committee (IEC), GMC Baramulla. He has been the secretary general of the Association of Radiation Oncologists of India (North Zone). At present, he is the vice chairman of the ethical committee of SKIMS Srinagar.

Dr. Maqbool is married to Shafiqa Rashid, who is a teacher and has supported Dr. Maqbool through the tough years of his life. His son is a software engineer working in Canada, and his daughter a doctor working at SMHS Hospital.

Dr. Mohammad Saleem Wani

Dr. Mohammad Saleem Wani is associated with a landmark in the history of medicine in Kashmir (i.e., renal transplantation). Dr. Saleem heads the only renal transplant unit operating in Jammu and Kashmir that has so far carried out more than four hundred successful kidney transplants (it has recently been started at GMC Jammu also). This landmark achievement has brought relief to hundreds of families and saved the state exchequer worth millions as the patients had to be referred outside for this procedure.

Dr. Saleem Wani was born in Dana Mazar, Safa Kadal, Srinagar, on February 7, 1962. He did his MBBS in 1986 from Government Medical College, Srinagar, and postgraduation in surgery from SKIMS Srinagar in 1993. Dr. Saleem was one of the few from Kashmir to get admission to MCh in urology from Banaras Hindu University, which he completed in 2001. He also subsequently did DNB in urology from the National Board of Examinations. He received the prestigious FICS in Urology from the International College of Surgeons, Chicago, Illinois, in 2006 and FACS in Urology from the American College of Surgeons in 2021.

Dr. Saleem was inducted into the faculty at SKIMS as an assistant professor in 2001, got promoted as associate professor and additional professor, and, eventually became the professor of urology in 2013. At present, he is the professor and head of the Department of Urology and heads the Kidney Transplant Unit at SKIMS.

Dr. Saleem has been instrumental in starting MCh course in urology at SKIMS. Currently, SKIMS is the only center in Jammu and Kashmir offering MCh Urology. Each year, four candidates join the training course through NEET (SS) Examination. Dr. Saleem is credited with starting minimally invasive laparoscopic surgeries and keyhole surgery like PCNL and lithotripsy at SKIMS. The urinary bladder and prostate cancer surgery have been a successful endeavor at SKIMS. Various complicated surgeries for urological cancers have been performed at SKIMS, which include the removal of cancerous urinary bladder and construction of a new bladder in young patients using small intestines. More than two hundred such cases have been performed so far at SKIMS.

Dr. Saleem has presented his work in UK, UAE, and US and bagged the Best Paper Award more than five times.. Under his able leadership, the infrastructure at the SKIMS Urology Department has been upgraded and mobile C-Arm and EMS lithoclast machines have been procured. Bio-polar TUR system from Olympus has been procured and made functional in 2019. HIVEC lab for bladder cancer was also started in 2019; 3D laparoscopy system Rubina and advanced urodynamic lab were also started.

Dr. Saleem has more than seventy publications in various national and international journals. He has been a guide to fourteen candidates for MS in general surgery and ten candidates who have done or are pursuing MCh in urology at SKIMS. He is the principal investigator for the ICMR project on invasive bladder cancer. Dr. Saleem has strived consistently to upgrade the Department of Urology to international standards and to relieve the distress of patients suffering from urology-related diseases. In recognition of his services in the field of medicine, he was conferred the State Award in 2013.

Dr. Saleem is working on Cadaver Transplant Program so that kidneys are transplanted from brain-dead patients to those who are desperately waiting for a donor. This is a mammoth project and requires social, political, and administrative efforts. Dr. Saleem has involved himself in awareness programs regarding kidney transplantation and motivating relatives and general public to donate kidneys to the patients in need so that the patients in need of a transplant are helped.

Dr. Muneer Khan

Dr. Muneer Khan is a dynamic surgeon who is one of the first Kashmiri doctors to specialize in urology and has become an inspiring figure for many young surgeons to pursue this challenging superspeciality. He is a doctor who, helped to provide urology services to the people of Kashmir at SMHS Hospital, Srinagar, and also build his own facility in the private setup.

Dr. Muneer Khan was born in Srinagar in 1951. He did his MBBS in 1976 from Government Medical College, Srinagar; MS in general surgery from Government Medical College, Srinagar, in 1981; and MCh in urology in 1987 from AIIMS New Delhi. He was greatly inspired by Prof. Mahmooda Khan during his training years. He was inducted into the faculty of Government Medical College, Srinagar, in 1983 as a lecturer in surgery, became an assistant professor in 1990, and was promoted as an associate professor in 1998. He retired as the professor and head of the Department of Surgery, GMC Srinagar.

Dr. Muneer Khan is considered to be a bold and talented surgeon who, in spite of working in a hospital setup that had no superspeciality urological services, introduced urology superspeciality in SMHS Hospital, Srinagar. He has been a pioneering urological surgeon who has excelled and left an indelible mark in providing urological services to the people of Kashmir Valley and beyond. Dr. Muneer Khan has many firsts to his credit. Dr. Khan holds the distinction of being the first laparo-surgeon of Jammu and Kashmir who started laparoscopic surgery in Kashmir in 1994. He holds a special interest in retroperitonoscopy. He also holds the distinction of starting ureteroscopy and PCN in Jammu and Kashmir in 1989 and 1990, respectively.

Dr. Muneer Khan is a member of a dozen national and international urological and surgical associations/societies. He holds executive membership in NZ-USI. He has served as president of NZ-ASI (from 2004 to 2005). He has delivered many invited guest lectures and presented his data and experience at various national and international conferences. He has been the invited faculty in various workshops conducted by AIIMS and NZ-International College of Surgeons, held at the prestigious AIIMS New Delhi and other institutes of repute. He has published his data related to laparoscopic surgery and urological surgery in many national and international journals, and many of his studies compare the conventional operative procedure with the laparoscopic procedures. Dr. Muneer Khan has organized more than six national and international conferences in Srinagar and managed to get the faculty from reputed institutions for deliberations and discussions in spite of challenging times in Srinagar.

Dr. Muneer Khan has been the external examiner for MS (general surgery) and MCh (urology) at various institutions across the country including AIIMS (New Delhi), Banaras Hindu University (BHU), Baba Farid University, and ASCOMS (Jammu).

Dr. Muneer Khan was nominated by Economic Times as an "Inspiring Urologist for 2022" and invited to participate in the conclave in New Delhi, India. For his exemplary services, he has received Bharat Shiromani Award and Rashtriya Gaurav Award.

Dr. Muneer Khan is the founder of Kidney Hospital, which is a superspeciality hospital mostly dedicated to the management of kidney diseases. With his efforts and commitment, it is a teaching hospital imparting superspecialist training in urology.

Dr. Murtaza Chishti

It was a proud moment for all Kashmiris when a Kashmiri cardiac surgeon, Dr. Murtaza Chishti, performed the maiden heart transplant surgery at Mahatma Gandhi Medical College and Hospital (MGMCH) in Jaipur, Rajasthan. Under the supervision of Dr. Chisti, a significant page in the medical history had been written at MGMCH. The doctor became an instantaneous hero and was praised by the media, and state's Chief Minister Vasundra Raje and Health Minister Rajendra Rathore extended thanks and applause to Dr. Chishti.

Talking over phone from Jaipur to the press in Srinagar, Dr. Chisti expressed his gratitude to his team and hospital administration for achieving the feat. "It couldn't have been possible for me to do it alone without the support of my wonderful team and administration. Indeed, it was a big achievement in my medical career," he said. Working as the chief consultant cardiac surgeon and director of organ transplantation in Mahatma Gandhi University of Medical Sciences and Technology, Dr. Chisti said the operation was performed in almost five hours. "Being the first operation of its kind, I had to do a lot of home work. I also went to United States for a month to get special training before performing the operation," he said.

Dr. Chisti said they were able to harvest a heart from an eighteen-year-old resident of Sanganer after he was declared brain dead following a road accident. "I am out of words for the generosity showed by the deceased family to agree to donate his organs. Their kindness saved people who otherwise had no hope of survival," he said. The family members of the deceased person donated two kidneys, liver, and heart to four different people.

This brilliant cardiac surgeon, was born in Baramulla, Kashmir. He completed his MBBS from the University of Kashmir in 1981, and in 1987, he was awarded MS in general surgery by the University of Kashmir. He did his MCh in cardiothoracic and vascular surgery from Sree Chitra Tirunal Institute for Medical Sciences and Technology, (SCTIMST) Trivandrum in 1990. SCTIMST is a center of excellence for cardiac and neurosciences, and the training in this institute helped him to become what he eventually became—an exceptional cardiac surgeon. After completing the degree, he later moved to United States. He was awarded a fellowship in cardiothoracic surgery from St. Mary's Hospital, USA; Royal Perth Hospital, Australia; and Prince Henry and Prince of Wales hospitals, Australia. Dr. Chisti served in Prince of Wales Hospital in Sydney, Australia, for three years.

Dr. Chishti joined Fortis Escorts Heart Institute, New Delhi, where he practiced for seven years honing his skills and perfecting his technique. He had his reasons for not returning to Kashmir after vigorous training. "I would have liked to serve in my own homeland rather than practice somewhere else but after I returned from US in 1993, Kashmir was in turmoil and there was no scope for growth," he said. He said the dearth of infrastructure and lack of political will from successive J&K governments compelled him to move outside Kashmir to pursue his career.

Dr. Murtaza is an expert in adult cardiac surgery and has performed more than six thousand complex cardiac surgeries. He was awarded a certificate of excellence from the Rajasthan Government for his outstanding contribution to organ transplantation. His works have been published in various reputed journals related to cardiology and thoracic surgery. His area of specialization includes total arterial revascularization, complex and reoperative coronary surgery, surgery of the aorta, mechanical circulatory support, and heart and lung transplantation.

Asked whether he would return to the valley, Dr. Chisti outrightly rejected the idea, saying there was no infrastructure for doctors in the state to prove their caliber. "I don't see any hope of my return. There is still a lot that needs to be done by the government to lure the doctors, who are practicing across India and abroad, back to the Valley," he added.

With more than thirty years of experience, Dr. Murtaza was associated with various hospitals of repute such as Sigma Heart Institute, Fortis Escorts Heart Institute, and Kota Heart Institute. He is one of the best cardiac surgeons in India and one of the most sought after as well.

The history of heart transplantation in India includes two alumni of GMC Srinagar, but, unfortunately, the facility is not available in Kashmir!

First successful heart transplant in India—state/union territory (UT) wise

S. no.	State/union territory	Name of the surgeon	Year
1	New Delhi	Dr. P. Venugopal	1994
2	Tamil Nadu	Dr. K. M. Cherian	1995
3	Kerala	Dr. Jose Chacko Periappuram	2003
4	Telangana	Dr. Alla Gopala Krishna Gokhale	2004
5	Karnataka	Dr. P. V. Rao	2008
6	Rajasthan	Dr. Murtaza Chishti	2015
7	Maharashtra	Dr. Anvay Mulay	2015
8	Andhra Pradesh	Dr. Alla Gopala Krishna Gokhale	2016
9	Madhya Pradesh	Dr. Anil Bhan	2018
10	West Bengal	Dr. K.M. Mandana and Dr. Tapas Raychaudhury	2018

Shroff S, Mittal K, Navin S. "Heart transplantation in India-—looking back as we celebrate 25 years of the transplant law." *Indian J Thorac Cardiovasc Surg.* 2020; 36 (Suppl 2): 215–223.

Dr. Muzaffar Ahmad

A primitive dispensary in the heart of Srinagar just adjacent to Dastgeer Sahib, Khanyar Srinagar bore a sick look. It looked more like a stable for horses than a health-care unit. I never thought in my childhood that it could ever be upgraded or transformed. However, it did undergo a transformation and got converted into a hospital that catered to the needs of people from Downtown Srinagar. The massive transformation of the allopathic dispensary of Khanyar, Srinagar, to a full-fledged Gousia Hospital happened under the eye of a visionary director, Health Services, Kashmir, Dr. Muzaffar Ahmad. It became a landmark health-care facility for Downtown Srinagar. Modern equipment along with surgical facilities including laparoscopic surgical facilities at Gousia Hospital were started for which doctors were deputed for training to AIIMS, New Delhi. In the very heart of Srinagar, another hospital—namely, Jawahar Lal Nehru Memorial Hospital (JLNM)—underwent transformation. Dr. Muzaffar Ahmad planned the construction and establishment of a five-hundred-bedded new JLNM Hospital with the state-of-the-art equipment and latest operative and laboratory services. Trained manpower and qualified doctors were posted to these newly created health-care facilities. He encouraged in-service doctors to undergo superspeciality training (i.e., DM and MCh courses) despite resistance from the administration. He increased the pool of superspecialists and provided them with all the facilities so that they could provide tertiary care services to the people. This move destressed the overburdened hospitals of Srinagar—namely, SMHS Hospital and SKIMS. The vision and zeal of Dr. Muzaffar brought about a transformation in the health-care scenario of Srinagar City. Dr. Muzaffar has received the prestigious Dr. BC Roy National Award from the honorable President of India for his outstanding work as a doctor and for his contribution to medical science at the state level and national level.

This energetic and able doctor was born in Zainakadal, Srinagar, in the family of famous Hakim Ahmadullah (Amma Hakim), who was a well-known Unani physician of his time and had two sons: one, Dr. Muzaffar's father, Qudratullah, educated for a degree in Unani medicine; and second son, Dr. Hafizullah, the famous chest physician who is profiled elsewhere in the book. Dr. Muzaffar Ahmad received his education from CMS Biscoe School, Srinagar, and after passing his twelfth class from SP College., he joined Government. Medical College Srinagar for MBBS. Later, he completed his post-graduation in internal medicine.

During his registrarship in internal medicine, Dr. Muzaffar Ahmad was assigned the job of looking after Chittaranjan Mobile Teaching-cum-Service Hospital initially as the medical officer and subsequently selected as assistant professor/deputy medical superintendent. He was promoted to the post of medical superintendent in the pay and status of a professor. Chittaranjan Mobile Teaching-cum-Service Hospital was an institution in itself for imparting training and teaching to medical students and interns in the rural setting. During his tenure in the mobile hospital, the diagnostic and operative facilities along with the bed strength of one hundred beds made this mobile hospital known nationally and globally. It was even recognized for the externship of medical students from UK, Australia, Japan, and other countries. This mobile hospital had the distinction of being a research institute of ICMR and WHO. Besides the Ministry of

Health, the Ministry of Women and Child Welfare earmarked it for training and research in the area of ICDS. Dr. Muzaffar utilized this scheme (mobile teaching hospital) to provide health-care services in the far-flung areas of Kashmir, covering the areas of Uri, Gurez, Tangdar, Chokibal, Sogam, Kupwara, and Handwara in Kashmir, far-flung areas of Ladakh, including Drass, Sankoo, Zanskar, Nobra, Kargil, etc., and in Jammu Division, Ramgarh, Baspur, Suchetgarh, Budhal, Thanamandi, Kapran, Gool Gulabgarh, etc., and other such backward areas where the services in the district and subdistrict hospitals were not available. The diagnostic services like various laboratory tests, radiological services, including X-ray, ultrasonography, GI endoscopy services, etc., were provided, and senior faculty from medical colleges of Srinagar/Jammu would provide services by rotation. A number of research papers were published based on the surveys conducted in the far-flung areas. Research on hypertension supported by ICMR was also carried out. The training was imparted to youngsters from remote areas in radiology (X-ray and USG). Laboratory technicians and pharmacists from these far-flung areas were also trained. Male and female multipurpose workers and sanitary supervisors were trained for the award of diploma in the field in which they were trained.

Dr. Muzaffar Ahmad has been a visionary and, as medical superintendent planned the construction of three-hundred-bedded GB Panth Cantonment General Hospital. Initially, it was planned as a general hospital but subsequently got converted into a pediatric hospital. This hospital started in Sonwar in the campus of the old Cantonment Hospital and became one of the major hospitals in the valley.

During the turmoil in the valley, Dr. Muzaffar Ahmad was assigned the responsibility to look after the health services of Kashmir as director of Health Services (January 1998). He held this post for more than twelve years and was elevated to the status of the director general. His posting in the Health Department was quite challenging as the health system in Kashmir had completely collapsed with non-functional peripheral hospitals. The district hospitals were providing only OPD services with the referral of patients to the major hospitals of Srinagar. The majority of health-care facilities worked from privately rented buildings. Dr. Muzaffar Ahmad planned a major infrastructural development in the Department of Health for Kashmir on modern lines. He was responsible for the construction of primary health centers with adequate accommodation and residential facilities for doctors, nurses, and paramedical staff. There was an expansion of subdistrict and community health centers for the first time in the history of Kashmir. The district hospital buildings with robust infrastructure were conceived, planned, and constructed during the tenure of Dr. Muzaffar Ahmad. This revolutionized the Department of Health and revived the peripheral health-care setup. The district hospitals that hardly had seventy beds were converted into four-hundred-bedded hospitals. These hospitals were constructed in Baramulla, Anantnag, and other districts. It may be worth mentioning that it was his vision that facilitated the starting of medical colleges in Baramulla, Anantnag, and Handwara. He had planned ahead of their conversion into medical colleges. The latest equipment including CT scan machines were procured for the district and some subdistrict hospitals. Dialysis facilities were made available at the district level for which he encouraged and deputed postgraduate doctors for DM in nephrology and other specialties outside the state.

For improving maternity and child-care services in the valley, Maternity and Child Hospitals at Anantnag and Sopore were established, and advanced maternity care services at Wayel, Lar, and other distant places were also provided. Besides the infrastructure buildup, essential equipment for diagnostic and operative facilities were provided. Intensive care units for neonates at the district level were established. Ultrasonography facilities were provided even at the primary health centers in rural areas, and doctors were imparted short-term training to help deal with the emergencies and to decrease dependence on tertiary-level hospitals of Srinagar. Equipment for advanced anesthesia services in the newly constructed hospitals and latest machines for critical care were provided. Free cataract surgery using the technique of phacoemulsification was introduced in the mobile eye unit of the directorate. This was started before it started in the medical colleges of the state.

Regional Institute of Health at Dhobiwan, Tangmarg, was also the brainchild of Dr. Muzaffar Ahmad. This training institute for capacity development of medical officers, paramedical, and other staff was rated as one of the best training centers in India with facilities of IT, excellent library facility, along with residential facilities for resource persons who would come for imparting training to the staff working in the health department. WHO established a collaborative center for the surveillance of noncommunicable diseases, and a large number of periodicals and publications were published in addition to a quarterly journal. Training on BCLS and ACLS was initiated in this institute for doctors and other staff with the help of doctors and nurses from California who would provide the requisite training.

To overcome the shortage of anesthetists and obstetricians in the Health Department, 150 in-service doctors were deputed for undergoing diploma in anesthesia and gyne-obstetrics to SKIMS and GMC Srinagar outside the preview of the Board of Professional Exams (BOPPEE). This initiative provided manpower in all the district and subdistrict hospitals.

Dr. Muzaffar was instrumental in starting the College of Nursing and schools for paramedical training in the Health Department. It was during his time as the director of health that emergency medical services were conceived, and he provided more than 450 ambulances and 120 supervisory vehicles to various health-care institutions.

Dr. Muzaffar Ahmad has authored six books on public health, medical emergencies and disasters, and has more than 140 publications in national and international journals. He had the distinction of being a member of the Executive Committee, chairman of Teachers' Qualification Committee, and chairman of Ethics Committee of the Medical Council of India. He has worked as the vice president of the National Board of Examination, where his contribution to the formulation of syllabi for various streams and starting of DNB "Family Medicine" and DNB in other streams has been appreciated. He has been a member of the Drug Technical Advisory Group, Government of India. He has been a member of national programs of RNTCP (TB)/Leprosy besides being a member of the National Taskforce on HIV/AIDS and NRHM. He is a visiting professor and expert in the Ministry of Health, Malaysia; Fujita Gakuen University, Japan; GW University, USA; and many other internationally reputed universities.

Dr. Muzaffar, after his superannuation, joined the WHO as a senior consultant for emergencies and humanitarian crises where he contributed to humanitarian response for emergencies in South Asian countries. He was selected as a member of the National Disaster Management Authority of India (NDMA) with the status of union minister of state under the chairmanship of the honorable prime minister. As a member of NDMA at the national level, he looked after public health emergencies, medical preparedness for mass casualty management, chemical industrial disaster management, community-based disaster management, NGOs coordination, school and hospital safety, and mitigation at the national level. He contributed to the formulation of more than eight national guidelines on the important subjects of disaster management (i.e., the role of NGOs in disaster management, community-based disaster management, emergency management exercises, retrofitting, school safety, hospital safety, preparedness for pandemic beyond health, national action plan for chemical safety, etc). For the first time in India, he planned and conducted emergency management exercises in various states in collaboration with experts from the USA and the UN agencies besides capacity development workshops, programs, simulation exercises, and training on mass casualty management and public health emergencies.

Dr. Muzaffar is credited for planning and launching of “National School Safety Project” in India and also the formulation of guidelines for minimal initial service packages for maternal care during disasters in partnership with UNFPA. Dr. Muzaffar Ahmad also worked on guidelines for chemical terrorism, biological disasters, biological terrorism, and management of dead during disasters.

In recognition of his contribution to the development of emergency and disaster medicine in India, he was awarded a fellowship by the Royal College of Physicians of London (FRCP London). For starting a faculty development program under the UK-India collaboration project, he was awarded the Fellowship by the Royal College of Physicians Edinburgh and also by the Royal College of Physicians and Surgeons of Glasgow. He is a fellow of the National Academy of Medical Sciences of India (FAMS) and a fellow of the American College of Physicians. He is the recipient of many medals and awards for his distinguished services. He received Sriram Award for the best publication by the National Academy of Medical Sciences. He is the recipient of Dr. R. V. Rajan Oration Award in 2010. He was awarded for his outstanding service by the National Academy of Medical Sciences, awarded for the service for humanity in the earthquake (2005) by Indian Institute of Public Administration, and received Dr. M. D. Sharma Award for his contribution in public health by the Indian Association of Epidemiology.

He also received the Lifetime Achievement Award from Indo-Global Health International Society in 2014 and received the Disaster Risk Reduction Excellence Award in 2022..

Dr. Muzaffar is presently working on the projects of public health emergency management, emergency and disaster medicine, the impact of climate change on health with special reference to the impact of the "heat wave in metro cities of India" and upon the initiatives for reducing the impact of air pollution. He is working on competency/skill-based medical education and project formulations, management, monitoring, and evaluation besides capacity building and training of professionals in public health emergencies, mass casualty management, and noncommunicable diseases.

Dr. Muzaffar is the national advisor of UNICEF helping states in the development of plans and building up capacity for public health emergency management in coordination with CDC Atlanta, USA, and other national and international agencies. He is on the board of many prestigious universities and bodies including Public Health Foundation of India. He has the distinction of being the leading resource person/specialist in the area of public health emergency management at the national and global level.

Dr. Nisar Ahmad Chowdri

In the times of conflict and chaos at SKIMS, a few people held the fort and continued their work with honesty, dignity, and grace. They held together the academics that was in shreds, the innovation that was forgotten, and worked hard with the intent to help and cure the patients. One such name in surgery synonymous with gentle mannerism and competence is Dr. Nisar Chowdri, who has been a pillar of SKIMS surgery. He fitted the role that was granted to him and in the absence of staff worked wherever he was asked to work.

Dr. Nisar was born in Srinagar and did his MBBS from GMC Srinagar. He was bright and hardworking and bagged the first position in anatomy and passed ENT with honors. He did his MS in surgery from SKIMS in 1988. He received fellowship from various renowned associations, including the Associations of Surgeons of India (FAIS), the International College of Surgeons (FICS), the Association of Colon and Rectal Surgeons of India (FACRSI), the Association of Minimal Access Surgeons of India (FMAS), and the fellowship from the American College of Surgeons (FACS). Dr. Chowdri holds important portfolios/ prestigious executive posts in these associations and is well-known for his surgical expertise and contribution to academics.

Dr. Nisar Chowdri is a keen researcher, and two of his research articles were named among the one hundred best papers from India in the past decade (Indian Surgical Literature: The Top 100 Papers, *IJS* 68 (1); 11–16, January–February 2006).

With these articles, SKIMS got a place among the five best institutions of the country. He has more than ninety research papers published in various reputed national and international journals. His research papers have been published in high-impact journals (i.e., *British and American Journal of Plastic Surgery, Annals of Plastic Surgery, Burns, International Journal of Trauma, World Journal of Surgery, Human Genomics, BMC Cancer, World Journal of Surgery*, and *Postgraduate Medical Journal*).

Many of Dr. Chowdri's papers received the Best Paper Award at various national and international conferences. His paper titled "Intra and Post-Operative Intra-Lesional Corticosteroid Therapy for Hypertrophic Scars and Keloids" was awarded the best paper in the Fifty-Seventh Annual Conference of the Association of Surgeons of India, 1997. Another paper titled "Primary Closure of Common Bile Duct over Endo-Nasobiliary Drainage Tube," presented at the Twenty-Fourth Annual Conference of Northern Chapter of Association of Surgeons of India at SKICC, Srinagar, June 3–5, 2004, received the Best Paper Award, and his paper on "Stapled Haemorrhoidectomy," presented at the Asian Federation of Coloproctology in September 2009, Goa, India, also fetched him the Best Paper Award. Dr. Nisar has coauthored more than eight books and written many book chapters. His latest book, titled *Benign Anorectal Disorders: A Guide to Diagnosis and Management*, has been published by Springer in 2016. Dr. Nisar Chowdri innovated some new surgical procedures that have been highly appreciated and accepted at national and international levels, including

- Z-lengthening and gastrocnemius muscle flap for severe postburn contractures of the knee (*International Journal of Trauma*);

- intralesional corticosteroid therapy for childhood cutaneous hemangiomas (*Annals of Plastic Surgery*);
- closure of CBD over ENBD tubes (*World Journal of Surgery*);
- tube ileostomy as an alternative to a conventional ileostomy and pouch intubation for ileal pouch perianal fistula (*Journal of Colorectal Diseases*).

Dr. Nisar introduced the modern surgical stapling technique and "stapled pouch surgery" for the first time in the state. Dr. Nisar has delivered more than sixty talks/lectures, including invited guest lectures and orations at various national and international conferences. He has been an organizer and a co-organizer of many national and international conferences.

After working extensively in plastic surgery and general surgery and contributing immensely to the academics and research there, Dr. Nisar established a new superspeciality, Department of Colorectal Surgery in SKIMS. It is running a two-year fellowship course in colorectal surgery, and the department is set to start MCh. SKIMS will be among the first few institutes in India to have this course..

Dr. Nisar has guided and helped many budding surgeons to fulfil their dream of becoming exceptional surgeons. He is a calm, patient, and extremely dedicated surgeon. He does things in his own style, meticulously, always aiming perfection. He is a teacher of skills to the youngsters, never losing his calm in the worst scenario. His colleague and his taught, Dr. Fazal, the professor of surgery at SKIMS, has the following to say about him: "I have known Prof. Nisar A. Chowdri since 1991 when he was appointed as a faculty in the department of Plastic Surgery. He was appointed as a faculty member at a very young age. He had the charisma of being a great academician, a great researcher and a system builder. All admired his commitment and dedication to the system as a wonderful teacher. I was a

Junior Resident at SKIMS in 1991 and always respected him as a great teacher. When I was recruited into the SKIMS faculty in 2001—our bond strengthened as we worked together in General Surgery. We travelled together, worked together towards our goal of establishing a State Chapter of ASI and the Division of Colorectal Surgery at SKIMS. The Colorectal Surgery division has become a brand in the whole country because of the quality work performed and high-impact research publications from the department. He gives the youngsters a space to grow and is lovable because of his down-to-earth nature. His commitment and sincerity has earned him the place of the 'President Association of Colorectal surgeons of India.'"

Dr. Nisar Chowdri is a brilliant and innovative surgeon. He has served SKIMS unselfishly without craving for a position. His ever-smiling face and his helping attitude have made him a darling of SKIMS.

Dr. Nisar Ahmad Tramboo

Silently pursuing his dream of making SKIMS Cardiology as one of the best cardiac centers of India, Dr. Nisar has guided his team to accomplish this dream. He has braved difficulties, fought the odds, and achieved his goal. Through the years of turmoil, he has waded through harsh currents supporting his colleagues to achieve the best for SKIMS.

Dr. Nisar has been an asset to the valley in general and SKIMS in particular. It takes determination and iron will to deliver good consistently in a land of inconsistencies. Born in Baramulla in 1958 to Mr. Ghulam Hassan Tramboo, Dr. Nisar received his initial education at St. Joseph's School, Baramulla, and Government Higher Secondary School, Baramulla. Dr. Nisar pursued his dream of becoming a doctor in 1981 from Government Medical College, Srinagar. He did his MD in general medicine from Government Medical College, Srinagar, in 1986 and DM in cardiology from PGI Chandigarh in 1991. Dr. Nisar was inspired by his teachers, especially Professor Mehraj-ud-din, who, according to him, handpicked him from the crowd and pushed him to pursue cardiology. He was appointed as assistant professor in cardiology at SKIMS in 1993, promoted as associate professor in 1997, and became professor of cardiology in 2010. He headed the Department of Cardiology at SKIMS from 2014 to 2020.

An astute clinician and interventionist, Dr. Nisar is known for his academic excellence. I remember his patience and ability to moderate mortality meets for "one full year" without break at SKIMS. His ability to dissect cases and his focus on "introspection" had no match. His skillful cross-examination of different cases presented to him unveiled a "clinical wizard" in him.

Dr. Nisar has more than thirty publications in national and international journals and has guided postgraduates and postdoctorals in general medicine and cardiology. He has published some of his research papers in the *American Journal of Cardiology* and the *American Journal of Medicine*. Dr. Imran Hafeez, his student and a junior colleague, has been greatly inspired by Dr. Nisar and has the following to say about Dr. Nisar: "Dr. Nisar has been there as a pillar for his colleagues and scholars alike, inspiring newcomers like me right from the first day of our endeavors at the prestigious institution of SKIMS. Being my research guide and teacher since 2005 he has been thoroughly professional in his attitude towards clinical medicine and Cardiology alike. I always look towards him as an honest person, upright professional, sincere clinician and a true guide. Intervention was his passion and he worked up to the hilt so that the SKIMS cardiology can compete with other institutes of national repute. And he has greatly succeeded in his endeavors. He has performed a significant role in improving the interventional cardiac care at SKIMS and taking our department to a new high. I pay gratitude to his steadfastness and wish him best of luck for his future endeavors. I am pretty sure that wherever he works he is going to excel and create a team that can compete at national and international levels." Dr. Nisar has transformed the Department of Cardiology, SKIMS, and was instrumental in getting the postdoctoral course (DM cardiology) recognized by MCI. SKIMS Cardiology is one of the best-performing cardiac centers in government setup, and Dr. Nisar may be to a large extent credited for it.

Dr. Nisar always wanted to serve his own people and wanted to establish a state-of-the-art cardiology team at SKIMS, which he believes he achieved. He believes the best colleagues for him have been all those who worked with him tirelessly to save lives and to build the Department of Cardiology at SKIMS. This includes his fellow faculty members, technicians, helpers, and sanitary aids. All these, according to Dr. Nisar, were instrumental in delivering the best treatment to the patients. Dr. Nisar practices cardiology in Srinagar and lives with his wife and three daughters in Srinagar.

Dr. Omar Javed Shah

One of the versatile surgeons who founded a department and created facilities for curative and palliative surgical management of patients with hepatobiliary and pancreatic diseases, Dr. Omar has done a remarkable job in putting the valley of Kashmir onto the global map as a region where treatment for such diseases is readily available. Innovation, defined as the introduction of something new, whether an idea method or a device, is synonymous with Dr. Shah. He is well known for developing new techniques and updating the old ones so as to give maximum benefit to the patients. The procedures developed and popularized by him are known for their speed and safety. He is a creative surgeon, an energetic administrator, and an active researcher. Born in Srinagar to Ghulam Nabi Shah and Rasheeda Begum on September 21, 1959, Dr. Omar is third among four children. Nurtured by his parents and surrounded by love, he grew up to enjoy a happy childhood with his siblings, devoting himself to his studies and indulging in sports, especially cricket.

After completing his MBBS from Government Medical College, Srinagar, in 1982 and MS in general surgery from Sher-i-Kashmir Institute of Medical Sciences Srinagar in 1988, he did his senior residency and registrarship in SKIMS and GMC, respectively. This done, Dr. Omar was recruited as a lecturer in the Department of Surgery, Government Medical College, Srinagar, and worked there from 1992 to 1994. After his initial stint as a consultant surgeon in GMC, he was selected as an assistant professor in the Department of Surgery, SKIMS, in 1994. He believes that he owes a lot to his teachers, especially Prof. H. U. Zargar, Prof. Mehmooda Khan, Prof. Mir Nazir, and Prof. Nazir A. Wani, and attributes much of his success in hepatobiliary surgery to his guide and mentor, Prof. N. A. Wani. The year 2005 saw him being made the founder head and professor of surgical gastroenterology at SKIMS.

Dr. Omar was instrumental in laying the foundations of the rare superspeciality of surgical gastroenterology at SKIMS. This was the first such department in Jammu and Kashmir and fifth in North India. Much acclaimed as a hepatobiliary and pancreatic surgeon, he is a fellow of the International College of Surgeons (FICS) and also a fellow of the Association of Indian Surgeons (FAIS). For his outstanding contribution to the field of surgery in the region, he was honored with the prestigious Fellowship of the Royal College of Surgeons Edinburgh (FRCS) in 2020.

Dr. Omar has served in various prestigious positions in SKIMS—as dean of medical faculty (January 10, 2018–December 31, 2021), as the director and ex-officio-secretary to J&K Government (January 11, 2018–October 9, 2019), SKIMS. Pertinent to mention: he has to his credit 112 research papers published in outstanding international and national journals.

Observing the difficulties faced by families of patients needing surgical treatment for portal hypertension, Dr. Omar developed a special interest in this field and is credited with introducing an innovative technique of splenorenal shunt (Omar's technique). This technique simplified the intricacies of the technically demanding and cumbersome "central splenorenal shunt," which translated into positive ergonomics. The mean operative time, as well as the mean blood loss, were grossly reduced, and the long-term results were encouraging. Thus, SKIMS became a focal point in the region for patients needing such treatment. The technique is a modification of Linton's shunt and Cooley's shunt, and the credit for bringing it into the global limelight goes to the legendary professor Denton Cooley. This innovative approach has been critically acclaimed in the famous textbook titled *Mastery of Surgery* by Joseph Fischer and is now a widely used technique in parts of South America, the Middle East, and some parts of Russia. ("A Simplified Technique of Performing Splenorenal Shunt (Omar's Technique)," *Texas Heart Inst J.* 2005: 32 (4): 549–554).

Besides portal hypertension, Dr. Omar developed a keen interest in the diseases affecting pancreas. He is credited with getting SKIMS Pancreatic Surgery at par with any center of excellence worldwide by making SKIMS a high-volume center for such surgery with a remarkable rate of success. He also introduced a new technique of pancreaticoduodenectomy (PD) and compared its results with the classical Whipple procedure. The results were heartening; significant differences were observed in terms of reduced operative time, operative blood loss, and the need for intraoperative blood transfusion. This technique allows fast, safe, and virtually bloodless dissection for exposure of the superior mesenteric and portal veins during the early steps of PD, which is normally a difficult and tedious procedure carrying an inherent risk of major venous injury leading to substantial blood loss. Moreover, with the lucid exposure and vascular control provided by the technique, vascular resections and reconstruction became very easy. This approach found international recognition and was accepted as one of the six methods for performing pancreaticoduodenectomy (*British Journal of Surgery*, 2018; 105: 628–636; *Annals of Surgery* 2019; 270 (5): 738–746). This innovation found favor with John Cameroon, the renowned pancreatic surgeon. With its application over time, hundreds of patients needing pancreatic surgery got benefited, and SKIMS gained international repute. In a nutshell, Dr. Omar brought successful pancreatic surgery within the reach of common masses.

Another feather to his cap was the introduction of a new technique for palliative surgical decompression of an obstructed common bile duct, the hepaticocholecystoduodenostomy (HCD), which was compared with the established Roux-en-Y choledochojejunostomy for the decompression of the biliary tract. This study was published in *Ann Saudi Med.*, 2009 September–October; 29 (5): 383–387 ("An Innovative Original Technique"). The technique in comparison is far more effective, patient-friendly, and less expensive. The ease with which this procedure can be performed translates into better post-operative outcome. Thus this procedure became popular among surgeons worldwide (*Pancreatic Cancer: The Role of Bypass Procedures,* in the book *Pancreatic Cancer, Cystic Neoplasms and Endocrine Tumors.* Editor: Hans G. Beger, A. Nakao, J. P. Neptolems, Shu Y. P., Michael G. Sarr, pp. 83–93, Wiley Blackwell, 2015).

With over 102 citations, an innovative approach proposed by Dr. Omar and his team revolutionized the management of Mirizzi syndrome, an affliction much more prevalent because of the abundance of gallstone disease, in Kashmir Valley and South-Asian countries. This new breakthrough got published and helped in laying the guidelines for the management of this complex disease ("Management of Mirizzi Syndrome: A New Surgical Approach," *Australian and New Zealand Journal of Surgery* 2001; 71: 423–427).

Dr. Omar has been quoted in major textbooks of medicine including *Harrison's Principles of Internal Medicine, Bailey and Love Surgery*, and various gastrointestinal surgery books. Kangri cancer, a condition peculiar to Kashmir, was brought to the international arena and published in the twenty-third edition of *Bailey and Love* by a photo courtesy of Dr. Omar (pp. 148). Omar's modification of Linton's shunt finds a mention in *Fischer's Mastery of Surgery* 5th *Edition*, pp. 1366. The occurrence of the rare anomaly of preduodenal portal vein and its implication in liver transplantation finds a mention in the third edition of the *Textbook of liver transplantation* by Drs. Busuttil and Klintmalm.

Dr. Omar has contributed photographs of the ectopic pancreas, annular pancreas, and mucocele appendix in "Essential Surgical Practice" (*Higher Surgical Training in General Surgery* in the 5th edition, pp. 801, 802, and 932). In *Blumgart's Surgery of the Liver, Biliary Tract and Pancreas*, 5th Edition (pp. 1029, 1031, and 1034), his contribution to biliary ascariasis like the post-cholecystectomy biliary ascariasis, postoperative biliary ascariasis, and biliary ascariasis in pregnancy has been referred. He is credited with reporting the first case of anterior splenic vein in humans. A classical picture depicting a parotid tumor has been preserved in the illustrative section of the Royal College of Surgeons of England Library. Dr. Omar is on the editorial board of many reputed international journals, including the *World Journal of Gastrointestinal Surgery* and *Case Reports Hepatology*, and also serves as an editor of the *International Journal of Hepatobiliary and Pancreatic Diseases* (IJHPD) and is a reviewer for numerous international journals.

Dr. Omar has organized more than two-dozen conferences in SKIMS on GI surgery and pancreatic, liver, and bile duct diseases. As dean and director of SKIMS, he was instrumental in starting many PG and postdoctoral courses and getting recognition for many courses from MCI (now NMC). To effectively monitor the starting of various courses by SKIMS University and to seek their recognition from NMC, an MCI/NMC cell was created for smoothening the entire process and putting all NMC-related affairs under a single roof.

Dr. Omar is a considerate and humble human who derives a lot of pleasure in helping others, especially the sick and helpless. He lives with his wife, two children, and a grandchild in Srinagar. He is actively involved with his patients at his private clinic, 'The Surgeons'. He wishes SKIMS is able to meet health-care challenges and transforms into a world leader in the next decade. For that goal to achieve it needs to transform medical education and expand research.

Dr. Parvaiz Ahmad Koul

If you are looking for the perfect combination of clinical acumen, research, and academics in a Kashmiri doctor, Dr. Parvaiz Koul leads the group as he excels in all three fields. People like me trying to put his massive CV in words for the book land up in hung computers and out-of-ink printers because neither computers can bear the load nor can the printers print the massive work that Dr. Parvaiz Koul has been doing as an internist, a pulmonologist, a geriatrician, and an infectious disease specialist in Kashmir.

Dr. Parvaiz Koul was born in Downtown Srinagar on March 9, 1959. He received his initial education from Srinagar and has been exceptionally brilliant in his studies. He did his MBBS in 1984 from Government Medical College, Srinagar, and MD in internal medicine from SKIMS in 1988 (first batch). He was a registrar in medicine at SKIMS till May 1991 and was inducted into the faculty at SKIMS as an assistant professor of internal and pulmonary medicine in 1991. After serial promotions as associate and additional professor, he became professor and head of Internal and Pulmonary Medicine in 2008. It is true that institutions outlast individuals, and individuals who work in the institutions do not lose—but their work survives and flourishes through the institution that they work on. However, there is a "dependency factor" operable for many individuals who work tirelessly for an institution and get associated with its every milestone—Dr. Parvaiz Koul is one such individual, and SKIMS is one such institution!

Dr. Parvaiz Koul is considered to be the backbone of SKIMS from its founding years, through its years of glory, gloom, and struggle. He has always been there either at the front pulling the cart, in the middle stabilizing it, or at the back cushioning it. It is difficult to narrate what Dr. Parvaiz Koul is to SKIMS as we are yet to witness an era where the "Parvaiz factor" is not there.

Dr. Parvaiz Koul has traveled far and wide learning, teaching, and gaining expertise in the areas that needed attention at SKIMS. Dr. Parvaiz Koul received ACP Fellowship in pulmonary medicine in 2005 and worked as a fellow at Northshore-Long Island Jewish health system in New York, USA. He was trained in pulmonary, critical care, and sleep medicine with a focus on sleep medicine at the LIJ Health System Sleep Center. His training in sleep medicine helped him to set up a "Sleep Lab" at SKIMS. He is a fellow of the American College of Chest Physicians (2010) and a fellow of the Royal College of Physicians, London, United Kingdom (2012).

Dr. Parvaiz Koul diversified the Department of Internal Medicine at SKIMS and created sub-specialities of geriatrics, infectious diseases, rheumatology, besides expanding pulmonary medicine and introducing emergency medicine as a separate speciality. Dr. Parvaiz Koul has been involved in varied activities related to the development, expansion, and research promotion at SKIMS. His role has shifted from time to time, but his goal has remained the same—to achieve the best for SKIMS. He has been a member of various committees, including the Purchase Committee, Dean's Committee, Library Committee, and Selection Committee—every time stretching himself to work toward creating something new and something better for SKIMS. As a coordinator for the purchase of equipment at SKIMS (2011–2016), he was instrumental in updating and expanding the infrastructure of almost all the departments and laboratories at SKIMS (which had been affected by the decade-long turmoil)—getting them the best equipment and bringing them at par with the best institutions of the country. He has been the chief of "Human Resource Development" (2012–2020) at SKIMS and has analyzed and evaluated the need versus the demand aspects of human resources at SKIMS—a novel initiative unheard of in any other health-care institution of Jammu and Kashmir. He has been the registrar of academics, SKIMS, constantly improving the academic environment and updating teaching programs to bring them in line with the best institutions of the country. He has been the chief of Clinical Research, SKIMS (2014–2020), and has managed to get grants for innumerable research projects from national and international grant agencies.

Dr. Parvaiz Koul is an acclaimed academician and has been an external examiner for MBBS, MD (internal medicine, pulmonary medicine), and PhD in various reputed institutions/universities of India, including Maulana Azad Medical College-New Delhi, University of Rajasthan, University of Gujarat, and the prestigious All India Institute of Medical Sciences, New Delhi. He has been an accreditation and infrastructural inspector for the DNB program of various institutions. He has mentored more than fifty postgraduates in MD medicine and allied specialities as a supervisor or cosupervisor.

Dr. Parvaiz Koul has been the chairman of the State Task Force/Core Committee, RNTCP Program, J&K (2014–2021), and nodal officer, HIV/AIDS, JK SACS (2005–2021). He is the governing body member of the Indian Chest Society and editor in chief, *Lung India* (official organ of the Indian Chest Society). Besides being a member of more than two dozen national and international organizations and associations, he is the governing body member of the Indian Society for Bronchology (Joint Secretary 2016–2019) and the Geriatric Society of India. He has been instrumental in launching JK chapter of many national organizations and is the chairperson of the Indian Chest Society, Indian Society for Critical Care, and general secretary of Association of Physicians of India (since 2004).

Dr. Parvaiz Koul has presented his phenomenal work on influenza, respiratory infections, hydatid disease, interstitial lung disease, COPD, etc. at various international conferences in the USA, Germany, UK, Indonesia, Saudi Arabia, Dubai, Canada, and Australia. He has participated in hundreds of national-level conferences, symposia, and seminars held in various parts of the country as a guest faculty (including in the virtual mode). With an RG score of 53.95, an H-index (Researchgate) of 68, and 72,051 citations, Dr. Parvaiz Koul is one of the highest-cited researchers of India. He is listed in Stanford University's database of the top 2 percent of global researchers (2020), and Elseveir's top 2 percent of global researchers, (2021). He has been a part of the "hypoxia research on HIF" that was awarded the Nobel Prize for Medicine in 2019. He has more than three hundred research publications indexed in PubMed and is the coauthor on one of the four papers that won the prize (Nature Genetics 2014). He has been a recipient of many awards including SAMA Oration Award at NAPCON in 2018; the Distinguished Services Award for Influenza Vaccination, Influenza Foundation of India, APACI, GSI 2016; Bill and Melinda Gates Award for ICID 2016 at Hyderabad; the Honor Scroll, Geriatric Society of India for contribution to the development of Geriatric Society of India; Pfizer Human Initiative 2004 Award (international fellowship); etc. He is a peer reviewer for more than two dozen international journals, including *BMJ* and *Lancet*.

In collaboration with Dr. Stephen Walsh, Royal Free Hospital (UK), Dr. Parvaiz Koul received a grant of £76753 for the study of "Renal Tubular Acidosis in Kashmir and Its Possible Link with Malaria Resistance" from the St. Peter Trust for Kidney, Bladder and Prostate Research. Dr. Parvaiz had a collaborative partnership with Chest Research Foundation, Pune, India, for conducting a study on peak flows in Indian Adults (PERFORM study). He has been the PI (principal investigator) for the Burden of Lung Disease BOLD study in collaboration with Imperial College, London. He has been PI for a multicentric international study on COPD funded by Wellcome Trust, UK. He also is the PI for the ILD registry of India.

Dr. Parvaiz has led the research on the study of influenza in Kashmir in collaboration with national and international agencies focusing on surveillance and pattern of influenza in Kashmir under the aegis of the India Influenza Program and CDC, USA. As the PI for the influenza surveillance in Srinagar, Dr. Parvaiz Koul established a network of data-generating labs that contributed to the description of influenza in India and documented the patterns of circulation of influenza in the country, which, despite being in the northern hemisphere geographically, exhibited a southern hemispherical pattern of influenza circulation. This documentation was a revealing experience and was the basis for the changed recommendation for vaccine timing in India. As a principal investigator/lead researcher, Global Influenza Hospital Surveillance Network (GIHSN), SKIMS, became the only India site of the GIHSN network. Dr. Parvaiz and his team were responsible for contributing to the GIHSN network data on influenza in hospitalized patients, and the data generated thereof was responsible for many high-impact publications from the collaboration. For his tremendous work and contribution to influenza studies, Dr. Parvaiz Koul has held many prestigious positions at the global level related to influenza study groups, which include the vice chair, MENA-ISN Influenza Stakeholders Network, and collaborator, Global Burden of Disease, Institute of Health Metrics and Evaluation, USA. He has also been the vice chairman of the Middle East North Africa Influenza Stake Holders Network (2021). Dr. Parvaiz Koul has many collaborative research projects with the

University of Utah, Salt Lake City, USA. He has done studies on the genomic links of Kashmiris and broken the myth that Kashmiris and Jews have a genetic link.

Dr. Parvaiz Koul has the honor of publishing in *Nature*, *Nature Medicine*, and *Nature Genetics* and is the only medical professional from Kashmir with such an honor. He has the highest number of publications for any medical professional in the country. Dr. Parvaiz Koul reached the pinnacle of his career as he was chosen for the post of director at SKIMS, competing for it at the national level with the best in the field. He is shouldering this huge responsibility since January 2022, and the expectations about reclaiming the glory of SKIMS are brightened.

When asked about his contributions to the field of medicine, Dr. Parvaiz Koul says, “I am a doctor researcher and did my bit, I want youngsters to outdo and outperform me.” He further says, “My objective is to motivate youngsters so that besides being good clinicians they develop an interest in clinical research. I hope the milieu of research improves in the developing world so that our research is viewed as credibly as from the developed world.”

It is almost an impossible task to put the profile of Dr. Parvaiz Koul in these words—a book on him wouldn’t do justice either. However, for inspiration and stimulation, his profile links may help.

Profile links:

https://www.researchgate.net/profile/Parvaiz_Koul
https://scholar.google.com/citations?user=Ukl8X1cAAAAJ&hl=en&oi=ao.

Dr. Shabir Iqbal

The high incidence of cleft lip and palate anomaly in Kashmir is a problem of great magnitude. It leaves families devastated. These children suffer from recurrent infections and feeding difficulties. Later on in life, children get issues related to speech and appearance. Parents and children go through continuous trauma as surgery is undertaken in multiple stages. Ask the parents about the trauma they go through and your heart will ache.

In September 2012, Kashmir was in news for the wrong reason. A child with a cleft lip and palate anomaly was abandoned in a childrens' hospital. Where there is a difficulty, God sends relief too. The child was rescued, adopted, and operated free of cost by Dr. Shabir Iqbal under Smile Train Program in January 2013. The child needed many procedures, which were done to ensure that child had good looks and good speech. I am sure if the parents of the abandoned child knew how their child became after treatment, they would not have abandoned her. Cleft lip and palate is scary for parents, but not when people like Dr. Shabir Iqbal are around. Kashmir has an increased incidence of these anomalies, but people like Dr. Shabir Iqbal here work day in and day out to set right the anomaly that thousands of children suffer from. Dr. Shabir corrects their anomaly, counsels their families, and works hard to give them a normal life.

Dr. Shabir Iqbal is a cleft lip and palate repair master. When I showed a photograph of one of his patients to an expert in the US, he said, "The child is lucky, she has got the perfect procedure at the perfect time. We in the US do not do better than this."

This humble, hardworking, and meticulous plastic surgeon would be seen in the operating room at SKIMS working with tedious grafts, dissecting vessels in microvascularization procedures, releasing tough burn scars and contractures, reconstructing body parts (i.e., nose and ear), and dealing with ugly Kangri cancers and skin cancers. He helped many men and women who had lost their limbs in accidents and fixed them back and actually saved them from the misery of losing a limb. The procedure would last for hours, and this surgeon would be doing his job quietly and diligently.

Dr. Shabir Iqbal involved himself in the painful reconstruction of bear maul injuries, that are so common in mountainous areas of Kashmir. The affected patients are usually poor people who are mauled beyond recognition and cannot afford treatment elsewhere.

This plastic surgeon of extraordinary talent and patience was born on June 9, 1955 in Sopore to Mr. Ghulam Mohammad Dar and Azi Begum. He did his matric in 1971 and MBBS from Government Medical College, Srinagar, in 1983 and thereafter went to PGI Chandigarh for his MCh in plastic surgery, which he completed in 1991. Together with Dr. M. A. Darzi, he was the founder member of the Department of Plastic Surgery at SKIMS. As a faculty member at SKIMS, he was greatly appreciated for the brilliant work that he did. Known for his patience, perseverance, innovation and love for perfection- Dr. Shabir gave to SKIMS some of its proudest moments when he achieved the seemingly impossible! He resigned from his position as an additional professor in 2007 to serve patients in private. However, he was a restless teacher and joined Government Medical College, Srinagar, Plastic Surgery, where he helped to establish and buid another department of Plastic Surgery creating the facilities and performing complex surgeries.

Dr. Shabir has authored many papers in reputed national and international journals and presented his work at various forums; one titled "Nitroglycerine in Flap Ischemia" and the other titled "Burn Contractures of Foot" won him the Best Paper Award. Dr. Shabir has published in reputed journals (i.e., *Burns, Annals of Plastic Surgery*, and *American Academy of Otolaryngology*). His publications have found mention in the *Year Book of Plastic Reconstructive and Aesthetic Surgery* (1996).

Dr. Shabir has been the project director, Smile Train operating at Modern Hospital, Srinagar, since 2007. All cleft lip and palate cases are done free of cost at Modern Hospital by him and his team. Dr. Shabir is without a doubt the best plastic surgeon that Kashmir has produced. He has rendered a service for which the entire community is indebted to him. Dr. Shabir's skill, innovation and love for aesthetics have made him the unmatched "master" of plastic surgery.

Dr. Shahida Mir

From its glorious years, the Government Medical College, Srinagar, went through its darkest era in the '90s that affected the quality of education, research, patient care activities of SMHS and Associated Hospitals, cultural events, sports, and other activities for which Government Medical College, Srinagar, was famous. The lull was so hard to break, creeping back to normal seemed a difficult task, and getting that shining streak seemed a distant dream. Here, again, a woman with her team came to restore all that Government Medical College had lost—its charm, its beauty, and its top position in academics and patient care.

Dr. Shahida Mir, the dynamic gynecologist and obstetrician who took over as the principal of Government Medical College, Srinagar, in 2009 and worked hard not only to restore the glory of Government Medical College, Srinagar, but also to remake it better, reshape it, reform it, and rebuild it.

Dr. Shahida Mir was born on July 2, 1953, in Rajbagh, Srinagar. She is the daughter of Mir Ghulam Hassan, who retired as secretary, Legislative Council. She studied at Mallinson Girls School, Srinagar, and was very bright in studies. She passed her matric in 1969 with flying colors. She joined Government Medical College, Srinagar, in 1972. She was an all-round student excelling in sports as well as in studies. She proved her excellence in sports and received the Best Lady Athlete Award in 1973 at the Government Medical College, Srinagar, sports event. Dr. Shahida completed her MBBS in 1976 and was adjudged the Best Outgoing Graduate among females.

She pursued her postgraduation in gynecology and obstetrics and completed MS in gynecology and obstetrics in 1982. Gynecology and obstetrics was a challenging branch, which was star-studded with the likes of Professor Girja and Prof. J. A. Naqshbandi when Dr. Shahida joined it as faculty. With her hard work and commitment, however, Dr. Shahida made a space for her in this star-studded department. She became professor and head of Gynecology and Obstetrics in 2000 and continued in this position till 2009. She became principal, Government Medical College, Srinagar, in 2009 and retired as the principal, Government Medical College, Srinagar, in 2011.

Dr. Shahida is an expert gynecologist and obstetrician who performs all kinds of surgeries. She regards herself as lucky because she worked under the guidance and mentorship of Prof. Wazira Khanum for a long time, whose dedication, hard work, helpful nature, and honesty helped her to grow as a surgeon and face the challenges as a professional initially and an administrator later on.

Dr. Shahida is one of the most successful principals of GMC Srinagar who undertook the tough task of starting superspeciality facility in the superspeciality hospital associated with GMC Srinagar. GMC Srinagar had for long remained static and stagnant so far as its expansion of superspeciality and subspecialty services was concerned. Dr. Shahida, however, changed the scene and lifted the lid off the inertia that had stalled this important developmental milestone. Under her leadership, the superspeciality services were started in cardiology, neurology, nephrology, and gastroenterology. It was a difficult task to work towards getting the required infrastructure,; getting the high-end equipment, and recruiting the manpower to make the dream of transforming a general hospital into a super-speciality hospital come true. She worked towards the transformation of cardiology into interventional cardiology with the commissioning of a 'one of its kind' cardiac intervention laboratory. She worked hard for this dream to be realized. She established a separate sub-speciality of traumatology, where patients of poly-trauma were treated under one roof without them being shuttled from one department to another.

The tremendous burden of psychiatric diseases in the valley stimulated Dr. Shahida to work toward a Center of Excellence in Psychiatry for which funds worth Rs 30 crore were sanctioned in her tenure. The Hospital for Psychiatric Diseases was also modernized with open wards, modified ECT, a modernized biochemistry lab, and a *Sarai* for the families of the inmates. Land for a modern institute of ophthalmology was acquired, which was a long pending demand of the Ophthalmology Department, GMC Srinagar,. The Department of Radiation Oncology was modernized to tackle the increased burden of cancer patients and to provide these patients with much-needed specialized care. The Dermatology Department was modernized, and the hair transplantation facility started during her tenure. The research was promoted in biochemistry, and the department received grants from the Biotechnology Department for various research activities. GMC's quest for newer departments like Physical Medicine and Rehabilitation was also addressed by providing land for the same. The old building of GMC Srinagar was refurbished and modernized during her tenure. She paid attention to minute details of all the projects.

The Golden Jubilee of GMC Srinagar was celebrated with pomp and enthusiasm after decades of silence. GMC alumni of the past from all over the world gathered in Srinagar and participated in a gala event lasting for days to make the event a success. It was nostalgic to hear the prominent alumni recount their experiences and share their dreams for GMC Srinagar. While it brought back the memory of nostalgic years, it took out GMC from a big slumber. This event highlighted the qualities of Dr. Shahida as a dynamic leader who worked to restore the glory of Government Medical College, Srinagar.

Dr. Zaffar Abass, the multi-talented faculty member at GMC who has a keen eye on the happenings in GMC Srinagar, comments in his editorial of *KASHMED* (2011), "Possibly the last of the superstars (in her own way) is the present Principal of this college. Nobody can take it from her that she has got the college out of the deadly, destructive inertia that had set in before she took over."

Dr. Shahida is actively practicing postretirement and wants to work more towards alleviating the suffering of infertile couples. She lives with her husband, Prof. Qazi Masood, in Srinagar. Her children work abroad. Dr. Shahida visits them but prefers to be in Srinagar working here for the welfare of the people.

Dr. Shariq Rashid Masoodi

It is difficult for me to write about a colleague who, without a doubt, is one of the most impressive faculty members in the SKIMS of today. An endocrinologist by profession, a researcher by passion, an educationist by desire, a master of statistics, a computer wiz kid, an education reformer, an innovator, an event manager, a humorist, a mountaineer, and a man with countless qualities and characteristics—his very presence in an institution is a blessing and honor for all who get to work with him. Every day, the institution grows with him. At SKIMS, I have not witnessed an academic exercise of which he was not a part or a scientific event to which he did not contribute. He is a modern man with traditional values, a bird on a flight with SKIMS in sight, a problem solver, an architect, a builder, and what not. God has invested heavily in him. He is Dr. Shariq Rashid Masoodi—the man behind many great things that SKIMS does!

Dr. Shariq was born in Sopore, the famous "Apple Town" of Kashmir, in February 1963. His father, late Mr. Abdul Rashid Masoodi, a schoolteacher, wanted him to study Arabic. But his mother, Zubeda Bano, a homemaker, always wanted him to become a doctor to care for her as she always used to be unwell. He himself wanted to become an inventor, a scientist and do something new. He received his early education at the nearby Government Boys Middle School Jamia Qadeem, Sopore. He later on went to the Government Higher Secondary School, Sopore, and the Government Degree College, Sopore. He was selected for MBBS in November 1982 and completed his MBBS from Government Medical College, Srinagar, in 1987. In college, he was considered to be bright and brilliant. He was very much interested in sports especially hockey. In GMC, he was introduced to trekking, a passion that he continues today. He was greatly influenced by Dr. Mohammad Sultan Khuroo ever since he saw the latter using a hammer to check the tendon jerks of his younger sister. After passing MBBS, he wanted to become a surgeon and, in December 1989, joined as a house surgeon in Surgical Unit IV, headed by Dr. Misgar. He found he was not passionate enough about surgery and later changed his mind. He joined medicine at SMHS Hospital, Srinagar, Dr. Durrani's unit.

Dr. Shariq joined SKIMS in September 1990, when he got selected for MD medicine and worked under Dr. Khuroo and other doyens of medicine there. He did his MD in medicine in 1992 under Dr. Bashir Ahmad Butt, the head of the Department of Physical Medicine and Rehabilitation. He was awarded first prize in the postgraduate research presentation for his research work on the role of exercise in the management of low back pain in 1993. He passed DM in endocrinology from PGI Chandigarh in December 2003, under the guidance of the legendary Dr. R. J. Dash, the first DM endocrinology in the country. He stood first in MD medicine at SKIMS Srinagar and DM endocrinology at PGI Chandigarh. He was inducted into the faculty at SKIMS as a lecturer of endocrinology (post-redesignated as assistant professor later) in 1995 and worked closely with Dr. Abdul Hamid Zargar, his mentor in endocrinology. Dr. Zargar is always appreciative of the work that Dr. Shariq did with him and admits that the tremendous work done by the Department of Endocrinology, SKIMS, would not have been possible without the role that Dr. Shariq played. He became an associate professor in 2001, additional professor in 2005, and, finally, professor of endocrinology at SKIMS in 2010. He worked as the in-charge head of the Department of Endocrinology from 2009 to 2011. As the HOD, his main achievement was starting of DM endocrinology program at SKIMS.

Practicing endocrinology in a private setup is very lucrative, as a large chunk of our population suffers from endocrine-related disorders. Dr. Shariq had a passion for this subject and never ignored his role as a physician, a teacher, a researcher, and an educator. He became everything but a private practitioner that would have given him money and fame.

Dr. Shariq has guided more than sixty postgraduate, doctoral, and postdoctoral students. His research interests are varied. He has authored 222 papers. He has been an author or coauthor of some of the phenomenal research that has taken place at SKIMS, especially research related to endocrinology. Many of his papers presented at various conferences have received the Best Paper Award. He received the AV Gandhi Award (2004) for Excellence in Endocrinology at New Delhi, which carried a gold medal, a citation, and a cash reward of Rs one lakh. He has received the DBT-CREST award (2013) for cutting-edge research enhancement and scientific training.

Dr. Shariq has done extensive research on thyroid disorders and has been instrumental in bringing the attention of health-care authorities to the problem of iodine deficiency and hypothyroidism in Kashmir. The work on diabetes, childhood diabetes, prediabetes, and obesity, published from SKIMS for which he has been an important contributor, is appreciated throughout the world, Dr. Shariq has directly or indirectly contributed to that massive work.

Dr. Shariq is a well-known academician and was a visiting professor at the University of Maryland School of Medicine in 2014. He has served as the founder and chairman, Ethical Committee of SKIMS; subdean, Academics, SKIMS; and coordinator, Medical Education Unit of SKIMS. Moreover, as an editor, *Journal of Medical Sciences*, SKIMS, he helped in the indexing process of the journal and the creation of the journal website. Besides mesmerizing talks at national and international conferences, he delivers lectures to create awareness in the community about lifestyle disorders, diabetes, nutrition, vitamin D deficiency, osteoporosis, and hypertension. He has a great fan following on social media as people follow his posts related to healthy diet and other aspects of lifestyle modifications. Dr. Shariq is a doctor who fulfills the criteria of an "ideal doctor"!

Dr. Shiekh Aejaz Aziz

Dr. Aejaz was born on February 21, 1956, to Mr. Sheikh Abdul Aziz and Salima Aziz in Srinagar, Kashmir. He did his MBBS from GMC Srinagar in 1981. He was a postgraduate in the Department of Internal Medicine at Government Medical College, Srinagar, from 1985 to 88 under the mentorship of Professor Allaqaband. He completed his very well-conducted research on "Role of Treadmill Cardiac Stress Testing in Evaluating Patients with Chest Pain with Normal ECG for Ischemic Heart Disease," for which he was awarded MD (internal medicine) from GMC Srinagar in 1988. Although Cardiology interested him, he found the speciality of medical oncology relatively unexplored and very challenging.

Dr. Aejaz completed DM (medical oncology) from Dr. MGR Medical University, Chennai Tamil Nadu, in 1992 after securing a rank in the entrance test on an All-India basis. He came back to Kashmir and served in SKIMS Medical Oncology in various positions. It is pertinent to mention here that Dr. Aejaz was pained to see the increasing number of cancer patients in the valley who were desperately looking for respite for their illness. When Dr. Aejaz joined SKIMS, there was neither infrastructure nor enough faculty to tackle the burden of cancer cases. He worked as consultant (lecturer) in the Department of Medical Oncology, SKIMS, Srinagar, from 1993 to 1997. He was promoted to the senior positions at SKIMS and worked there from 1997 to 2000. He was awarded Fellowship in Pediatric Hematology-Oncology at St. Jude Children's Research Hospital, Memphis, USA, in 2000. He was also awarded UICC-Fellowship in Bone Marrow Transplantation from Imperial College (School of Science and Technology, Hammersmith Hospital, London, UK) in 2001. Despite great job offers from abroad, he preferred to stay back in Kashmir and was appointed as professor and head, Department of Medical Oncology, SKIMS, in April 2012, and he continued to serve as professor and head of Medical Oncology, SKIMS, till his superannuation in 2018.

Dr. Ajaz's research work is quoted in *A Textbook of Cardiovascular Medicine* by Eugene Braunwald, in the chapter "Cardiotoxicity of Antineoplastic Agents (5FU)," chapter 69, page 2243, by P. Zipes and Peter Libray, 6th edition (2001), WB Saunders. He has contributed chapters to the book *Medical Emergencies*, edited by Prof. Mohamad Yousuf. Dr. Aejaz has authored more than one hundred publications in many national and international journals and has worked on a project on multiple myeloma funded by ICMR. He is a reviewer for many reputed journals of oncology. For his exemplary work to tackle cancer, Dr. Aejaz is included in "Marquis (USA) Who's Who," *World Encyclopedia*, 15th edition, and *Dictionary of International Biography*, 27th edition, of International Biographic Center, Cambridge, UK. Dr. Aejaz is included among the most outstanding people of the twentieth century of the IBC, Cambridge, UK. He is also the International Man of the Year 1999–2000 of the IBC, Cambridge, UK. He was awarded Rashtriya Gourav Award (2007), by Mr. Bisham Narayan Singh, former governor of Tamil Nadu and Andhra Pradesh. He was awarded third prize at the International Symposium on Renal Cell Carcinoma organized by the Medical Council of Goa and Tata Memorial Hospital Mumbai in March 2012.

Dr. Aejaz pioneered peripheral stem cell hematopoietic transplantation (PBSCT) in the Jammu and Kashmir. The first case of PBSCT was performed on a patient with multiple myeloma in the Department of Medical Oncology, SKIMS, Srinagar, under his supervision. Dr. Aejaz organized many international conferences and symposia, including the International Symposium on Genomic Instability and Cancer, jointly organized by SKIMS, Srinagar, Ohio State University, USA, and the University of Kashmir, in Srinagar on July 22–26, 2007. He also organized the Annual Conference of the Indian Society of Medical and Pediatric Oncology (ISMPOCON 2009 Srinagar) in Srinagar. He has attended more than one hundred conferences and presented his work in many national and international forums including in the US.

Dr. Aejaz has been an external examiner for MBBS, MD (medicine), BSc, and MSc MLT (immunohematology) and was appointed as external examiner for DM (medical oncology) examination, by All India Institute of Medical Sciences, New Delhi (AIIMS).

Dr. Aejaz has been the founder and executive secretary general of the Cancer Society of Kashmir (NGO). This NGO did a lot of work to help people with cancer and also rendered help in the early detection and treatment of cancer by conducting mass screening in remote areas of Kashmir. Dr. Aejaz is a life member of the Indian Society of Oncology, a life member of the Indian Society of Medical and Pediatric Oncology, a life member of the Indian Oncology Network (ICON), a member of the New York Academy of Sciences, USA, and member of the American Society of Clinical Oncology ASCO (2006). Dr. Aejaz Aziz was instrumental in starting the DM course in medical oncology. DM in medical oncology is a very competitive stream and is a dream desire for superspeciality aspirants throughout the country.

Dr. Aejaz is the chairman of the Shama Foundation (NGO). This foundation is an organization engaged in helping female patients with cancer, providing help to girls in meeting marriage expenses, helping women to pursue Islamic studies, helping them to pursue higher studies like MPhil/PhD and providing scholarships for the same.

Dr. Aejaz interestingly has been fond of water sports and is a life member of J&K Water Sports Association and a life member of J&K Kayaking and Canoeing Association. He is a keen golfer and a life member of Kashmir Golf Club. Dr. Aejaz lives with his wife and two sons in Srinagar. He currently sees patients at Ramzana Hospital, where he runs an oncology clinic. Dr. Aejaz is married to Ms. Safia Aejaz, has two sons, and lives with his family in Srinagar.

Dr. Showkat Ali Zargar

When the Srinagar floods of 2014 submerged a greater part of the city, a man was struggling to get into an ambulance with his family from the interiors of Rajbagh in the early morning hours. The man knew the fate of the house he had constructed. Calm and relaxed while the water was roaring into his area, he went to the place where he actually belonged . . . Sher-i-Kashmir Institute of Medical Sciences. He stayed there in one of the quarters and took care of the hospital amid the crisis caused by the deluge. Sick patients shifted from other hospitals were looked after, those injured and struggling for lifesaving drugs and support were catered to, help teams were sent to the submerged undergraduate SKIMS Medical College, and whatever equipment could be salvaged was salvaged. Faculty and staff were kept on high alert to fight any eventuality. This was all when his own home was in water, with everything submerged and spoiled. He worked harder in those stressful times, many times conducting hospital rounds in the early morning hours or late evenings. That is the man of the moment—Dr. Showkat Ali Zargar, a renowned gastroenterologist who was the director of SKIMS when it faced a crisis of a mammoth proportion. Dr. Showkat Ali Zargar possesses the rare combination of an excellent researcher, a brilliant academician, a clinician of repute, and a very effective and successful administrator. He is known as a man who possessed a vision for SKIMS and attempted to transform it into an institution of international standing.

Dr. Showkat Ali Zargar was born on May 24, 1954, in Srinagar, Kashmir. He did his MBBS from GMC Srinagar in 1976 and MD in general medicine from GMC Srinagar in 1981. He did DM (gastroenterology) from Postgraduate Institute of Medical Education and Research Chandigarh (PGIMER) from 1986 to 1988. While undergoing training for DM gastroenterology at PGI Chandigarh, a new classification of "Caustic Burns" was described by him, which is universally followed and has great diagnostic and therapeutic implications. This work was published as three in high-impact journals (*Gastroenterology* 1989, 97: 70207; *Gastrointestinal Endoscopy* 1991, 37: 165–9; and *American Journal of Gastroenterology* 1992, 87: 337–41).

Dr. Showkat did a phenomenal work on biliary ascariasis under the tutelage of Professor Khuroo. In 1985, he, along with Prof. M. S. Khuroo, described biliary ascariasis in Kashmir with its natural history and detailed clinical aspects, and these findings were published in high impact journals ("Biliary Ascariasis: A Common Cause of Biliary and Pancreatic Disease in an Endemic Area." *Gastroenterology* 1985, 99: 418–22, and "Therapy of Biliary Ascariasis and Its Rationale.: *Gastroenterology* 1987, 93: 668). The landmark paper from India on biliary ascariasis came from the joint work of Dr. Khuroo and Dr. Showkat A. Zargar published in *Lancet* in 1990 (Khuroo MS, Zargar SA, Mahajan R. "Hepatobiliary and Pancreatic Ascariasis in India." *Lancet* 1990, 335: 1503).

Dr. Showkat worked on hydatidosis of liver. In 1991, Dr. M. S. Khuroo and Dr. Showkat had the distinction of describing for the first time nonsurgical treatment for liver hydatid cysts by percutaneous route in a series of twenty-one patients, which evoked intense interest by other centers, and this became an established mode of treatment for hydatidosis. (This work was published in *Radiology* 1991, 180: 141–5, and *Gastrointestinal Radiology* 1992, 17: 41–45).

Dr. Showkat Ali worked as one of the founding members of SKIMS. He joined SKIMS as a senior resident in gastroenterology and became one of the most dynamic professors and an outstanding head of the department. The work of Dr. Showkat Ali Zargar on extrahepatic biliary obstruction published in *Hepatology* and *Gastrointestinal Endoscopy* threw new light on extrahepatic portal venous obstruction and its management. His work on the diagnosis on fine needle aspiration cytology of gastroesophageal and colonic malignancies was published in *Gut* and *Acta Cytologica* ("Endoscopic Fine Needle Aspiration Cytology in the Diagnosis of Gastro-Esophageal and Colorectal Malignancies." *Gut* 1991, 32: 745). Dr. Showkat has presented his work at many national and international conferences, and many of his papers have received the Best Paper Award for the quality research work that Dr. Showkat has done.

As the director of SKIMS and ex-officio secretary to the government, his work brought a new hope for SKIMS. He exerted his maximum during that fruitful tenure. He would personally visit each ward, the emergency, all the labs and interact with the staff, patients, attendants to know the deficiencies and address all the issues on the spot. He paid attention to each department. He was responsible for the diversification of all the specialities and subspecialties in medicine and surgery. He created many new departments and added a workforce to the departments that were already existing. One hundred twenty more beds were added to SKIMS. Kidney transplantation was speeded up by creating a new kidney transplant unit. The number of kidney transplants being done weekly was increased so that the waiting time of patients for kidney transplants decreased. Stem cell/autologous bone marrow transplantation became a regular feature at SKIMS. A three-phase expansion of the Accident and Emergency Department was done. From twelve beds, the strength of ICU beds went to forty-two. To cater to the dearth of nursing staff, technical personnel, and other paramedics, the intake capacity of students for these courses was increased with the addition of MSc and PhD courses in nursing.

Dr. Showkat Zargar is a reviewer for more than ten journals and is on the editorial board of more than a dozen journals. He was the editor in chief and founder editor (2010–2014) of *Journal of Digestive Sciences*, peer-reviewed journal of the Society of GI Endoscopy of India. He has got grants as a principal investigator for many ICMR and DBT-sponsored projects. He has mentored scores of MD, DM, and PhD students from SKIMS and other universities. He has been an examiner to many prestigious institutions and was on the selection panel of many national institutions and national bodies. Under the leadership of Dr. Showkat Ali, SKIMS was successful in getting an unprecedented number of centrally sponsored schemes. SKIMS obtained grants of Rs 158 crore via various schemes, which resulted in considerable improvement in patient care. Dr. Zargar's contribution has been that of a good pleader. Some of these schemes are

- Advanced Cancer Diagnostic Center,
- State Virology Lab,
- State Cancer Institute,
- Regional Geriatric Center,
- Bioinformatic Center,
- State Research Lab,

Dr. Showkat is a dynamic leader and an excellent gastroenterologist. He continues to see patients and do procedures in his private clinic. He is a straightforward person who does not mince words about the facts. He is a tough taskmaster and able doer of seemingly impossible things. He lives with his wife in Srinagar.

Dr. Upendra Kaul

Kashmiri Muslims and Pandits—- both communities had to bear the brunt of trauma as Kashmir suffered decades of conflict. There was a breach of trust between the two communities. More elements worked towards discord than towards harmony. The result was that the two communities were pulled apart, so much away from each other that there was hardly any communication. It was a pain to see the two communities who had lived together for centuries as brethren drift away from each other. However, there were sane voices and sincere people who felt the pain at the loss of togetherness that Kashmir had always boasted of. One such man is Dr. Upendra Kaul, who held together broken hearts without prejudice and tried to heal them. With his cool temperament and caring heart, he became a darling of Kashmir. He did not refuse treatment to anyone based on religion or association but worked towards a mission of healing broken hearts and putting together broken parts. Dr. Upendra Kaul, or U Kaul (as Kashmir calls him), is the man who embraced Kashmir in his arms when Kashmir was in pain and is working now with all his sincerity towards a healthy and peaceful Kashmir.

Dr. Upendra Kaul is one of the first cardiologist of Kashmiri origin and one of the pioneers of interventional cardiology in India. He is the chairman and dean of academics and research at the Batra Hospital and Medical Research Center, known for his expertise in procedures such as percutaneous cardiopulmonary bypass, rotational and directional atherectomy, coronary stenting, and percutaneous laser myocardial revascularization.

Dr. Upendra Kaul was born in Srinagar in 1948. His father, Mr. Prem Nath Kaul, who had studied in Lucknow, decided to move to Delhi for a job. Dr. Upendra Kaul and his mother followed him. Recounting his days from school, Dr. Upendra Kaul says, "My school and college life was spent in Delhi and saw failures and self-corrections. The 2 months of the summer vacations spent in the valley every year kept me in touch with my roots. The two places I enamored the most were Kani-Kadal, my aunt's (Masi's) house, on the river bank, and my father's place of birth village Hawal near Pulwama."

Dr. Kaul graduated in medicine (MBBS) from the Maulana Azad Medical College and continued his studies at the same institution to secure MD in internal medicine in 1975. He did DM in cardiology in 1978 and is the first DM(cardiology) of Kashmiri origin. Dr. Kaul had a sense of deep attachment to his mother and his motherland. By becoming a cardiologist, he fulfilled the dream of his mother, who herself wanted to serve patients as a nurse. Her role model was Florence Nightingale. He wanted to join the Sher-i-Kashmir Institute of Medical Sciences (SKIMS) and serve the people of Kashmir, but the administration at that point of time did not take his request seriously, and he did not succeed in getting an opening at SKIMS. He was disappointed but did not lose hope and continued with his academic pursuits at PGI Chandigarh, GB Pant Hospital, and, finally, AIIMS in New Delhi.

Dr. Kaul obtained advanced training in interventional cardiology from Australia during 1983–84. He served the All India Institute of Medical Sciences (AIIMS) as a professor of cardiology and has been a member of the faculty of the Post Graduate Institute of Medical Education and Research Chandigarh, GB Pant Hospital, New Delhi, Batra Hospital and Fortis Health Care, NCR. He was the executive director and the dean at Fortis Health Care, New Delhi, till 2017. Dr. Kaul is a former president of the Cardiological Society of India and the SAARC Cardiac Society. He is a fellow of the American College of Cardiology and the National Academy of Medical Sciences (NAMS). He has published over 450 medical papers and won the Medtronic Award for the Best Scientific Paper in 1983.

Dr. Upendra Kaul received the highest Indian award in the medical category, Dr. B. C. Roy Award in 1999. The government of India awarded him the fourth-highest civilian honor, the Padma Shri, in 2006, for his contributions to medicine in India. He is also a recipient of the Dr. Thapar Gold Medal in 1970, the Searle Award of the Cardiological Society of India in 1986, the Shakuntala Amir Chand Prize of the Indian Council of Medical Research in 1987, and the Press India Award in 1992.

Despite the fact that he got international recognition in his profession, he always felt a vacuum in his life. The burning desire of working in Kashmir was always a part of him. In the most testing period of the valley in the 1990s when all systems collapsed there, he did his best to help sick patients from the valley coming to AIIMS for treatment. During the same period, he helped the members of the Pandit community who had to migrate to Delhi and NCR by getting them jobs in various sectors. Looking at the faith Kashmiris had in him and the dedication with which he was treating them, the CM of Jammu and Kashmir at that time gave him the opportunity of seeing patients in the government-owned Kashmir Nursing Home at the Gupkar Road. Thereafter, he would go regularly to see patients in Srinagar and helped in initiating the angioplasty programs in SKIMS and also in a private hospital, Khyber Medical Institute. He was a frequent visitor to SKIMS for training their consultants in complex angioplasty cases and the use of new devices. SKIMS honored him with the annual award on Founder's Day in 2012. About this initiative, Dr. Kaul says, "This gave me some happiness but not satisfaction." Dr. Kaul's departed mother, Gauri, who was his greatest inspiration always, had a lingering desire to have a small home in the valley. He eventually fulfilled that by making a house "Gauri Manzil" in Srinagar in 2013. It was not easy to swim against the tide. A Pandit trying to come back to Kashmir was considered amateurish. Many Muslim friends, however, supported him in this initiative.

In 2020, after visiting North Kashmir, Kupwara town, and Machil valley, along with his friends Azaz Rashid and Nasir Lone, he identified several deficiencies in the health-care system. It was decided to do health camps in different districts under the banner of "Gauri Healthy Heart Project." The feedback from these camps was that less than half the patients with hypertension had their BPs controlled to acceptable limits. Inadequate treatment, nonavailability of medicines at the health centers, inability to afford costly medicine, and poor motivation were the main reasons. Likewise, more than one-third of diabetics were uncontrolled diabetics when the random sugar assessment of these people was done. Glycosylated Hb to assess the level of control was very rarely done, and facilities for this test were hardly available. The newer drugs like SGLT2 inhibitors (Dapagliflozin or Empagliflozin) were rarely prescribed. Lack of awareness among the doctors working in these areas and cost being the important issues. After recording these startling findings, Dr. Kaul's group decided to open a cardiac center with all advanced noninvasive facilities in Srinagar, which would cater to the needs of patients of most districts. The setup "Gauri Heart Center" started functioning in April 2021. Besides ECG, it has facilities like echocardiography, stress tests, head-up tilt test (HUTT), and ambulatory BP monitoring facility. Facilities for blood biochemistry and point-of-care biomarkers for diagnosing heart failure and thrombotic conditions like NT-proBNP, ST2, troponins, D-Dimer, etc. are also available. The reports of biomarkers are available within fifteen minutes to help in the proper management of these patients. A team of doctors, dietary counselors, and technicians are available throughout the day till 8:00 p.m.

Under this foundation, funding was obtained for putting up telemedicine units in remote areas like Machil, Kupwara, and isolated townships like Jagti in Jammu. These centers helped needy people. The foundation has initiated health camps, extending the higher level of investigations for the needy people identified by local Panchayats and administration without charging them. To begin with, three districts in the valley (Tangdar, Uri, and Pulwama) and three in Jammu (Reasi, R. S. Pura, and Katra) were identified. Gauri Kaul Foundation has set up three more centers in Jammu and Kashmir:

(a) Machil, near LOC, District Kupwara;
(b) Jagti Migrant township, near Nagrota Jammu;
(c) Hawal, Pulwama (ancestral place of Dr. U. Kaul).

The work on Prasad Joo Khan Memorial Center (named after Dr. Kaul's grandfather) in Hawal Pulwama is complete. The center is well equipped with facilities for providing health-care facilities in cardiology, medicine, general surgery, and gynecology. It will be serving the residents of the districts of Pulwama, Shopian, and Kulgam. This is a dream coming true for Dr. Kaul.

The work in others districts will follow. Besides an OPD, a telemedicine facility is also available with trained personnel in these centers. This is very useful during the harsh winter months when some of these places get totally cut off from the nearby medical centers. Indian Oil Corporation (IOC), Oil and Natural Gas Corporation (ONGC), and Astra Zeneca have generously helped finance these projects through their corporate social responsibility (CSR) funds. Currently, the mission of Dr. Kaul's foundation is “No More Heart Attacks” by spreading measures to be taken by the public at large by organizing public awareness programs and talking about the important modifiable risk factors and a stress on how to prevent the adverse factors. Counseling regarding the modification of diet and regular exercise is also done. The foundation does this at the district level in association with local administration and Panchayats. Print and electronic media are used to propagate these messages.

Dr. Kaul has treated people from all walks of life, which include the common villagers, highly placed bureaucrats, politicians, and even separatists. He has been associated with personalities as diverse as Mian Bashir Larvi of Wangat, Kangan, and Sathya Sai Baba of Puttaparthy, Andhra Pradesh. He has not refused treatment to anyone. The National Investigation Agency (NIA) grilled him after the NIA sleuths misread his use of medical jargon to mean a hawala transaction.

This journey of seven decades has been a long one for Dr. Kaul and satisfying too since it has him back to his roots and the holy soil of the place of his birth—the enchanting valley of Kashmir. Dr. Kaul always feels that he owes to give back whatever he can to the people of his place of birth, Kashmir.

(This profile is based on the information provided by Dr. Upendra Kaul and also on one of his write-ups in the local daily Greater Kashmir titled “A Nostalgic Journey” dated May 28, 2022).

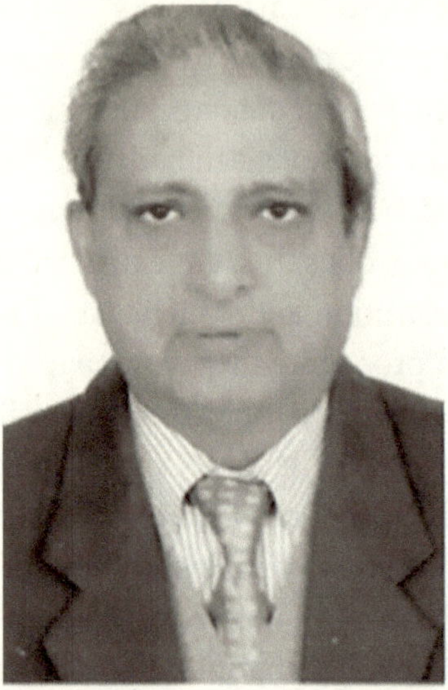

Dr. Ghulam Hassan Malik—the nephrologist from SKIMS who published excellent research on renal failure following trauma (*Nephron*)

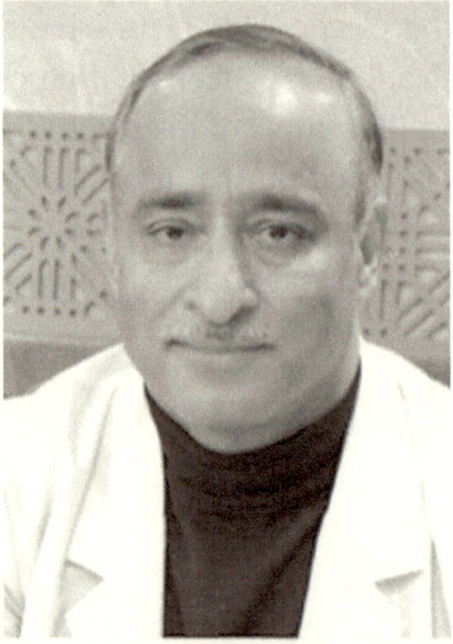

Dr. Parvaiz Ahmad Koul—renowned researcher who has done an outstanding work on influenza and pulmonary hydatidosis (Hi index 69)

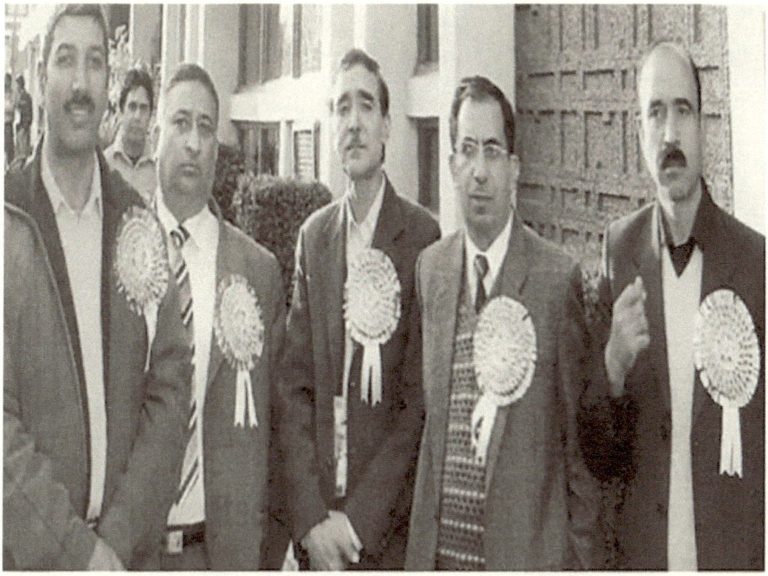

The custodians of SKIMS who dominated an era
and held its flag high in a difficult time.
(From L to R) Dr. Showkat A. Zargar, Dr. Sheikh Ajaz,
Dr. Khurshid Iqbal, Dr. Mushtaq, Dr. A. H. Zargar (In
the background, Dr. A. G. Ahangar is also seen.)

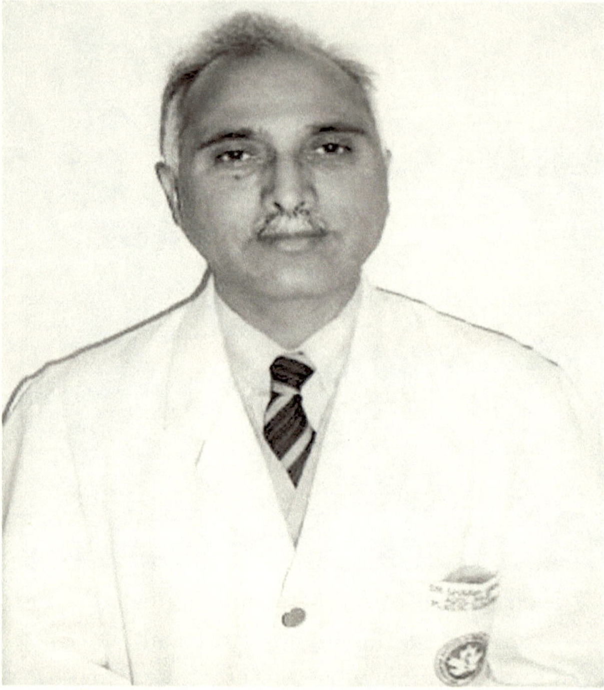

Dr. Shabir Iqbal—the plastic surgeon who changed the face of modern aesthetics in Kashmir.

The Path Breakers

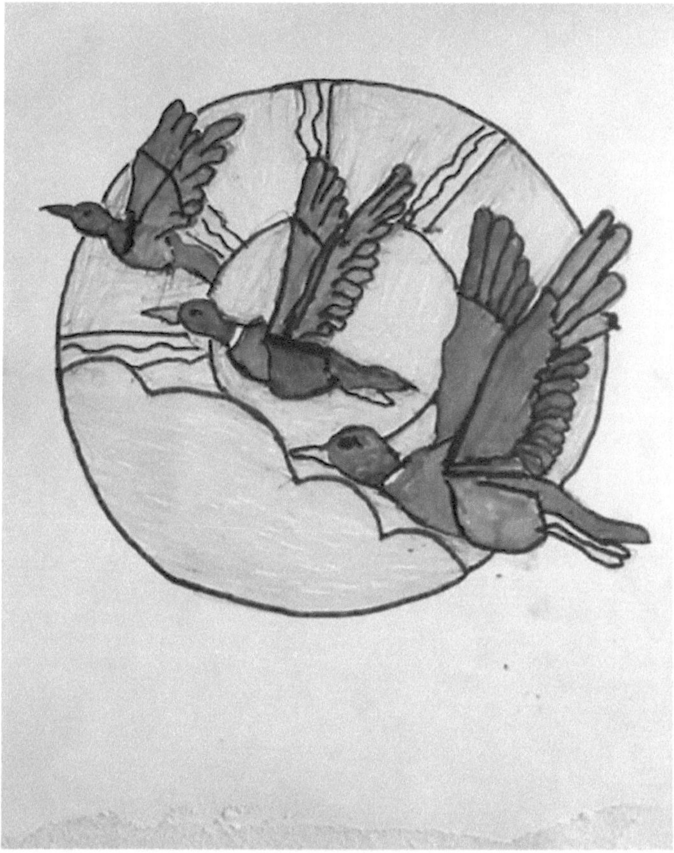

Art by Dr. H. A. Durrani

Contributions of Nonresident Kashmiris (NRK)—International Medical Graduates (IMG)—to Health Care in the USA

(Prof. Faroque A. Khan)

Immigrants to the USA have played a pivotal role in developing and advancing all aspects of life in the USA and beyond. Over the past sixty-plus years, immigrants from Asia/Africa have played a significant role in health-care delivery in the USA, and, before that, it was the European immigrants who helped. In fact, many of the major academic centers in the USA were established and staffed by these European immigrants—for example, Dr. Osler at Johns Hopkins University in Maryland and many others.

The civil rights movement spearheaded by the Afro-American community played a significant role in changing/ending many policies, which allowed more equitable access for non-European immigrants to come to the USA. I, along with other NRKs profiled in this book, was the beneficiary of the civil rights movement. The focus of this chapter is the role of Kashmiri physicians in the USA. From the first batch of GMC in 1965, six individuals took the ECFMG exam in New Delhi, and, to the surprise of many faculty at GMC, all six passed and received scores, which mirrored the final grades in the MBBS exam.

For me, personally, that was "proof" of the high-quality education we received at GMC in spite of the lack of many support facilities—for example labs. It was the combination of experienced teachers and students selected on merit that resulted in academic excellence. The medical curriculum around the world is undergoing changes, and, as an educator, I often emphasize the importance of selecting motivated dedicated students guided and taught by seasoned committed compassionate teachers.

By and large, immigrants in general and physicians in particular have done well in the USA; some have excelled in their respective fields, and some have even gone beyond—doing the extraordinary—and helped uplift the community at large. Few are profiled in this book. What is the secret recipe for this success? Perhaps the following example will answer this question.

Case study: A young Muslim IMG from Algeria came to the USA on a three-month scholarship. His education in Algeria was in French, and he barely spoke English. He had an "idea" that he presented to his Jewish boss, Dr. Siegelman, who responded by encouraging him to study it further. Well, to everyone's surprise, Elias Zerhouni's idea of measuring the calcium content radiologically in pulmonary nodules resulted in a radical change and improvement in managing the common problem of the solitary pulmonary nodule. Elias continued his training at Johns Hopkins University. He replaced Dr. Siegelman as chair of the Radiology Department, was promoted as dean for research, and eventually was appointed by Pres. George W. Bush on May 15, 2002, as the fifteenth director of the National Institute of Health—the largest research organization in the world. When asked to comment on the secret of his success, Dr. E. Zerhouni said, "I don't think there is any country in the world like the US where different people from different countries are accepted and welcomed as members of a society and as good citizens. The tolerance and support I have received is a continuing inspiration for me, both as an American and as a Muslim." (1)

My comment: Elias had a good, responsive mentor, a supportive environment/community, and an inquisitive mind with a willingness to work honestly and diligently.

Profile of IMGs in USA: Based on AMA Masterfile. Ref: IMGs in the US Physician Workforce Paper, 2009 edition.

In 2009, out of 902,053 physicians, 228,665 IMGs received medical degrees from 127 countries, accounting for 25.3 percent of the total physician count.

- IMGs make up approximately 25 percent of the US physician population.
- The heaviest concentration of IMGs is in New Jersey (45 percent of doctors), New York (42 percent), Florida (37 percent), and Illinois (34 percent).
- The largest national group is from India (20.7 percent of the total).
- Among the top four primary specialities, the IMG population represents 37 percent of total physicians in internal medicine, 28 percent in anesthesiology, 32 percent in psychiatry, and 28 percent in pediatrics.
- The total physician population increased by 350,386 between 1970 and 1994 (or 104.9 percent), while IMGs accounted for over one-fourth (27.8 percent) of this increase by gaining 97,359 physicians.
- In this twenty-four-year period, non-IMGs grew by 91.4 percent, while IMGs increased by 170.2 percent.
- In 1980, IMGs accounted for 20.9 percent of the total physician count of 467,679, while that percentage

> climbed to 22.6 percent of the total count of 684,414 physicians in 1994.

IMGs showed significantly greater representation among active practicing physicians in four specialities: internal medicine (39 percent), neurology (31 percent), psychiatry (30 percent), and pediatrics (25 percent). IMGs in GME showed significantly greater representation in five specialities: pathology (39 percent), internal medicine (39 percent), neurology (36 percent), family medicine (32 percent), and psychiatry (31 percent; all $P<.001$). IMGs make up nearly a quarter of the total GME pool and practicing physician workforce, with a disproportionate share, and larger increases over our study period in certain specialities. (Ref 4) https://www.ncbi.nlm.nih.gov/pmc/articles/PMC5901803/

Challenges Faced by IMGs

Responding to the unique needs of IMGs and the program directors, particularly in states with a large percentage of IMGs, the American College of Physicians (ACP) asked me to prepare a report, which led to the publication titled *International Medical Graduates in US Hospitals—A Guide for Program Directors and Applicants* (Ref2). We wanted to know the views of both the IMGs in training and the program directors and also invited the comments from well-known educators. Few excerpts follow:

Prof. Faith Fitzgerald—Consider the IMG's situation: new language, new technology, new population of patients, new drugs, new laboratory units, sometimes new attitudes to be adopted, new hierarchical structures of authority to be learned and discarded, and new epidemiology of disease to be assimilated. (For example, a recent graduate from India who was serving as a house officer in California initially diagnosed malaria in anyone with a fever. And why not?) (xvii ref 2).

In a survey of 150 trainees, Dr. Farida Khan found the IMG trainees had substantial difficulty addressing the following issues when they started training—medical ethics, HIV counseling, medical genetics and clinical epidemiology, the US medicolegal system, and adjusting to the role of nurses in the health-care team (page 31-ref 2).

All training programs in the USA undergo a vigorous inspection to maintain accreditation. Dr. Michael La Combe was an inspector for a medicine training program that had predominantly IMGs as trainees. He was so impressed with what he saw and encountered that he wrote a seminal article titled "International Hero," published in *American Journal of Medicine*. With the author's permission, we reproduced the article in our book. After describing his interview with the Nigerian, Chinese, Egyptian trainees, Dr. Lacombe marvels at how the program director has impacted these trainees by developing specific culturally sensitive orientations for these "foreign" trainees. The result in the words of a consultant in the program: "What the program director has done through the years is to make every one of them proud of their heritage, made them identify with it, cling to it, yet helping them in every way that he could to adapt to English and the American way of life. The effect has been twofold: they are happy, secure, and self-confident and therefore, great workers and great doctors and secondly some of them return home." (page 34-ref 2 & ref 3).

In my preface for the book, I shared some of my initial challenges dealing with abbreviations and cultural differences—a man with chest pain is admitted with R/O-MI, CAD, ASHD, HCVD. Having had no experience with abbreviations at GMC, you can imagine my anxiety after encountering this note.

I was called from the ER to deal with a patient who has severe abdominal pain because of the "SS" crisis—having never seen or read about sickle cell disease in Kashmir, one can imagine the tension and anxiety I felt.

Having trained in the British system where we address the nurse as "sister," imagine my shock when I addressed the charge nurse as sister and her response was "Honey, don't call me sister; you and I know we are not related. We may develop a relationship, but not as brother and sister" (xi.-ref 2).

An IMG has much to learn and absorb and that too rather quickly.

NRK Contributions in US Health Care

Like IMGs from other countries, NRKs have followed several pathways in the USA. Few, after completing training in the USA, returned to Kashmir: Drs. G. Q. Allaqaband, Zahoor Ahmed, Mahmooda Khan, Rachpal Singh, and others I am not aware of. Several have come for short-term training and returned to Kashmir: Drs. G. M. Malik, Parvaiz A. Koul, MMA Kamili, Samia Rashid, Khurshid Aslam Khan (medicine), Mukhtar Siddiqui (radiology). Many others have been sponsored by NRKs for short-term training in various disciplines. I mentioned the ones I was personally familiar with; however, the majority of the NRKs did not return to Kashmir, and the reasons are many. To cite my personal example, after finishing our training, my wife, Arfa, and I were planning to return to Kashmir in early '70s. We had a good job offer; however, my father advised us against returning, his reason related to the ongoing political uncertainty in Kashmir and his concern that our training and talents would not be fully utilized in Kashmir.

To summarize the role of NRK in the USA,

a) Patient care—Significant percentage of NRK chose a clinical practice in their respective fields, many serving in underserved areas of the country. Some helped develop unique programs, which helped improve access to care for individuals with limited or no health insurance. One such NRK, Dr. Shagufta Yasmeen, is profiled in the book.

b) Research: A minority of NRKs chose the academic track with a focus on research. A few of them are profiled in this book: Hamid Band, Prediman K. Shah, Romesh and Nancy Khardori, Iftikhar Kullo, Raffit Hassan, Riyaz Bashir. Details of their accomplishments are in the individual profiles.

c) Innovators and entrepreneurs: Dr. Fayaz Shawl represents an example of an innovator who utilized the opportunity provided with the advent of invasive cardiology and developed expertise in invasive cardiology, resulting in his becoming one of the world's leading invasive cardiologists.

d) Professional and other organization leadership: Dr. Tanveer Mir completed her tenure as chair of the board of regents of the American College of Physicians in May 2016. ACP, with 140,000 members globally, is the largest speciality organization in the world, a unique distinction and recognition for Dr. Mir's outstanding contributions to ACP. Dr. Khalid J. Qazi, in addition to his professional work, was key in developing an active Islamic center in Buffalo and also became a voice and face for the Muslims in New York through his work in Muslim Public Affairs Council and other organizations. Dr. Abdul R. Mir played a key role in developing and sustaining the Islamic Society of North America, the largest Muslim organization in the USA. These are a few examples of the contributions of NRK to national organizations in the USA.

American College of Physicians (ACP) and GMC Alumni Contributions: In 1915, an idea was promulgated by a

German-born physician, Dr. Heinrich Stern, who, along with six colleagues, convened and established the ACP, which now consists of 140,000 masters, fellows, members, associates, and students. IMGs make up a third of ACP's overall membership. Their experience and understanding of other medical education systems, health-care environments, and cultures have influenced patient care, the profession as a whole, and the college. IMGs have served in various committees, as council members, as chapter governors, and as regents and officers.

GMC alumni have had a significant role and impact within ACP. Four have been awarded mastership in ACP, a unique distinction bestowed on less than 1 percent of all internists: Dr. Mohd, Sultan Khuroo, Dr. Khalid J. Qazi, Dr. Tanveer Mir, and Faroque A. Khan, all are profiled in this book. Dr. FAK served as regent of ACP from 1995 to 2001, and Dr. Tanveer Mir served as chair of BOR for 2015–2016.

Additionally, three GMC alumni were the recipients of the ACP International Exchange Program fellowships: Dr. Parvaiz A. Koul, 2004; Dr. Khursheed Aslam Khan, 2006; and Dr. Samia Rashid, 2013–2014 (Ref 4, Chapter 13).

I focused on ACP since I am quite familiar with it. Other medical and speciality organizations have also had IMGs play a significant role as members and as leaders.

GMC and NRK—All the NRKs wish and desire GMC to shine, GMC alumni receive quality medical education at minimal expense, and most NRKs have the desire to contribute to the well-being of GMC, so the obvious question comes up: Why has that not transpired to the maximum? I can only relate to my personal experience in my dealings with GMC and the health-care leaders over the past fifty plus years—for example, in 1987, as president of the Islamic Medical Association of North America, I had proposed to have the first international convention of IMANA in Srinagar, but permission for this was denied.

To summarize:

Political uncertainty: The ongoing uncertainty in Kashmir has adversely impacted medical education. The exodus of minority faculty and the security concerns of students and remaining faculty have clearly had a detrimental effect on the quality of education. The civil service rules, in my opinion, also adversely impact the management of GMC. The principal/dean often stays for short periods, which does not allow long-term planning or strategizing. In 1986, I applied for the position of chairman of medicine at Nassau County Medical Center. I was interviewed by the search committee composed of leading NCMC staff and the chair of medicine from Stony Brook. After a long grilling process, background checks, I was finally offered the job, and I stayed at NCMC for twelve years from 1987 to 1999, enough time to see the results of my efforts. Later on, I learned from some members of the search committee that there were twenty-nine applicants and all except me were US medical graduates. The point I am trying to make is that GMC and other institutions in Jammu andKashmir may consider adopting an alternate method of recruiting senior management folks and allow them some time and freedom to develop and improve health care at GMC and other institutions.

With globalization and improved access and communication, with some dedicated organizational effort both at GMC and in the USA, many initiatives are possible, utilizing the expertise and skills of NRK's in the USA and the faculty at GMC with the eventual goal of enhancing medical education and training at GMC, which will enhance and improve the overall health-care delivery in Jammu and Kashmir. I am cautiously optimistic that the GMC alumni association will serve as a catalyst for making this possible.

References

1. Khan, F. "Profile of Dr. Elias Zerhouni: A Contemporary Muslim Scientist." *Journal of Islamic Medical Association*, vol. 37, 2005, page 43–44.
2. Khan, F. and S. Lawrence, editors. *International Medical Graduates in US Hospitals: A Guide for Program Directors and Applicants (Ref2)*, published by American College of Physicians 1995.
3. La Combe, A. M. "International Hero." *American Journal of Medicine*, 1993; 95: 329.
4. Tooker, J. and D. Dale D., editors. "Serving Our Patients and Profession: A Centennial History of the American College of Physicians 1915–2015," published by *ACP.* ISBN 978-1-934465-99-8.
5. Awad A. Ahmed, et al. "International Medical Graduates in the US Physician Workforce and Graduate Medical Education: Current and Historical Trends." *Grad Med Educ.* 2018 April; 10 (2): 214–218.

A word from me!

Kashmir, in spite of decades of conflict, has moved ahead as regards health care. From an era of sweeping epidemics to an era of "phenomenal work on epidemics," Kashmiris have not lagged behind. Kashmiri doctors have proved their mettle here in Kashmir, in the America, or in the UK. We should be thankful to Dr. Faroque Khan—that he has collected inspiring stories of Kashmiri doctors who have done an enormous amount of work and contributed so much to the humankind. It has been a marathon effort on his part to put together so many profiles. Dr. Faroque is the leader who knows what to do and when.

The scenario in Kashmir has changed and yet not changed . . . Kashmiris still chase medicine as the first career choice. However, GMC Srinagar is not the only institution producing doctors now. Many more medical colleges have come up in the valley, and many Kashmiri youngsters are graduating from Bangladesh and other countries in the neighborhood. There are so many aspiring to go to US, UK, Canada, and Australia. Not bad, really . . . Doctors like Prof. Faroque Khan and Prof. K. J. Qazi have helped many Kashmiri doctors in the past with their careers in the US. In the younger lot, Dr. Khurshid Guru has sponsored many doctors from Kashmir for a short-term fellowship, but more efforts are needed as Kashmir continues to produce more doctors aspiring to work abroad. We need these efforts as residency in the US is getting more difficult—for there may be many Fayaz Shawls or P. K. Shah's waiting in the line for some extraordinary work . . . It is obligatory on part of NRKs to help them achieve their dreams. As I note in most of the profiles from our colleagues from abroad, most attribute their success to the teachers and mentors here in Kashmir who built their strong foundations in medicine. Those strong foundations were laid by our teachers . . . I wish those values and principles set by them are retained in the present generation medical teachers and professionals working in Kashmir. In the book, for example, there is an account of how a professor in GMC Srinagar inspired his student to excel in Harvard.

There has been an effort by nonresident Kashmiri doctors like KASHMER for many health-related initiatives including procuring ambulances and equipment for various institutions of the valley. Kashmir education initiative (KEI) sponsored by nonresident Kashmiri doctors for promotion of quality education to deserving poor but bright children of the valley is a well-thought and well-implemented initiative. The work done deserves all the applause. I do see many of my friends and colleagues carrying home some catheters, a pediatric laryngoscope, a core biopsy needle, a slide for discussion, or some material for teaching every time they come home for a vacation. Every gesture counts, and every effort matters.

Someone asked me as to why Kashmiris, especially Kashmiri doctors, do so well outside. I thought for a while for this reply. Kashmiri doctors run a race with hurdles here . . . it is a race nonetheless. And, when they work outside, they see no hurdles and thus run their races fast and outshine the rest. Kashmir has a lot to do with what they become outside Kashmir. The inspiring teachers, the innocent yet desperate patients readily offering themselves for learning, the relatively free education, and the Dua's and sacrifices of their loved ones especially parents go a long way into making them successful in an alien land. I know how many parents shuttle between US/UK and Kashmir to do babysitting while the children build their careers . . . or suffer alone in a conflict zone, never recalling their children home or falsely reassuring them about their well-being.

It is important for NRKs thus to invest their time and energy in Kashmir. Important for them to pay back their home, important for them to train manpower in Kashmir, important to involve themselves in "correction" rather than criticism, and my request to the NRK's is do not stop to teach and train your colleagues in Kashmir.

I think the Chinese proverb holds true:

"If you give a man a fish, you feed him for a day. If you teach a man to fish, you feed him for a lifetime."

And do not restrict your visit to GMC Srinagar only; there are many new medical colleges and hospitals that might benefit from your expertise.

NRK doctors are profiled at the end of the book . . . though I know their accomplishments demand that they be profiled at the top. But most of them are humble enough and quite satisfied that they are behind their teachers and mentors. Kashmiris working anywhere in the world hold Kashmir very dear to their hearts, and for Kashmiris back home, Kashmiris doing well outside is always a source of pride and prestige. Hope through this book we retain that mutual love for each other.

I understand the longing of NRK's for their beloved homeland. Here is a small poem by Agha Shahid Ali for them:

A Call

I close my eyes. It doesn't leave me,
The cold moon of Kashmir, which breaks
into my house
and steals my parents' love.
I open my hands:
empty, empty. This cry is foreign.
"When will you come home?"
Father asks, then asks again.
The ocean moves into the wires.
I shout, "Are you all happy?"
The line goes dead.
The waters leave the wires.
The sea is quiet, and over it
The cold, full moon of Kashmir.
Aga Shahid Ali (The veiled suite)
Rumana

The list from US

1. **Dr. Abdul Rauf Mir**
2. **Dr. Arfa Rasool Khan**
3. **Dr. Faroque Ahmad Khan**
4. **Dr. Fayaz Shawl**
5. **Dr. Hamid Band**
6. **Dr. Iftikhar J. Kullo**
7. **Dr. Khalid Jahangir Qazi**
8. **Dr. Khurshid A. Guru**
9. **Dr. Mian Mohammad Ashraf**
10. **Dr. Nancy (Misri) Khardori**
11. **Dr. Noor Ali Pirzada**
12. **Dr. Parvez Ahmad Mir**
13. **Dr. Prediman K. Shah**
14. **Dr. Raffit Hassan**
15. **Dr. Riyaz Bashir**
16. **Dr. Romesh Khardori**
17. **Dr. Shagufta Yasmeen**
18. **Dr. Suhail A. Shah**
19. **Dr. Tanveer P. Mir**

From UK and Middle East

20. **Dr. G. M. Din**
21. **Dr. Ghulam Jeelani Mufti**
22. **Dr. Ghulam Rasool (Gulzar) Mufti**
23. **Dr. Mohamed Abdullah Sofi**

Young sensations

24. **Dr. Noor Ul Owase Jeelani**
25. **Dr. Rizwan Romee**

Dr. Abdul Rauf Mir

Abdul Rauf Mir was born in Srinagar, Kashmir, in a renowned family, sixth of the seven siblings. His father, Ghulam Mohiuddin Mir, in addition to participating in his family business, served his community in various positions, including as secretary, Department of Revenue, J&K. His mother, Zaiba, was the daughter of the prominent community leader and religious activist Mr. Abdul Aziz Bhat, who passed away when Dr. Mir was a toddler, likely from a cerebral stroke and uncontrolled hypertension. He was inspired to pursue a career in medicine by the premature loss of his mother and by the remarkable service he observed certain clinicians provide their patients, including his maternal uncle Dr. Ghulam Ali, who was the first Kashmiri ophthalmologist.

Dr. Mir received his primary education at the CMS Tyndale Biscoe School. He excelled academically as well as in sports. At the age of fifteen, one year after matriculating, Dr. Mir, along with four lifelong friends, established the Jammu and Kashmir Mountaineering and Hiking Club. After the mandatory two-year premed at SP College, he joined GMC in 1962 at the age of sixteen, in the fourth batch of the newly established Government Medical College.

Two years after graduating from GMC, he was selected to receive formal mountaineering training at the Indian Mountaineering Institute in Darjeeling. His mentors there included the late Tensing Norgay (who accompanied Sir

Edmund Hillary on his historic summit of Mount Everest), Sherpa Gombu (the first person to summit Mount Everest twice, a record he held for twenty years), and Colonel Singh (the first, and at that time only, Indian national to summit Mount Everest).

Dr. Mir graduated from GMC in June 1967. He has fond memories of participating in dramas, interclass sports competitions, and was one of seven students selected for a college-financed tour of India (which included a breakfast with then prime minister of India Indira Gandhi at her residence in Delhi). After completing his internship and a brief period in Jammu, he joined the medical unit headed by the renowned physician and master clinician Dr. Ali Mohammad Jan. Dr. Mir, along with one classmate, was selected as the first batch for an MD (postgraduate course in medicine) at GMC, Srinagar. Under the tutelage of Prof. Zahoor Ahmad, he studied peptic ulcer disease in Kashmir. His research required the use of upper GI endoscopy. While the first flexible endoscope in J&K had been purchased over a year earlier, it had remained under lock in Ward 6 of SMHS Hospital. After a monumental effort, in 1970, Dr. Mir was able to secure the use of the flexible endoscope and help establish a GI lab in a side room of Ward 3 of SMHS Hospital and contributed towards the era of GI endoscopy in J&K (previously, endoscopies were performed by the ENT staff using a rigid metallic scope).

In the same week in 1971, Dr. Mir received invitations to pursue two lifelong dreams: an invitation to participate in an international group's planned ascent of Mount Everest and an offer to pursue specialized training in nephrology in the United Kingdom. Dr. Mir elected to pursue his opportunity to become a nephrologist and, in June 1971, started as a senior house officer in medicine and nephrology in Liverpool, UK, which he pursued further in the USA at the University of Missouri in Kansas City, Missouri. He was appointed as the lecturer in medicine and later a clinical professor in medicine and nephrology at the University of Missouri School of Medicine and also at the School of Health Sciences, both in Kansas City. From 1975 until his retirement in 2009, Dr. Mir practiced as a nephrologist with Midwest Nephrology Consultants, where he was the founding director. He is boarded in the speciality of internal medicine and subspecialty of nephrology and has published several papers on topics in clinical nephrology and transplantation. In his professional capacity, he serves various community organizations including as a board member of the Midwest Transplant Network since 1986 and member of the Ethics Committee of the National Kidney Foundation.

In Kansas City, Missouri, Dr. Mir invested heavily in the development of a Muslim community. When he arrived in 1972, there were very few Muslims, no Muslim community, and no mosques. . To participate in his first Eid prayer after arriving in the US, Dr. Mir had to drive over two hundred kilometers to Manhattan, Kansas, where the campus of Kansas State University was located and a group of international students had organized an Eid prayer. That fall, he attended his first annual convention of the Muslim Students Association in the US. That experience led to a life membership in the organization and inspired the establishment of a formal Muslim community in Kansas City called the Islamic Society of Greater Kansas City, which began its activities in a rented space in a local church. After many years of planning, fundraising, and organizing, a mosque was built and formally opened in March 1981. Dr. Mir played a key role in the creation of the ISGKC, the building of the first mosque in Kansas City, and the development of the Muslim community in Kansas City for over four decades, including a full-time Islamic school. In 1989, he became a founding member of the Interfaith Council of Greater Kansas City. In 2008, he was instrumental in establishing the Midwest Islamic Council and received its Legacy Award in 2013. At a national level in the US, Dr. Mir serves as a founder and a member of the Development

Foundation Board of the Islamic Society of North America. He is also a life member of the Islamic Medical Association of North America, which he served as president from 2002 to 2003 and served on its board of regents as well. He established a free community health clinic in Kansas City in 2014.

During Dr. Mir's yearly summer visits to Kashmir, he regularly provides free medical consultations, participates in ward rounds, and lectures at SMHS and SKIMS Hospitals. Most remarkably, he succeeded in the initiation of kidney transplantation at SKIMS in July 1999 performed by a team headed by surgeon Dr. Tajammul Fazili, the nephrology group headed by Dr. Salim Najar and the superb backing of then director Dr. Mehraj-ud-Din. Regrettably, despite multiple attempts and detailed expert planning, a time-consuming and cherished dream of establishing a world-class tertiary care hospital, by a group of nonresident Kashmiri friends, in Srinagar could not come to fruition. However, he firmly believes that a physician is uniquely qualified to influence many a sphere of the community in a very positive manner.

Dr. Mir married Naseema Jan Hakim in 1973. He currently lives in Northern Virginia in the US with his wife. He has three children and four grandchildren.

Dr. Arfa Rasool Khan

Arfa Rasool is the second of six children—four girls and two boys. Her father, Dr. Ghulam Rasool, was the legendary surgeon of Kashmir, and her mother, Ruqia, was the key force in inculcating the importance of higher education in her children, something she herself was unable to accomplish. She created and ensured an appropriate home environment for this to happen, which resulted in four doctors: Arfa, Rabia, Ayaz as GMC alumni, and Zahida as the alumnus of Lady Harding, Delhi. Besides this, the other children became accomplished professionals; Ajaz became an engineer, and Abida a physicist/businesswoman.

Dr. Arfa R. Khan has several unique accomplishments to her credit; she joined GMC in the first batch in 1959 and set all kinds of academic records, graduating as the first valedictorian of GMC in 1964. In addition to her academic excellence, she served as a class representative, general secretary, and was the All-Round Best Athlete for 1960. She also participated in the college dramatic society. In his letter of recommendation, Principal Lt. Col. S. Kaul wrote, "She is one of the very intelligent and hardworking doctors of GMC and I am sure she will be an asset to any institution she may work in." Professor Kaul's prediction was right on target.

After marriage to her classmate Faroque Khan, ARK migrated to the USA in 1966 and obtained training in radiology at Long Island Jewish Medical Center (LIJMC) in New York, where she remained till her retirement, initially as an instructor and later on taking charge of the Thoracic Radiology Division. In 2015, at an awards ceremony, her department chairman Dr. Larry Davis stated, "The Department of Radiology at North Shore LIJ Health System wants to congratulate Dr. Arfa Khan on her incredible achievement—45 years of service to the health system and especially Long Island Jewish Medical Center. She has been indispensable to the department. We are all very proud of her accomplishments."

The CEO Michael Dowling, in his letter of congratulations celebrating her forty-five years of service, wrote, "Our employees are our greatest asset. It is the talented, creative and hardworking people like you who set us apart from other organizations." Indeed a remarkable accomplishment of having worked in the same institution for decades and getting recognized for this service.

In March 2018, ARK retired after fifty years working at LIJMC first as a trainee (1967–1970) and later as a consultant (1971–2018) and chief of Thoracic Radiology. She retired as professor emeritus at the Zucker School of Medicine at Hofstra/Northwell and continued giving lectures to the radiology residents till 2020. Her retirement was celebrated at a large gala event attended by family, friends, and colleagues.

Dr. Arfa Khan is a nationally and internationally known thoracic radiologist as well as a researcher. She is dedicated to excellence in patient care and has stayed on the cutting edge of new technologies. She has trained generations of radiologists and has been a role model to all. She has won the department's Resident Teaching Award several times.

When asked to comment on the impact of ARK, one of the graduates, Dr. Karen Song, currently on the faculty at Johns Hopkins Medical School, stated, "I had the good fortune of getting to know Dr. Arfa Khan during my Radiology Residency at LIJMC. From the moment I met her, Dr. Khan has inspired me to strive to be the best radiologist I could be, she has been an outstanding role model as a successful woman in medicine. She helped shape my decision to become a thoracic radiologist. Dr. Khan prioritized resident lectures and had an extensive interesting case and teaching file that was available to residents as needed. She initiated the Chest Case of the Week, which was a weekly activity in which interesting cases were either hung on a view box or distributed electronically. Residents participated by submitting their responses including a differential diagnosis privately, and then Dr. Khan would review the case in chest conference. The resident with the greatest number of correct responses would win a certificate and an award—typically funded by Dr. Khan—at the end of the academic year at graduation. This is just one example of the creative ways in which Dr. Khan made learning thoracic radiology fun and challenging."

Dr. Khan has had extensive research interests during her career, including pulmonary emphysema, solitary pulmonary nodule, pulmonary embolism, and lung cancer screening. She has over two hundred published articles, presentations, and scientific exhibits to her credit. On a personal level, Dr. Khan is loved by all of her residents and coworkers, which is due in no small part to her warm and friendly demeanor.

At the national level, ARK was a founding member of the Society of Thoracic Radiology and a regular participant at its annual meeting. She also chaired the chest panel of ACR Appropriateness Criteria and served as the American Board of Radiology examiner. She contributed her expertise and knowledge internationally and commenting on her role in improving the standards of radiology in Saudi Arabia. Dr. Sven Larsson, the director of imaging at King Fahd Medical City, noted, "She has through the years volunteered her services in teaching our radiology residents, conducting board review courses and her yearly visit is one of the highlights for our department. Prof Arfa was the initiator and co-organizer for our first International Cardiothoracic Imaging Conference here in

Riyadh in 2012 which was a great success. I am forever grateful for Prof. Arfa's unsurpassed commitment to our department and our radiology residents."

Responding to the need for providing proper religious education to her children, she, along with a few other like-minded parents, founded the Islamic Center of Long Island (ICLI), which has now developed into one of the leading progressive Islamic centers in the USA. She served as a volunteer Sunday school teacher for ICLI and also as one of its first female executive committee members and currently is a member of its board of trustees.

ARK also played a major role in contributing towards the development of the Islamic Medical Association of North America, where she served on the executive committee and as a member of its board and was a regular contributor as a speaker at its annual national and regional meetings.

ARK has contributed in several educational initiatives at GMC in Kashmir, including on-hand training in CT-guided lung biopsy. She mentored Dr. Mukhtar during his short-term training in radiology at LIJMC and has contributed towards the development of mental health services in the valley. After the floods of 2014, ARK participated in many meetings and helped towards relief work in Kashmir.

On a personal level, she celebrated her fifty-seventh wedding anniversary with her husband and batch mate at GMC, Faroque Khan, on April 16, 2023. They are blessed with son, Arif, a world-renowned pediatric ophthalmologist, and his wife, Seema, a lawyer; daughter, Shireen, a youth transition counselor; and grandkids, Hasan and Leena. Given her outstanding contributions, an Arfa Khan named scholarship was established in 2020 at the Kashmir Education Initiative in Kashmir, which supports both undergraduate and postgraduate students. Currently, ARK is enjoying her retirement with family and friends.

Dr. Faroque Ahmad Khan

It was the early '90s, and I was a medical student at Government Medical College, Srinagar. Life was tough; there was pain, killing, and scare all around Kashmir. For those of us studying medicine, there was double trouble- the burden of medical studies and the stress of turmoil; I wanted to express my pain—cry for all that I had lost. Health care was gasping, college was just surviving, but I didn't know whom to ask—to fix it! With external turmoil, the internal turmoil became unbearable, but as I was getting into a higher professional, there was no time for me to cry my heart out. I became a machine gradually, remembering, recollecting, and rehearsing the difficult chapters of medicine and surgery.

And then it changed one day. It was 1999, and I came across a notice on the college notice board. Someone in America wanted an essay on any aspect of health care in Kashmir. I wrote my essay—a sentimental one about the plunder of health care in Kashmir amid turmoil and highlighted the agony of Kashmiri patients. I forgot all about the essay—for a couple of months—when, one day, I was informed that my essay titled "Kashmiri Patients—Innocent or Ignorant" had won AFK (Arfa and Faroque Khan Foundation) sponsored Dr. Ghulam Rasool Memorial Award. I attended the award ceremony. An immaculately dressed gentleman with a clear voice gave the Dr. Ghulam Rasool Memorial Oration. I was called to the stage—a young postgraduate, I was praised for my essay and presented a cheque for seventy-five dollars. I was bursting with happiness—someone had read my essay, appreciated my views, and encouraged me. The man who delivered Dr. Ghulam Rasool Memorial Oration was Dr. Faroque Khan, professor and chairman of Medicine at Nassau County Medical Center, New York. He helped me to pen my thoughts and took a transcontinental flight to honor me—there were six more students who were honored with me.

With this award, unknown happiness returned to me. Hitherto clogged, my mind started opening. I began to write more. I rejoiced as my essays were adjured the best by AFK foundation for three consecutive years. From here onward, I wrote under the pseudonym of Umimaryam and later on gathered enough courage to own my writings in newspapers and journals. I had found an outlet; my thoughts had found a channel—and thanks to Dr. Faroque Khan for giving me an opportunity to find my love. After a year or two, Greater Kashmir held an essay competition on the Kashmir imbroglio. I was no Kashmir expert, but I wrote my own tale—I won an impossible second prize worth Rs 10,000/-. This was huge for a doctor sitting amid writers who were experts on Kashmir! The day came in my life just because Dr. Faroque Khan had encouraged me to write and write!

There was this initiative by Dr. Khan in Kashmir of the '90s—a Kashmir that was bleeding, and there were many more initiatives. He organized a couple of international conferences in Kashmir in collaboration with Kashmiri doctors, and he patronized Government Medical College Srinagar and arranged short training courses for Kashmiri doctors in the US to keep them abreast with the latest advancements in medicine and help them to improve their skills. Our dusty and desolate library at Government Medical College got its first computer through Dr. Khan. The world had marched ahead, and Dr. Khan was keen to see his alma mater having something basic, and he worked hard to get it.

This able son of soil assumed the role of a patron, a guide, and a teacher for all those Kashmiris who were fleeing their troubled motherland and seeking to launch their careers as doctors in the US. Prof. Mohammad Yousuf's ex-head, Department of Medicine, GMC, calls Dr. Khan "a global asset who made a significant contribution to the world of medicine and held out a helping hand to his own Kashmiri doctors when they needed him. GMC Srinagar is proud of one of its ablest students and Kashmir too is proud of its son."

Dr. Khan was born in Udhampur in 1942. He did his schooling from Presentation Convent/DAV High School and SP College. He was a bright, meticulous, and hardworking student, tailor-made to undertake a journey towards becoming a doctor. He joined Government Medical College, Srinagar, in 1959 and completed the course in 1964 as the student of the first batch. His illustrious father, Mr. Ghulam Hassan Khan, a Harvard qualified engineer who held many important portfolios in Kashmir, was instrumental in inculcating in him a vision for the exploration of a world beyond Kashmir, benefitting from the science and technological advancements of a brighter world and at the same time keeping an eye on one's "roots." Heeding to his father's advice, he qualified ECFMG in 1965. The journey of Kashmiri doctors in the US begins with Dr. Khan when he and his wife, Dr. Arfa, arrived in the USA in May 1966, a month after their wedding. Their choice of selection of training positions was determined by the prevailing circumstances. The good news was the availability of numerous training positions in almost all fields because of the lack of an adequate supply of US graduates, many of whom were being conscripted for Vietnam war duty. The not-so-good news was that there was hardly anyone around who could guide them. Dr. Khan did his internship in 1966–1967 at Barberton Citizens Hospital, Ohio, and his residency in 1967–1970 at Queens General Hospital in NYC.

While at QHC during his second year, he was on a rotation to the Pulmonary Service, and towards the end of the rotation, he was called to the office of the chief. Such calls usually spell trouble; however, he was pleasantly surprised when Dr. Nathan Seriff, the chief of the Pulmonary Service, offered him a fellowship in pulmonary medicine, although Dr. Khan's initial choice was GI, Dr. Seriff, a great mentor and teacher changed his orientation. After finishing pulmonary training, Dr. Seriff offered him a job as an attending physician, with major administrative responsibilities involving the supervision of Drs. Lamberta, Epstein, and others who had been his teachers. Recalling his interaction with his teachers, Dr. Khan says, "Up to June 30 1972 I was student/trainee and on July 1st 1972 I was 'managing/supervising' my teachers, I had lots of hesitation in asking my teachers to follow the new rules and regulations as we were busy developing a modern teaching service, they—former teachers, great clinicians—were willing, cooperative, helpful and supportive. In fact, Dr Epstein a great expert in TB management gifted me his entire teaching file of X-rays when he retired and I used it during my teaching sessions at QHC and later on at NCMC as chair of medicine. This is reflective of the systems in the USA where by and large talent gets recognized and everyone benefits."

Dr. Faroque Khan—a competent doctor, a compassionate human being, and a visionary leader—evolved into one of the most famous names Government Medical College, Srinagar, had ever produced. The chair of Medicine at Stony Brook, Dr. Harry Fritts, encouraged Dr. Khan to apply for the position of chair of Medicine at Nassau County Medical Center. He was selected from among twenty-nine candidates; all of whom except Dr. Khan were US medical graduates. Dr. Khan was at NCMC from 1987 to 1999, responsible for the training of ninety-nine internal medicine trainees and fellows in twelve medical specialities. At Nassau County Medical Center, he played a father figure role for Kashmiris seeking to find residency and fellowships in the US.

Dr. Faroque did a remarkable work on Quinolones and was a pioneer in introducing ciprofloxacin in patients with respiratory tract infections. He became an expert on the subject and shared his experience globally, generating over $1 million for his department in Queens Hospital Center, which helped to launch the careers of many doctors—some of them from his alma mater.

As a member of the American College of Physicians, he helped it to overcome the bias and discrimination against international medical graduates (IMGs). After a lot of hard work, he was successful in authoring a book, *IMGs—Guide for Applicants and Program Directors*, which was published by ACP in 1995. His commitment and innovative approach to tackle various problems was acknowledged, and he was elected regent of ACP and served it from 1995 to 2001—the first IMG to hold that position. He helped open new avenues for ACP in countries like Saudi Arabia and Jordan. Dr. Khan became a powerful voice in ACP—the largest medical speciality organization with more than 120,000 members globally—and was bestowed the mastership in ACP in 1994.

Dr. Khan and his influence beyond America was apparent when he was approached to treat King Fahd of Saudi Arabia in 2005 when Dr. Abdullah Amro, the CEO of King Fahd Medical City (KFMC), requested him to join his team as a consultant at KFMC. Dr. Faroque shared his expertise and helped to develop the institution by recruiting top-notch faculty, developing a research program, and advising on facilities and infrastructure. Dr. Abdullah Amro, recalling his contribution to health care in Saudi Arabia, says, "From the first encounter I was very much impressed with Dr. Khan's medical, leadership, and personality capabilities. He worked on a few extremely important projects.

He helped us in recruiting the best medical staff and establish the medical bylaws. He helped us in arranging summer studies for our medical students in the United States. He also helped the medical college at KFMC to build the international relations. He was behind the idea of establishing an ACP Chapter in Saudi Arabia. He was able to invite pioneers in the medical field to visit Saudi Arabia and help in improving the image of the Saudi Heath care system."

Dr. Faroque Khan stayed in Saudi Arabia for five years and helped many institutions in Saudi Arabia in planning their teaching and training of medical students and faculty. At KFMC, he arranged training of nursing students from Kashmir's Bibi Halima Nursing College. Each year, ten to fifteen nursing students from the said college received practical hands-on training at KFMC in a highly advanced center, and, since 2009, over sixty students have graduated and returned to Kashmir with a broader and better feel for the profession. The nonresident Kashmiri doctors happily supported the program.

Dr. Khan has served as the President of IMANA (Islamic Medical Association of North America) and is presently overseeing its international initiatives. The organization's commendable efforts encompass acts of charity, medical help, and help rendered at the time of disasters . Dr. Faroque has helped to generate resources for this organization and has played a key role in the success of this organization. In 2011, he helped set up an International Collaborative Program between IMANA in the USA and KSA with the transfer and sharing of knowledge. Dr. Faroque oversaw the publication of a book regarding the first fifty years of IMANA titled *Serving Faith, Profession and Community.* Under his leadership, IMR/IMANA was selected as the winner of the 2016 ACP Rosenthal Award.

A devout Muslim himself, Dr. Khan authored a book titled *Story of a Mosque in America*, which was published in 2001. He enriched the cosmopolitan environment of New York (Long

Island) with his community service and interfaith dialogues. The reason this book was written was, while Muslims on an individual basis were doing their part in explaining the faith of Islam to non-Muslims, the management at ICLI felt that there is need for an institutional effort to present the true image of Islam, which embodies peace, justice, and moderation, with a focus on the role of the mosque. This book provides that story, a journey that was fulfilling and challenging.

Dr. Khan talked about peace in a place threatened by war; he talked about love when hatred had become the order of the day, especially post-9/11. With Rabbi Jerome Davidson, he started a much-needed dialogue between Jews and Muslims in New York to bridge the gap between the two communities. Rabbi Jerome Davidson calls Dr. Faroque as a courageous community leader. The revered Rabbi says, "As the guiding spirit of the Islamic Center of Long Island, three decades ago in 1992 he and I met, together with a few lay people from each community, to establish one of the first, if not the first, on-going dialogue programs in the United States between a mosque and a synagogue. It was a time when American Jews and American Muslims were almost totally ignorant of each other, having no meaningful relationships and hardly aware of each other's presence in our two neighboring communities. There were certainly many Jews and Muslims who not only had no interest in such an alliance, they viewed it with fear and even antipathy. Yet, Faroque sensed the need for these two religious minorities to reach out to each other with understanding and friendship."

Dr. Khan has helped all, especially the needy, strangers, and those who had great dreams about America but were clueless as to how to achieve them. Vouching for his secular credentials is the touching story of Dr. Ashok Karnik, who was trapped without support in America once the war broke out in Kuwait. Recalling his struggles in the US, Dr. Karnik says, "Life plays strange games of ups and downs: in Kuwait, I was in a position when I had sponsored Dr. Khan as a Visiting Professor; two decades later, he was able to find my first job in USA when I was in need. What is more remarkable is, that, his behavior towards me did not change one iota during those 'up' and 'down' periods of my life. Some of his gestures during that period, such as his walking down to the car park with me to 'admire' my first car in the USA, a small Buick, which I am sure he did to boost my morale and allow me to use his Chairman's office, when, as a research fellow, I had no designated place to sit, have left an indelible mark on my memory and taught me many practical life-lessons. One rarely gets the pleasure and privilege of working with a colleague and a Chairman who makes your job a pleasure, a friend who stands by you in the time of your need, a physician, who by his own example, teaches you how real good medicine should be practised and who, as your mentor, literally helps alter the course of your life. Dr. Khan is such an individual. But above all, he is a fine man with wonderful qualities of heart and mind."

Continuing with my own story and my love for writing, I wrote a book *White Man in Dark*, purging out my experiences as a doctor and a medical student studying medicine in the worst phase of Kashmir's history. Our tragedies needed to be told to the world too busy with its own happenings. The book was received well by doctors and Kashmir experts. There was a calling in the book for all the nonresident Kashmiri doctors, reminding them about the homeland that was in tatters. Dr. Faroque heard about my book, got in touch with me, and purchased one hundred copies, distributing them for free among nonresident Kashmiri doctors in the US. Not just that; wherever he went, he distributed copies of the book among the intelligentsia and the elite.

Following devastating floods of 2014, the submerged GMC Srinagar robbed Dr. Khan of his sleep. He rushed to Kashmir with help from IMANA. He got in touch with the key folks in the administration and offered his advice and assistance. I saw him in a meeting of GMC alumni nearly fifteen years after I had seen him last. Same looks, same commitment—but in the attire of a fighter, sports shoes, jacket, and a cap. I heard him—there were pearls of wisdom flowing out of his mouth, and I was impressed yet again by Dr. Khan as he offered his help to the sinking alma mater. I couldn't help but admire the meticulousness of this great man—notwithstanding his silver eyebrows and snow-white hair, his aggressiveness to pursue a matter to a logical end was unmatched.

The thought of writing a brief autobiographical sketch of one hundred Kashmiri doctors struck me. I shared this thought with Dr. Khan and requested his coauthorship. He was quick to respond to my request and, in fact, gave the much-needed ignition to the project. The project was recognized as workable just because Dr. Khan is a part of it. What is my standing otherwise?

A generous man that Dr. Faroque Khan is, he wired a big amount of money to a student who couldn't afford admission to IIT and promised him a scholarship during his studies when he got to know about the poverty-struck bright boy from Kashmir who, otherwise, had to forgo his seat.

I know there are many people from Kashmir whom Dr. Faroque Khan has helped, many more whom he has inspired, many Kashmiri doctors who traveled to America struggling to launch their dreams and Dr. Faroque helped them realize those dreams, many lucky Americans whom he has taught and treated, and many more with whom he has talked "peace." I wish I could do justice while I attempt to write his profile. Dr. Faroque Khan is a better profile writer than me; he has written some jaw-dropping profiles of some of his colleagues in the USA, including a soul-touching profile of his illustrious father.

Dr. Faroque's life is an inspiration. He is notably the most outstanding face that GMC Srinagar has produced! Together with his brilliant wife, Dr. Arfa Khan, who is an accomplished radiologist, they represent a prototype of what a Kashmiri can do and how best he/she can help the people back home. Dr. Faroque is a family man; he has a son, Arif, a successful ophthalmologist working at Cleveland Clinic Abu Dhabi Specialist Hospital in Abu Dhabi, UAE; and a daughter, Shireen, who did master's in education in counseling psychology. Arif's wife, Seema, is an accomplished attorney, and they are blessed with two kids, Hasan and Leena.

Dr. Faroque has led a life many of us only dream about. About his life, he says, "I thank Allah for all the blessings He has bestowed upon me—loving caring nurturing family, an opportunity to learn and work in the USA, serving people of all faiths both in the USA and globally and mentoring many bright minds. I regret that individually and collectively we the NRK's were unable to do more for Kashmir's health care. Sadly, our proposal for building a modern hospital in Srinagar was not approved by the J&K government."

He wishes for a trouble-free Kashmir that has adequate health-care facilities and adequate training facilities for budding doctors.

Dr. Fayaz Shawl

Dr. Shawl is currently the director of Interventional Cardiology at Adventist Health Care White Oak Medical Center, Silver Spring, Maryland, as well as a clinical professor of Medicine at George Washington University School of Medicine in Washington, DC, USA.

Dr. Shawl was born at Shamaswari, Srinagar, near Fateh Kadal, son of a handicraft dealer Mohammad Saleem. He and his elder sister Farida burned the midnight oil to become doctors. He wanted to become a pilot, but after his father died at a young age from cancer of the stomach, he decided to become a doctor. When he was just thirteen years, after his father's death, he tried odd jobs to help the family. They had no income except support of Rs 100 a month from his maternal uncle, Mr. Habib-ullah Gundroo. His other siblings are Farhat (doctor in genetics) and Farooq. After the matriculation examination that he passed in second attempt, he studied at SP College for two years before heading to the Medical College.

Dr. Shawl received his medical degree from Government Medical College, Srinagar, Kashmir, in 1972. At the Medical College, he was an average student and enjoyed taking part in the cultural programs of the college and was awarded the Best Actor Award in the college plays with the final plays being shown at the Tagore Hall. He fondly recalls his first assignment as assistant surgeon at Shahdara Sharief (Dispensary) in 1973 when he had to work as a sole family doctor for over six thousand patients. To reach this remote location, he had to take a short flight (from Srinagar to Jammu), followed by a ten-hour bus ride to Rajouri, and, finally, a two-to-three-hour horse ride to Shahdara Sharief. The natives often called Dr. Shawl on weekends to arbitration. After a ten-month stay, Dr. Shawl took a longer plane ride to England in 1974 with barely fifty dollars in his pocket. He borrowed money to get a ticket to UK and completed his residency in England.

In 1977, Dr. Shawl moved to the United States and had to start from scratch and therefore started his internship in internal medicine at Prince George's Hospital. With his background of residency training in the UK, it was quickly realized by the chief of Medicine, Dr. David Goldman, that Dr. Shawl was far too brilliant and far too knowledgeable to benefit from further training in internal medicine. Therefore, the last two years of his residency were waived off, and he was advanced to a cardiology fellowship. He then completed his final cardiology fellowship at Walter Reed Army Medical Center, Washington, DC. As a final-year fellow, Dr. Shawl heard about the angioplasty live course given by Andreas Gruentzig, and, after many hurdles, he went to learn angioplasty from him in Switzerland and then started the program at Walter Reed.

Dr. (Major) Shawl brought the military into the balloon age when he performed the first PTCA in the United States Military (Army, Navy, Air Force) at Walter Reed Army Medical Center in 1981. Dr. Shawl got a lot of opposition from surgical colleagues in starting the angioplasty program at a time when there were only two physicians in the Washington, DC, area. Despite these oppositions, he and others continued to show both scientifically and technically the feasibility of this alternative method of treating coronary artery disease. Finally, it was 1982 when FDA approved the angioplasty procedure.

Dr. Shawl is a fellow of the American College of Cardiology, the American College of Chest Physicians, the American

College of Physicians, the American College of Angiology, and the Society for Cardiac Angiography and Interventions.

Dr. Shawl has played an active role in all aspects of interventional cardiology ever since he performed the first PTCA at Walter Reed Army Medical Center in 1981. While he has lectured widely on every topic of interventional cardiology, he has been a leading proponent and innovator in the development of the percutaneous approach (known as the Shawl technique) to cardiopulmonary bypass support in "high-risk angioplasty and cardiac arrest," performing the first percutaneous bypass-supported coronary intervention in the world in 1988. Since its invention in 1988, there has not been a single death in the Cardiac Catheterization Laboratory at Washington Adventist while Dr. Shawl performed coronary interventions. He has lectured on this topic and trained physicians throughout the world.

Dr. Shawl has been teaching through live demonstrations other techniques of interventional cardiology (including coronary, carotid, and other peripheral and noncardiac interventions like valvuloplasty, an ablative technique for IHSS, etc.) at Washington Adventist Hospital and all over the world. Such types of teaching seminars are done through satellite or local broadcasts live from the cath lab.

Dr. Shawl in collaboration with V. M. Kasim, chairman of Interventional Technologies Pvt, New Delhi, embarked on a mission of bringing interventional cardiology skills to South Asia in 1989. Commenting on this collaboration that transformed interventional cardiology in South Asia, Kasim, in a note of thanks, stated, "The first effort was in All India Institute of Medical Sciences in New Delhi in 1989 where you were able to demonstrate a CPS System very successfully. Since then there has been no end to the various workshops conducted by you, teaching budding Interventional Cardiologists how to perform intricate interventional procedures. I still remember the days and nights we spent traveling through Rawalpindi, Lahore, Karachi and then on to New Delhi. I cannot even recollect the number of cases you did and the applause you received from hundreds of cardiologists and physicians who were present in these workshops and meetings. In fact, without your help and assistance, Interventional Cardiology in this part of the world, would not have taken off and attained the proportion that it has reached today. It will be no exaggeration to say that our combined efforts (particularly yours) have been mainly responsible for bringing Interventional Cardiology to this stage that it is in India, Pakistan and Bangladesh. Before concluding this note, I cannot just think of any other person who has made so much of a contribution towards the progress of Interventional Cardiology in South Asia. Fayaz, all the credit goes to you, and I do hope you will continue to be associated with such educational programs in future."

A true innovator in working with the high-risk patient, Dr. Shawl was the first interventional cardiologist to use both the Eclipse Holmium Laser as well as the AngioTrax mechanical device (1999) for percutaneous transluminal myocardial revascularization in the investigational treatment of end-stage atherosclerotic heart disease (patients with no options). He did both procedures as part of research first in the world at New Delhi, India. He was also the first to perform the first mitral valvuloplasty in the Washington, DC, metropolitan area in 1985 and aortic valvuloplasty in 1986.

Dr. Shawl is a member of the renowned International Gruentzig Society and was recognized as one of the world's most talented interventionists in an interview for the *Journal of Invasive Cardiology* in April 2001 (JIC, vol. 13, no. 4, April 2001). He was acknowledged to have performed the most interventional procedures as a single operator (over nineteen thousand) in 2001 among any other interventionists in the world.

Currently, in pursuit of stroke prevention, the number-two cause of death, Dr. Shawl and others have pioneered the technique of carotid artery stenting. He performed the first percutaneous carotid artery stenting in this region in 1995. The results of this new avenue of endovascular therapy may challenge the accepted practice of surgical carotid endarterectomy. Having done over 1,100 carotid stent cases at Washington Adventist Hospital, using the present technique what he calls "meticulous technique" has resulted in a complication rate of < 0.5% in the last six hundred cases. He is also quite active in Structural Heart Program and performs "transcatheter aortic valve replacement" (TAVR) for patients with critical aortic stenosis as well as MitraClip procedure in patients who are deemed inoperable or "high risk" for conventional open heart surgery.

Dr. Shawl has a very active, accredited interventional fellowship program at Washington Adventist Hospital in association with the program at George Washington University Hospital in Washington, DC. He loves to "teach" interventional procedures in the cath lab. Dr. Shawl does not play any kind of sports and has no major hobbies except innovative research and development of innovative techniques in interventional cardiology. He has participated in over 140 research projects. Problems in interventional cardiology and difficult patient scenarios have kept him professionally challenged.

Dr. Shawl has authored over 150 leading articles, abstracts, editorials, and book chapters. He has also published a book entitled *Supported Complex and High-Risk Coronary Angioplasty.* Dr. Shawl has also received many awards for his innovative work in interventional cardiology. Some of his awards include the 2002 Innovators Award from the Alliance of Cardiovascular Professionals of the United States and Best Teachers Awards from Residents from the Maryland State Senate and the United States Congress (1992). Among other major awards Dr. Shawl received was the dedication of the Fayaz

Shawl Advanced Interventional Catheterization Laboratory at Washington Adventist Hospital in 1998. This unique event was attended by dignitaries from all walks of life. This unique recognition was bestowed upon Dr. Shawl for his innumerable contributions in the interventional cardiology. He is in fact considered a beacon for the advancement and teaching of interventional cardiac therapy. He received National Leadership Award from United States Congress in 2003. Dr. Shawl was also nominated as the International Health Professional of the Year (2003) by the Research and Advisory Board sitting at the International Biographical Center in Cambridge, England. This prestigious award is given to individuals whose achievements and leadership stand out in the international community. Dr. Shawl also received an award from the State of Maryland for his outstanding achievement and advancements in the field of cardiology. Dr. Shawl is also the only physician to be interviewed by *Insight"* on *The News Magazine*. In 2011, Dr. Shawl was recognized by the House of Representatives (United States Congress) as the world's foremost interventional cardiologist. He is also the founder of the "Dr. Fayaz Shawl Philanthropic Foundation", to treat impoverished patients. (Congressional Records, p. E469, vol. 157).

While the technical skills of Dr. Shawl are legendary, his interpersonal and doctor-patient relationships are best stated in a letter sent by a patient Leonard Ruben, who also happens to be a senior judge. Judge Ruben opined, "You are a living embodiment of the meaning of the Hippocratic Oath. I thank you, my children thank you and Ide thanks you for the quality of life you have afforded me. Your hands are golden, your mind that of a genius and your heart larger than the world itself." At this dedication of his cath lab, Dr. Richard Myler (who did the first human angioplasty in the world with Dr. Anreas Gruentzig—the inventor of angioplasty) wrote, "Charles Dotter and Andreas Gruentzig taught us the concepts of Intervention, you, have shown us what is possible with imagination, honesty, courage, enthusiasm, endless energy, patience, kindness and extraordinary talent." His teacher from Walter Reed Army Medical Center wrote, "I feel deeply honored to have had a small hand in your career development . . . your accomplishment in the world of Interventional cardiology, both as a clinician and as a researcher, have earned you the reputation as one of the World's leaders in the rapidly growing and critically important field of cardiovascular therapeutics."

To share his experience in the interventional treatment of cardiovascular diseases with an even broader population of physicians and patients who may not now have access to such techniques or facilities, Dr. Shawl established the Dr. Fayaz Shawl Philanthropic Foundation Inc., which has assisted many needy patients. During his frequent visits to Kashmir, Dr. Shawl brought supplies like coronary stents, catheters, etc. worth thousands of dollars and donated them to the SKIMS in Kashmir. His dream of developing a modern cardiac center in Kashmir did not come through, and, commenting on this disappointment, Dr. Shawl stated, "This was probably the saddest day of my life when I was not permitted to build the Hospital in Srinagar. I am in the process of selling the land I had brought for the hospital and proceedings will be given to charity."

When asked to recall some unique events from his illustrious career and the mentors/role models who influenced him the most, Dr. Shawl stated, "There have been many mentors who helped me to build my career. In the United Kingdom, it was Dr. Fletcher and then in the United States Dr. David Goldman to whom I remain indebted. I feel, the most key moment in my career 'personally fulfilling' was to marry my wife Gina. With her, I have a terrific daughter Isabella. I have two great sons David and Jonathan from my previous marriage. David is a Cinematographer in Hollywood and Jonathan is a Paramedic. I remain grateful to my Wife Gina and my kids for their support and love which keeps me going."

For medical students or young physicians, Dr. Shawl offered a few tips on how to establish a long successful and rewarding career. "The key is to work hard and take advantage of the opportunities that come your way," Dr. Shawl said. "That was helpful for me, and I have always found taking on new challenges to be very rewarding."

It's indeed a great honor to share a brief synopsis of Dr. Fayaz Shawl, a brilliant thinker and innovator blessed with outstanding technical skills.

Dr. Hamid Band

Hamid Band, MD, PhD, is the Elizabeth Bruce Professor of Cancer Research at the Eppley Institute for Research in Cancer and Allied Diseases of the University of Nebraska Medical Center (UNMC). He joined UNMC in November 2007, bringing with him his extensive experience on the leadership team of the NCI-designated Robert H. Lurie Comprehensive Cancer Center, a nationally renowned and highly funded cancer research program and an outstanding team of researchers.

At UNMC, Dr. Band served as associate director of Translational Research (until 2020) and currently serves as coleader of the Cancer Biology Program for the NCI-designated Fred and Pamela Buffett Cancer Center; director of the Center for Breast Cancer Research; a member of the Fred and Pamela Buffett Cancer Center Internal Advisory Council; member of the Eppley Institute Senior Leadership Committee; member of the Internal Advisory Board of the NCI Specialized Program of Research Excellence (SPORE) in Pancreatic Cancer; and member of the Promotion and Tenure Committee of the Eppley Institute. In his leadership roles, Dr. Band works closely with the cancer center director and other senior leaders to help sustain and expand basic science programs of the cancer center, promote collaborative projects between faculty in natural sciences and biologists/clinicians, facilitate translation of basic science discoveries into clinical interventions, develop and implement strategic goals of the cancer center; promote philanthropic and community outreach activities, develop strategies toward the goal of NCI designation as a comprehensive cancer center, recruit talented faculty to the institution, and mentor junior faculty. Dr. Band has been a part of the senior leadership team that has overseen the successful renewal of the NCI designation of the Fred and Pamela Buffett Cancer Center in 2011, 2016, and 2021 and oversees the ongoing expansion of the Cancer Campus at UNMC.

Dr. Band earned his MD in 1977 from the Government Medical College Srinagar, Kashmir University, India, graduating at the top of his class of 130. Following internship and residency in internal medicine and pharmacology, he elected to pursue research, receiving a PhD in immunology from the All-India Institute of Medical Sciences, New Delhi, India, in 1986. He trained as a postdoctoral fellow in immunology and an instructor in pathology and medicine between 1984 and 1989 at the Dana-Farber Cancer Institute, Harvard Medical School. He served as a member of the Faculty of Medicine as an assistant and associate professor and as a member of the Immunology Graduate Program at Harvard Medical School between 1989 and 2003. From 1992 to 2003, Dr. Band served on the faculty of the Division of Rheumatology, Allergy and Immunology at Brigham and Women's Hospital of the Harvard Medical School, now a partner of the Mass General Hospital-Brigham and Women's Hospital partnership. In 2003, Dr. Band joined Northwestern University as a professor of medicine in the Feinberg School of Medicine and as director of the Division of Molecular Oncology and Jean Ruggles-Romoser chair of Cancer Research at Evanston Northwestern Healthcare Research Institute and as professor of Biochemistry, Molecular Biology and Cell Biology at the Weinberg College of Arts and Sciences of Northwestern University. At Northwestern, Dr. Band served in senior leadership positions including the program leader of the Hormone Action and Signal Transduction

Basic Science Program, member of the Executive and Internal Advisory Committees, codirector of the SPORE in Breast Cancer, member of the Roadmap Committee for university-wide strategic planning, the advisory board of High Throughput Facility/RNAi Core, Advisory Board of Chicago Signal Transduction Society, Supra-departmental Search Committee for cancer-related faculty recruitment, and search Committee for Chair of Medicine. He served as a project coinvestigator with Drs. Vimla Band and Sam Stupp on the NCI Center of Cancer Nanotechnology Excellence (CCNE) at Northwestern University. Dr. Band was a member of the leadership team that helped obtain the elite status NCI renewal for the Robert H. Lurie Comprehensive Cancer Center in 2007.

At UNMC, Dr. Band holds secondary appointments as a professor of biochemistry and molecular biology, genetics, cell biology and anatomy, pathology and microbiology, and pharmacology and experimental neuroscience in the College of Medicine. He is also a preceptor of cancer research, immunology and infectious diseases, molecular genetics and cell biology, and other graduate programs. His experience in graduate training includes being a former member of the Graduate Committee on Immunology at Harvard Medical School, as well of two umbrella graduate programs and the NIH-funded Medical Scientist (MD/PhD) Training Program at Northwestern University.

Dr. Band has served as a member of the editorial board of the *Journal of Biological Chemistry* (1999–2007), the NCI Cancer Etiology Study Section (2000–2004), the NCI Program Project Parent Committee (2004–2007), and the NCI Molecular Oncogenesis Study Sections. Dr. Band has received a number of awards including the Distinguished Lecturer Award of the MD Anderson Cancer Center in 2005, the UNMC Distinguished Scientist Award in 2008, the UNMC Distinguished Leadership Award in 2015, and the "Pink Tie Guy" Award from the Susan G. Komen Foundation of Nebraska in 2015.

The major focus of Dr. Band's nearly thirty-three-year extramurally funded research program is the regulatory interactions between endocytic traffic and cell signaling with the goal of developing targeted cancer therapeutics and biomarkers, immune modulators for cancer therapy and autoimmune disease, and studies of cancer stem cells. Dr. Band has authored over 215 original articles and reviews in top-tier scientific journals, and his work is highly cited.

Dr. Band currently oversees an extramurally funded and nationally reputed research program with students, fellows, and other scientists that he advises. Dr. Band has mentored over six -dozen students, fellows, and junior faculty members in his laboratory, and many of his former trainees now hold leadership positions in academic and pharmaceutical/biotechnology corporations.

Overall, Dr. Band is a physician-scientist on a lifelong mission of helping to enhance our understanding of the biology of diseases toward the goal of alleviating human suffering, especially from cancer.

Dr. Iftikhar J. Kullo

Iftikhar Kullo was born in Saraf Kadal, Srinagar, Kashmir, to Ghulam Nabi and Ameena Kullo, the eldest of five siblings. Iftikhar (or Ifi as he is known to his friends and teachers in Kashmir) went to Presentation Convent, Woodlands, and Burn Hall for elementary, middle, and high school, respectively. He recalls his childhood as a particularly happy period with summers spent in Kashmir and winters in Jammu. His major influence growing up was his maternal uncle Ghulam Ahmed Ahanger, a secular intellectual who shaped his thinking and future direction. Iftikhar's passions as a student were literature and cricket, and his ambition was to become a writer. His uncle, a great admirer of Dr. Ali Mohammad Jan, pointed out that earning a livelihood as a writer would be difficult, but a vocation as a physician would allow him to serve the community, support himself, and pursue his interest in writing.

Consequently, Iftikhar entered a premedical track in the SP College of Science, Srinagar. In 1980, he entered the Government Medical College, Srinagar, and on completion of training received the Best Outgoing Graduate Award. Iftikhar's favorite subjects were physiology, pharmacology, and internal medicine. After internship, he served as a house officer in Dr. GQ Allaqaband's Ward 3 team in the SMHS Hospital. He also distinguished himself in sports, captaining the medical school cricket team and playing for Kashmir University.

After a nationwide qualifying examination, Iftikhar joined the Postgraduate Institution of Medical Education and Research (PGIMER), Chandigarh, in 1988, for postgraduate training in internal medicine. The institute, reputed for a fiercely academic atmosphere, provided a milieu that was transformative. Iftikhar's interest in vascular biology was fueled during this time while completing a research project in hypertension with Dr. B. K. Sharma. He was inspired by renowned teachers including Drs. Harinder Khattri (cardiology), Kartar Singh Chugh (nephrology), and Jagjit Singh Chopra (neurology). "The training in PGIMER was outstanding and has stood me in good stead. I am indebted to that institution and its faculty who inspired trainees to strive for excellence in academic medicine." In PGIMER, Iftikhar had the opportunity to take care of patients with diseases that he had not previously encountered including hepatic amoebiasis, neurocysticercosis, Takayasu's arteritis, and phosphorus poisoning.

Following PGIMER, Iftikhar sought further training in academic cardiovascular medicine in the US. In 1991, he took the ECFMG examination in Lahore, applied for an internship in the US, and was accepted to the Nassau County Medical Center, New York, by Dr. Faroque Khan. The academic environment in this institution was superb with master clinician-educators such as Drs. Donald Feinfeld, Christos Carvounis, and Faroque Khan. Caring for patients with the human immunodeficiency virus (HIV) infection, which at that time was at epidemic levels in the New York, left a lasting impression on Iftikhar. "Having trained in 'temperate' medicine in Kashmir, 'tropical medicine' in Chandigarh and 'HIV' medicine in New York, I felt my training in Internal Medicine was complete."

After the internship, Iftikhar was accepted into the clinician-investigator training program in cardiovascular medicine at the Mayo Clinic, in Rochester, Minnesota. During his two years of research, he studied the modulation of vascular function by dual angiotensin-converting enzyme and neutral endopeptidase inhibition as well as endothelial nitric oxide synthase (eNOS) gene transfer, with Drs. John Burnett and Tim O'Brien as mentors. A notable finding from his work was that adenoviral vector-mediated gene transfer of eNOS resulted in changes in vasomotor activity in an animal model. After the completion of clinical training in general cardiology and vascular medicine, Dr. Jamil Tajik, chair of the Cardiovascular Division at Mayo, recruited Iftikhar in May 1999. He established a practice in preventive cardiology and vascular medicine with a focus on heritable lipid disorders and early-onset coronary heart disease. Iftikhar credits Dr. Tajik for providing research time to junior faculty, which was pivotal in enabling him to obtain funding from the American Heart Association and eventually from the National Institutes of Health (NIH).

The NIH has continuously funded Dr. Kullo since 2003. His research on atherosclerosis in experimental animals and the molecular genetics of eNOS stimulated an interest in refining risk stratification for coronary heart disease using circulating biomarkers, noninvasive arterial assessment including endothelial function and arterial stiffness, and genetic markers of disease susceptibility. This led to several innovations at Mayo including the establishment of the Early Atherosclerosis Clinic in 2003, a novel cardiovascular marker risk panel for patients with a family history of coronary heart disease, as well as a panel for noninvasive tests of arterial function. Dr. Kullo received numerous awards including the Mayo Clinic New Investigator Award in 2006, authored more than 350 original papers, and has served on multiple NIH review panels including the Clinical and Integrative Cardiovascular Sciences (CICS) study section. He has mentored more than eighty research trainees/fellows/residents, many of whom have gone on to staff positions in various academic institutions around the country.

The current focus of Dr. Kullo's laboratory is implementing genomic medicine in clinical practice. He is the principal investigator in several National Human Genome Research Institute consortia including the Electronic Medical Records and Genomics (eMERGE) network, Polygenic Risk Methods in Diverse Populations (PRIMED) consortium and the Clinical Genome (ClinGen) Resource. In 2021, he was invited by the Hon'ble Xavier Becerra, Secretary of the Department of Health and Human Services (DHHS), to serve on the National Advisory Council on Human Genome Research of the NIH. As a council member, Iftikhar advises the DHHS and the NIH on genetics, genomic research, training, and programs related to the human genome initiative. Dr. Iftikhar J. Kullo was in news recently as he was nominated to the National Advisory Council on Human Genome Research (NACHGR) that the US National Institute of Health (NIH) runs. The orders were issued by Xavier Becerra, Joe Biden's secretary of health and human services (DHHS). Dr. Iftikhar will be part of the council till September 30, 2024. The NACHGR advises the US Department of Health and Human Services (DHHS), the National Institutes of Health (NIH), and the National Human Genome Research Institute (NHGRI) on genetics, genomic research, training, and programs related to the human genome initiative. Besides, the NACHGR performs second-level peer reviews for grant applications and determines the program priorities for NHGRI and the goals for the government's efforts in the International Human Genome Project (HGP).

"I am honored to serve on the National Advisory Council on Human Genome Research. Genomics is transforming biomedical research and I'm excited to have the opportunity to advise on the discovery and implementation aspects of genomic medicine to improve outcomes for our patients," Dr. Kullo said after his appointment to the National Advisory Council on Human Genome Research.

Iftikhar has three children, Aliya, Rehan, and Rauf, from his marriage to Dr. Salma Sayeed. All three were born in Rochester, Minnesota, and share a love for travel, sports, and their parental homeland of Kashmir. The extended family includes siblings Rafi, Shoukat, and Nusret and their families. His beloved sister, Sameena, passed away in 2021.

Dr. Iftikhar recalls his medical school days with nostalgia. He says, "I have fond memories of my medical school days. The situation at that time was peaceful; we had excellent teachers and an academic atmosphere. My friends included Drs. Mufti Mehmood, Javed Fazili, Sanjay Kaul, Abid Khan and Suhail Maqbool. My favorite teachers were Drs. G. H. Shah (Physiology), AK Raina (Biochemistry), Nirmal Raina and AH Fazili (Pharmacology). I owe a great debt to my medical school and to these wonderful teachers."

Twitter @iftikhar_kullo
Website: https://www.mayo.edu/research/labs/atherosclerosis-lipid-genomics/overview

Dr. Khalid Jahangir Qazi

Dr. Khalid Jahangir Qazi was born and raised in Zaina Kadal, Srinagar, Kashmir, along with his three sisters and a younger brother. His early education was in MPML Higher Secondary School, Srinagar, followed by premedical studies at Islamia College, Srinagar, where he excelled both in academics and sports. In 1963, he went to Government Medical College (GMC), Srinagar, and graduated with MBBS degree in 1968 with several honors including second position in internal medicine and third in class of 1968. He was the first postgraduate student of Prof. Syed Zahoor Ahmed under whose mentorship he obtained his MD degree in medicine from the University of Kashmir. He has fond memories of his peer postgraduates including Drs. Muhammad Amin, Sultan Khuroo, Manohar Lal, and Zaffar Mehdi. He was on faculty at GMC till his departure for the USA in 1976.

Dr. Khalid is nostalgic about his teachers including Professor Ayer and his lucid dissertations on embryology; Professor Goyal and his devotion to pathology museum; knowledgeable professor Kahali and the students' struggles to understand him; mercurial professor Syed Naseer Ahmed with devotion to all students; Professor Zahoor with his flair for scholarship; Dr. G. Rasool and Dr. Parmanik, the prolific surgeons; Professor Ahluwalia with meticulous attention to the lawns of the college; the inquisitive Dr. Harbajan Sigh; the passionate Dr. Girja Dhar; and Prof. Ali Jan, clinician par excellence, who passed away in his presence in Buffalo, New York. He was active member of Student "CASS" Union and one of the main organizers, with Prof. G. Q. Allaqaband and Prof. Hamid Durrani, of the First "Fun Fair" in School history. Along with Dr. Anwar Khan and Dr. Mohiuddin Subla, he was one of the key organizers of First International (Gastroenterology) Conference in Srinagar, Kashmir, under the patronship of Professor Durrani. He has loving memories of his classmates, staying in touch with many till today.

Dr. Khalid was especially honored to be invited as the keynote speaker in 2009 at the Fiftieth Anniversary of the College by the then principal, Dr. Shahida Mir. He has remained close to GMC and Kashmir throughout his life, assisting Kashmiri graduates with their training in the US and channeling relief and medical aid to Kashmir, on both sides of the cease-fire line. He spent significant time to establish GMC Alumni Association (GMCAA) and was appointed its international coordinator by the then principal, Prof. Rafiq Ahmed Pampori. He arranged and coordinated major fundraising and relief efforts following the disastrous floods in 2014 in cooperation with several alumni across the globe. These efforts continue till date.

In the US, Professor Qazi enjoys a distinguished career both in medical field and in community service. He has been the president, Medical Staff of the Catholic Health System (CHS) in Buffalo, New York. He has been on the faculty of the University of Buffalo Medical School since 1979, has been in the position of professor of clinical medicine, and has served with distinction on numerous committees. He has spent almost forty years at Sisters of Charity Hospital (SCH), which he considers his "second home." He served as chair of Medicine and program director for Internal Medicine Training for over fifteen years. He has trained hundreds of internists including many GMC alumni. Under his leadership, the training program attained national spotlight with superb resident achievements leading to consistent recognition by University of Buffalo for excellence in medical education. He had several research grants and is credited with over 110 publications (manuscripts, editorials, reports, posters). He is on the editorial board of and a reviewer for several reputable journals including *Annals of Internal Medicine*.

Dr. Qazi's election to the prestigious position of president of Medical Staff of CHS by his peers is a distinct honor and a remarkable tribute to his visionary leadership and commitment to excellence. Over the last three decades, Professor Qazi has played an active role and holds several important positions in American College of Physicians, culminating in prestigious Laureate Award in 2004 and Mastership Award in 2007, a unique honor bestowed upon less than 1 percent of the 130,000 members of ACP. Professor Qazi has served the Islamic Medical Association of North America for thirty-five years including as its president and the board of regents. He has chaired multiple committees for IMANA and serves as a member of the President's Council. IMANA has recognized him with several awards including its highest Ahmed Al-Kadi Award in 2014, named after one of the founders of IMANA.

Apart from his outstanding contributions as a physician and educator, Professor Qazi has passionately played pivotal role in establishing major organizations and programs for the benefit of the community. He serves on the board of directors of Muslim Public Affairs Council based in Los Angeles (MPAC), California, and is the founding president of Muslim Public Affairs Council of Western New York. MPAC promotes American Muslim identity and engages American Society on contemporary issues facing Muslims and to improve the understanding of Islam, while serving as a resource to government, media, and policy institutions. He has helped establish key programs aimed at ensuring civil rights of American Muslims and interfaith dialogue.

When asked to comment on the role he has played, the national president of MPAC, Salam Al-Marayati, states, "Khalid Jahangir Qazi is a devout family man, visionary community leader and effective organizer. He has established several interfaith, civic engagement and human rights causes. Khalid always impresses me with his meticulous planning. He is recognized by his community, by civic leaders and by government officials. He received an award from the US Attorney General, Eric Holder, for his outstanding volunteer community service. Dr. Khalid is busy every weekend, either at a charity event in Buffalo, a medical conference in Washington or at an Islamic convention in Los Angeles. Khalid has also made space for young leaders in our community to develop and play critical roles for our country."

With deep conviction in Islam, Professor Qazi is acknowledged as the first Muslim to advance interfaith dialogue in Western New York for which he was awarded the Brotherhood/Sisterhood Award of the National Conference of Christians and Jews in 1992. His vision led to the establishment and accreditation of Universal School, a full-time Islamic School in Buffalo. When asked to comment on his most fulfilling initiative from among his many impactful work for the community, Professor Qazi stated, "Apart from Universal School, the most fulfilling community achievements of my life has been to design and construct Islamic Center and establishing the Muslim Community Center for Western New York. I saw an opportunity and pursued it with my full personal dedication. Alhamdullilah, today, we have a vibrant Center, full to capacity and ready to be expanded. It's a dream come true!"

Professor Qazi, as a spokesperson for his community, has been extensively quoted and interviewed by local, national, and even international media outlets. He has received numerous citations locally and nationally including prestigious awards from US Departments of Justice and Homeland Security and was named Paul Harris Fellow of Rotary International. A recipient of the Leadership Buffalo Award and 2014 MPAC Lifetime Achievement Award, he received Buffalo News Outstanding Citizen of Western New York award and was honored with keys to Buffalo by the mayor in 2002, among many other recognitions.

In 2014, Professor Qazi retired from his position as program director, allowing him to devote more time with his family and his grandchildren. For him, this decision comes after the introspective period of Ramadan and performing the Holy Pilgrimage (Haj). Maintaining Kashmiri traditions and culture in his daily life, he lives with his wife, Tabassum, in Buffalo, New York. He is blessed with three children and six grandchildren, who are his joy and the center of his attention.

Dr. Khurshid A. Guru

A robotic surgeon who lives in Buffalo, New York, was returning home on September 18, 2015, after attending a medical conference in Bilbao, Spain, when he was told that a toddler on board the plane was in medical distress. The parents of the boy, a two-year-old, told Guru they had accidentally packed their son's asthma medication in their luggage. They were more than four hours into a seven-and-a-half-hour flight, and the child was crying and experiencing trouble in breathing. An oxygen meter showed that the toddler's oxygen level was alarmingly low, and his condition appeared to be deteriorating. Dr. Guru said he knew the little boy needed both oxygen and asthma medication, but the plane only came equipped with an adult asthma inhaler that requires the patient to breathe in the medicine. That is when Dr. Guru, who in his day job develops robotic surgical devices, switched on his creativity and cobbled together a makeshift nebulizer. The physician turned to items that he had on hand: an oxygen tank, a plastic water bottle, and a length of electrical tape. He hooked up the adult inhaler to a hole in the bottle and added oxygen through another opening he had made so the boy could inhale both simultaneously. To make it easier for the toddler to use his contraption, Dr. Guru modified his design by cutting a hole in a plastic cup and mounting it atop the bottle so that it could fit against his mouth and nose. About thirty minutes later, the boy began showing signs of improvement. By the time the plane landed, the two-year-old was playing with his mother as if nothing happened (abc NEWS September 24,2015). Dr. Guru said he decided to share the story to remind parents of kids suffering from asthma and the importance of keeping their medication at hand at all times. This innovator who could think out of the box in a plane to help a distressed kid is Dr. Khurshid Ahmad Guru.

Dr. Khurshid Ahmad Guru was born in 1968 in Srinagar, Kashmir; and is the son of famous cardiothoracic surgeon Dr. Abdul Ahad Guru. His medical education began at the University of Mysore at JJM Medical College, Davangere, India, and he completed his MBBS in 1994. Shortly thereafter, he completed his required rotating internship at the Medical City General Hospital in Manila, Philippines.

Dr. Khurshid moved to New York in 1994 to pursue further education and started a research assistantship in pulmonary medicine and critical care at the SUNY Stony Brook at Nassau County Medical Center. To understand the American clinical process, he started a first-year internal medicine residency in 1996. After completing this, he applied for a general surgery position at the combined program at Beth Israel Medical Center and Long Island Jewish Medical Center in New York. In 1998, he decided to take a detour and joined a nonaccredited Urology Clinical Fellowship at the VA Medical Center at Togus Maine. This fellowship involved covering over fifteen staff urologists from the Henry Ford Health System during their short weekly stunts at the VA Medical Center. This was a great opportunity to single-handedly handle the call as well as operate with excellent surgical teachers and learn from their variability in technique.

Dr. Khurshid began his residency in the Department of Urology of the Henry Ford Health System in July 1999. He was fortunate to experience and witness the robotic surgical revolution during his residency and also was the first formal robotic surgery fellow in his fifth clinical year. One of the greatest experiences he had was the option of traveling for three months to the prestigious Urology and Nephrology Center at El Mansourah University in Egypt. He spent three months attached to the legendary bladder surgeon Prof. Hassan Abol-Enein. On return, he had already decided that fighting bladder cancer would be his life crusade. He returned to the genius of Henry Ford Health System's robotic revolution and was blessed to incorporate both of these skills into his academic life as an academic robotic urologic surgeon. After his fellowship training, he accepted the position to become the first director of the Robotic Surgery at Roswell Park Cancer Institute in Buffalo, New York, in August 2005. About his experience in Rosewell Park, Dr. Khurshid says, "My position at Roswell Park is predominantly clinical and I spend 80% of my time managing complex urologic pelvic malignancies. My main clinical interest is in Bladder Cancer and roughly 70% of my practice is comprised of advanced bladder cancer. The remainder of my practice consists of patients with Prostate and occasionally kidney cancer. In the 9.5 years that I have been at Roswell Park, we have built one of the best robotic oncologic programs in the country and one of the finest robotic cystectomy programs in the world. Our approach has been cordial and multi-disciplinary and has improved our neo-adjuvant chemotherapy to over 60%. We also have performed 100% of our radical cystectomies utilizing a minimally invasive approach. I personally have performed over 435 Robot-assisted Radical Cystectomies with over 50% with an intra-corporeal approach and also completed over 850 robot-assisted radical prostatectomies. Being at the dawn of robot-assisted surgery allowed me to involve in developing training and investigating its safe application for bladder cancer. This opportunity has allowed me to grow my research portfolio quickly for both education and clinical outcome-based projects."

From 2005 to 2014, Dr. Khurshid developed the foundations of the robotic surgery program at Roswell Park Cancer, starting from its credentialing and privileging process to safe training processes. He expanded the team where currently over twenty surgeons engage in robotic surgery with a team of over fifteen nurses, operating room technicians, and three dedicated physician assistants who are engaged in robotic surgery and have performed over 2,500 procedures. Thirty surgical fellows have graduated who are practicing safe robotic surgery in their respective institutions. Dr. Khurshid has been involved in supervising the hands-on operative training for robotic surgery and chair the credentialing for robotic surgery at Roswell Park Cancer Institute. He has participated as an active member of the Surgical Quality Assurance Committee for several years and helped in the development of the quality metrics measuring surgical technique.

He has edited *Quality Book*, which reports overall clinical outcomes at Roswell Park Cancer Institute. He has also served on the Medical Staff Executive Committee that addresses and safeguards issues related to the medical staff at the institute.

Dr. Khurshid is also a key component of the fellowship program in training fellows in robot-assisted pelvic oncology especially reconstruction and redo-surgery. He mentors fellows from gynecologic and surgical oncology in principles of robot-assisted surgery and has mentored fellows in pursuit of their academic goals of developing a hypothesis, research pathways, and protocols to accomplish scientific results and their interpretation.

His introduction to global involvement began with him assisting the first live robot-assisted surgical procedure in Geneva, Switzerland, at the European Robotic Urologic Symposium (ERUS) when he was a robotic surgery fellow in 2004. These relationships build the foundation of his involvement with his colleagues at EAU and ERUS. This led to a partnership in teaching and developing a standardized program to popularize the technique of robot-assisted radical cystectomy across Europe. He has been a member of the group that has conducted successful courses in Europe since 2006. One of his major strengths has been the ability to render complex surgical procedures easy with clear straightforward surgical principles. He developed a simplified technique of spaces for the robot-assisted approach to radical cystectomy to make this procedure easy to teach. In 2009, he developed the Marionette technique for intracorporeal ileal conduit, which is now a well-accepted technique to perform this procedure. All his surgical fellows who have graduated under his mentorship have been able to independently perform robot-assisted surgical procedures. Dr. Khurshid has taken pride in developing and teaching the minimally invasive approach to bladder cancer for over a decade, thereby making this approach mainstream for patients suffering from a deadly disease with significant morbidity. His engagements with both national and international partners led to the establishment of the International Robotic Cystectomy Consortium, IRCC. At present, IRCC has sixty-nine member surgeons from thirty-seven institutions in sixteen countries. IRCC has to its credit publications that have addressed key issues related to RARC.

His partnership with the Virtual Reality Laboratory at the University of Buffalo School of Engineering and three years of extensive research resulted in the development of one of the first surgical simulators for robot-assisted surgery. The RoSS (Robotic Surgical Simulator) was spun into a start-up and now is managed by a California-based enterprise. Dr. Khurshid was able to develop a surgical training program and also published the first validated robot-assisted surgical curriculum—the Fundamental Skills of Robotic Surgery (FSRS). The RoSS is currently being used for safe surgical training outside the operating room at eighteen institutions in five countries. This surgical journey has also granted four patents filed with the US Patent Office.

Dr. Khurshid initiated a "mind-maps" project that evaluated the cognitive function utilizing EEG of trainees and experts in defining cognitive performance. He also got involved in assessing the true cognitive function of an expert surgeon and has been the lead in evaluating EEG-based findings of true surgical performance and different cognitive demands. He also developed an interest in evaluating the role of the surgical environment during robot-assisted surgery because of the remoteness of the surgeon to the patient. This led to the collaboration with the Human Factors Division at the Industrial Engineering at University at Buffalo Engineering School.

Dr. Khurshid had the honor of serving on two editorial boards: the Canadian Journal of Urology and British Journal of Urology International. He reviewed manuscripts for journals and also has been involved in writing several key editorials.

Dr. Khurshid has published more than one hundred peer-reviewed papers. He was also invited to write the introductory chapter on Robot-Assisted Urinary Diversion in the *Campbell Walsh Textbook of Urology*. Dr. Khurshid has received many awards, conducted workshops, conducted live surgical sessions, and been a keynote speaker in national and international conferences. He has been an innovator, has more than fifteen patents to his credit, and has devised new techniques and procedures.

He established a nonprofit organization, Guru Charitable Foundation, in 2007 in the state of New York. The purpose of this organization is to work to improve the quality of life in Kashmir by improving education and health care. Over two thousand economically challenged children have been educated in thirty-four government schools (primary, middle, and high) in BOSE System through the "Save the Future" education program since 2008. Some of the scholars have qualified into medical and engineering schools. He also established a craft center (knitting, embroidery *ari* work, cutting, and tailoring) in Sopore, which serves to train and educate dropout girls as well as widows to be financially independent. He established a grassroots program for breast cancer education and its early detection. Over three thousand women in rural Kashmir have been educated utilizing a house-to-house field education program (published in *Journal Breast* and MPH thesis on hookah and smoking trends in rural Kashmiri women—University at Buffalo Global Health Program—Zubair Butt, MD). Vision for all programs adapted from the Massachusetts State Eye Health Program for Children surveyed over fifteen thousand children in schools and provides them with free eyeglasses and eye care. This program also has provided free cataract surgery. The Guru Scholars program for health care has provided traveling observership for many faculty members from GMC, SKIMS, SKIMS-MC. The fields include pain and palliative management, colorectal surgery, head and neck oncology, medical ethics, physical medicine and rehabilitation, neonatology, interventional radiology, and pathology. The first AHA-certified ACLS program as Kashmir Life Support was also initiated. PGs and faculty from SKIMS, GMC, and the Department of Health Services Kashmir benefitted. As a founder of the Guru Foundation, he aims to establish a formal school and a college in Kashmir for better education.

Dr. Khurshid has elaborate research goals. Talking about these goals, he says, "My main research goals for the next five years are to establish a collaborative program between surgical technique, non-technical factors (operating room environment, team involvement), clinical outcomes and integration of industrial engineering principles in streamlining safe patient care. Secondly, I would like to engage in more basic science work in bladder cancer, especially in areas of metastasis after surgical removal after both radical prostatectomy and cystectomy. Thirdly I want to engage in the neuro-vascular mapping of the pelvis and its role in maintaining urinary and sexual function after radical cystectomy." Dr. Khurshid is working toward establishing Roswell Park Cancer Institute as one of the most comprehensive, innovative bladder cancer programs in the world.

Dr. Khurshid is a lover of the art, craft, and traditions of Kashmir. He and his wife, Dr. Lubna, have bought a ninety-seven-year-old vacant church in the US and converted it into a museum and library of art, culture, and history of Kashmir. The museum has over 1,500 paintings, books, and artefacts of Kashmir collected over the years by the couple. The work is a tremendous contribution to the history, culture, tradition, and handicrafts of Kashmir.

Dr. Khurshid is possibly the only Kashmiri to make it to the Reader's Digest influencers—in an article on "The Best Advice I Ever Got" by Lauren Gelman (June 1, 2015). Sharing twenty-one nuggets from the successful people in the world, Lauren rates this one from Dr. Khurshid as the best advice:

"I grew up in the northern Himalayan region of Kashmir. My grandfather would take all his grandkids for walks in his apple orchards, where he would pick apples that had been tasted by a bird and carve off the opposite side to give to us. I once asked, 'Why would you not offer the ripe-looking apple untouched by the bird?' I felt he was such a miser that he wanted to sell the 'good' apples instead of feeding them to his grandkids. He rolled his hand over my head affectionately. 'The bird would only eat one that is sweet, so I pick the best for you,' he said. 'Never assume; always ask.' This is my mantra in my personal and professional life." (*Readers Digest*, June 1, 2015).

Dr. Mian Mohammad Ashraf

Dr. Muhammad Ashraf Mian was born in Kashmir, India, and, like many pioneering physicians and surgeons of Kashmir received his medical education from King Edward Medical College in Lahore. He wanted to do big in life, and for this, he landed in the US in the late 1950s. He just arrived with five dollars in his pocket chasing his dream. The taxi ride interestingly was eight dollars, and he didn't know what to do when he would reach Memorial Hospital in Worcester for his residency. The taxi driver, sensing the unease of his passenger, said, "You keep your money. Welcome to America!" After this, there was no looking back for Dr. Ashraf. He returned the kindness that he received on his arrival to everyone he could.

After his residency, he trained as a cardiothoracic surgeon at Overholt Thoracic Clinic at New England Deaconess Hospital, then stayed at the hospital, where he was among the first physicians to perform open-heart and bypass surgery in Boston. "He had the reputation, really, of the master surgeon and had patients from all over the world," said Dr. Robert Berger, director of Clinical Research at Beth Israel Deaconess Medical Center. "He really took good care of his patients, and many of his patients stayed at his home, some of his patients traveled all the way from India and Pakistan not only for cardiac ailments but for any sort of medical treatment like people coming from India or Pakistan for kidney transplants and waiting in his home, or those recuperating from surgery or waiting for surgery. He built such a large international family with his magnanimity-a concept which is nonexistent today. Now, you operate and you leave. That wasn't his style."

Dr. Ashraf was a great mentor to his residents and medical students. At the hospital, he taught generations of surgeons. He was magnanimous with his time and talents. He loved his work and aimed for the ultimate technical excellence.

He founded the Happy Hearts Club, an organization that counseled heart patients about what to expect from the surgery and how to live their lives after cardiac surgery. He counseled his patients in the home and hospital. Dr. Ashraf was an accomplished heart surgeon when there were not many heart surgeons in the whole world. His career was unfortunately cut short because he was diagnosed with Parkinson disease at fifty years of age.

Dr. Ashraf had become involved with the Islamic Center of New England, which was in Quincy, before moving to Sharon. As president of the center, he helped find a new, larger location when the membership outgrew the mosque in a residential neighborhood in Quincy Point.

The people of Sharon, overwhelmed by his kindness and respect for all humans, came together at a horse-breeding farm in Sharon for laying the foundations of a new site of the Islamic Center of New England. Orthodox bishops, rabbis, and many people of different faiths came together for "peace." In an interview, which became later his favorite quote, he said, "I have never found a difference inside. Inside, everybody's got warm blood and a heart." His work forging congenial relations between the Islamic center and the residents of Sharon with its predominantly Jewish population drew national attention, and Dr. Ashraf was invited to a prayer breakfast at the White House. President Clinton later invited him to ride on Air Force One and accompany the presidential delegation to the signing of a peace treaty with Jordan.

His friends and colleagues call him an unusually kind man who would treat everyone equally no matter what race, religion, or status they had. People like him would be very helpful for the world of today. He died at the age of seventy-three, leaving behind his wife, his three daughters, and his son.

(The information for this write-up was gathered from Wickedlocal.com, June 10, 2009, titled "Dr. Mian M. Ashraf.")

Dr. Nancy (Misri) Khardori

Nancy (Misri) Khardori was born in Srinagar in a family where education was the most valued virtue. After finishing higher secondary education, she went on to complete premedical requirements from the Government Women's College, Srinagar. The same year, she was selected for admission to Government Medical College, Srinagar. This was a merit-based selection and happened before her sixteenth birthday. She graduated with distinction in obstetrics and gynecology and was among the top five students in the graduating class of 1972. She accepted the position of assistant surgeon in J&K Health Services. Her first posting was at a Primary Health Center (PHC) in Yaripora (near Kulgam). She was the first female physician to work in that village. She spent a year at SMHS Hospital, Srinagar, as a house officer in obstetrics and gynecology to complete a prerequisite for admission to postgraduate training (MD). Since she was left out of admission for postgraduate training in obs/gyn at her alma mater, she went to join MD in microbiology and immunology at the All India Institute of Medical Sciences (AIIMS), New Delhi. It was here her interest in basic sciences took off under the mentorship of Prof. A. Dasgupta (MD, PhD), who introduced her to cellular/molecular cell biology and immunology. Thus began her publication and research presentations record that started with salmonellosis, filariasis, and HLA typing in asthma. She worked as a junior faculty member at AIIMS following the completion of postgraduate training.

After moving to the United States, she worked as a postdoctoral fellow in microbiology and immunology at the Southern Illinois University School of Medicine. Her postdoctoral research area was cellular and antibody responses to *Histoplasma capsulatum*, a dimorphic fungus endemic in the Midwestern United States. She was the key person in raising high titer antiribosomal antibodies in rabbits against *Histoplasma capsulatum*, working with Ram Tewari (PhD) at the Southern Illinois University School of Medicine and Joseph Wheat MD from Indiana University School of Medicine. These would make it possible to detect Histoplasma antigen in the body fluids of patients that would previously go undiagnosed. This coincided with the largest documented outbreak of human histoplasmosis in and around the Purdue University campus in Indiana. Her work on Histoplasmosis resulted in major publications in leading microbiology and infectious diseases journals. These experiences carved the path for becoming a physician-scientist and practice bench to bedside medicine.

She entered a three-year residency training in internal medicine and won the best resident award after her first and third year of internal medicine training. She obtained certification in internal medicine from the American Board of Internal Medicine (ABIM). Her subspecialty training in clinical infectious diseases was completed at the University of Texas MD Anderson Cancer Center in Houston, Texas (under the mentorship of Dr. Gerald P. Bodey), leading to ABIM certification in the subspecialty of infectious disease.

Dr. Nancy's first faculty appointment was at the UT MD Cancer Center as a physician consultant/assistant professor of internal medicine in the subspecialty of infectious diseases and an adjunct appointment in basic sciences at the graduate school affiliated with the University of Texas at Houston. She started her independent research in the area of microbial adherence, biofilms, and device-related infections. The years at the world's largest cancer center provided Nancy with extensive and in-depth experience in infections in severely immunocompromised patients. In addition, she was involved in the work leading to the commercialization of liposomal amphotericin B and provided crucial data about the toxicity of the antifungal agent, Cilofungin. This was the first echinocandin studied for potential human use but for the side effects observed in the mouse model in Nancy's laboratory.

Southern Illinois University School of Medicine (SIU-SOM) at Springfield, Illinois, recruited her as an associate professor of medicine in the Division of Infectious Diseases and Microbiology/Immunology in 1989. She became the youngest faculty member in university history to receive tenure and rise to the rank of full professor. While she provided consulting services for all types of infectious diseases in a mixed patient population, she became part of the team providing care for advanced/nonhealing wounds and obtained certification in regenerative and hyperbaric medicine. She has continued independent research work (started at UT MD Cancer Center) on microbial adherence and device-related infections through the decades. Her laboratory has provided training in this area to a large number of physicians, PhD students, and postdoctoral fellows. The laboratory and clinical research were supported by extramural funds, and two patents were filed during that time.

Dr. Nancy has received the Best Teacher Award a record number of times from students, residents, and fellows and was inducted into the honor society AOA (Alpha Omega Alpha). She has been invited to serve on the NIH study section in the area of mycotic infections in immunocompromised hosts. In recognition of laboratory research and training of future physician-scientists, she has served on the advisory panel university MD, PhD Educators Council of Teaching Hospitals in Wisconsin and Illinois. She has been a member of twenty-two professional societies and a number of local, regional, national committees dealing with patient care, teaching, and research. She served on the test writing committee of ABIM (internal medicine), the National Board of Medical Examiners (NBME), and has been a charter member of the in-training examination committee for infectious diseases fellowship.

Dr. Nancy's research in the area of microbial adherence, biofilms, and device-related infections has won global recognition. She was among the early researchers to bring biofilms (from a phenomenon seen in nature) to the forefront in clinical infectious diseases. At the invitation of the Infectious Disease Society of America (IDSA), she has convened national symposia as part of continuing medical education for physicians. Having seen diseases like anthrax, smallpox, and plague in India and worked in research and diagnostic microbiology, she contributed to and edited a major book on bioterrorism preparedness in the aftermath of the 09/11 attack on US soil. She was invited multiple times by the American Society of Microbiology to hold national workshops on bioterrorism to educate health-care workers and laboratory personnel on the recognition and management of bioterrorism-related potentially fatal diseases. For her work related to public awareness in the area of infectious diseases, she received a distinguished author award from the Illinois Department of Public Health and the Illinois Public Health Association.

In 2011, Nancy moved to Eastern Virginia Medical School (EVMS), Norfolk, Virginia, as a professor of medicine/ infectious diseases and microbiology—molecular cell biology. She continued to teach both microbiology and clinical infectious diseases and provide consulting services in the areas of infectious diseases (including a large population with HIV infection), advanced wound care, and hyperbaric medicine. For the past three years, her focus has been to provide care to immunocompromised transplant patients including a large population of heart transplant recipients. The bench-to-bedside approach to patient care has enabled her to provide novel approaches/novel therapies for otherwise progressive and potentially fatal infections in very high-risk patient populations.

Dr. Nancy has been a prolific contributor to medical literature and has 456 publications in the form of original research papers, abstracts, invited articles, editorials, proceedings, and teaching aids. She has edited (by invitation) nine books besides serving as a guest editor for several volumes of *Medical Clinics of North America* and *Infectious Diseases Clinics of North America.* She has served as editor of *Year Book of Medicine* (Infectious Diseases Section) for seven years.

Dr. Nancy remains dedicated to her roots, family and friends. She carries a deep sense of gratitude to her teachers starting with those at the Government Medical College, Srinagar (Kashmir), and highly accomplished and inspiring mentors throughout her professional career. Three persons stand out through this long journey: Dr. B. K. Anand at GMC Srinagar, who transferred to her the passion for the science of microbes; Dr. Gerald P. Bodey at UTMD Anderson Cancer Center, who was the founder of the specialized branch of "Infections in Immunocompromised Patients"; and Dr. William Costerton at Biofilm Engineering Institute, Bozeman Montana (a Nobel Prize nominee), who provided the initial steps to launch her independent research.

Dr. Noor Ali Pirzada

Noor Ali Pirzada was born in Dalgate, Srinagar, Kashmir, to Mr. Ghulam Nabi and Khadija Pirzada and is the fourth of six siblings. He went to Burn Hall Higher Secondary School in Srinagar. He has fond and happy memories of his childhood living at the edge of the famous Dal Lake along the Boulevard. Playing cricket, listening to cricket commentary, reading, and listening to the BBC were some of his early passions. In his formative years, he was influenced by his parents, who were determined to provide the best education possible to their children, at the same time allowing them the freedom to make their own choices. Dr. Noor Ali recalls being fascinated very early on by physicians and their ability to treat and heal people.

After finishing high school, Noor Ali completed a year of premedical sciences at SP College, Srinagar. He entered the Government Medical College (GMC) in 1975. On completion of his training, he received the Best Outgoing Graduate Award. Other achievements in medical school included honors in pharmacology, obstetrics and gynecology, and pathology. He then served as a house officer under Prof. G. Q. Allaqaband in the Internal Medicine Department and went on to complete postgraduation in internal medicine. During this time, he was inspired and influenced by some outstanding physicians, including Prof. G. Q. Allaqaband, Dr. Mohammed Yusuf, and Dr. Sushil Razdan. Noor Ali has always considered Professor Allaqaband "one of the most outstanding clinicians and teachers he has encountered throughout his career" and credits his own teaching style and clinical skills to the influence of Professor Allaqaband.

After a national qualifying examination, Noor Ali was selected for specialization in neurology (DM Neurology) at the Postgraduate Institute of Medical Education and Research (PGIMER) in Chandigarh, one of the most prestigious and well-known medical institutes in India. Prof. Jagjit Singh Chopra, who was well known in India and abroad, led the Neurology Department at PGIMER. According to Dr. Noor Ali, "The training was tough, uncompromising, of an exceptionally high standard and one of the most rewarding and enjoyable periods of my academic life." During this time apart from becoming familiar with common and rare neurological diseases, he was exposed to sophisticated investigative techniques such as EEG, EMG, brain scans, etc.

Dr. Noor Ali subsequently came to the United States in 1991 and completed neurology residency at Hahnemann University Hospital in Philadelphia, Pennsylvania. His chair and mentor during this time was Prof. Elliott Mancall, one of the founding fathers of neurology in the United States. After finishing his residency, he went on to complete a fellowship in EMG/neuromuscular disease/botulinum toxin treatment at Duke University in Durham, North Carolina. At Duke, he trained with Dr. Donald Sanders and Dr. Janice Massey, two of the leading experts in the world in myasthenia gravis and other neuromuscular diseases.

After completing his fellowship, Dr. Noor Ali joined the Department of Neurology at the University of Toledo, College of Medicine (UTCOM), in 1996. Currently, he is a tenured professor in the department. He is the vice chairman of the department, director of the neurology residency program, and director of the EMG clinic and the chemo-denervation (botulinum toxin) clinic.

At UTCOM, he played a major role in establishing the neurology residency in 1998. His career has been consistently marked by a deep passion and enduring commitment to neurologic education and teaching. In 2008, he was selected as one of the neurology directors on the American Board of Psychiatry and Neurology (ABPN), one of the first international medical graduates to be awarded this honor. During his tenure, he served as the vice chair of the ABPN. As part of the examination committee of the ABPN, he was involved in writing questions for the national certifying examinations in neurology, vascular neurology, and neuromuscular medicine. For many years, he was also an examiner for the Oral Board Examination for Certification in Neurology. He has conducted educational courses for the American Academy of Neurology (AAN) and the American Clinical Neurophysiology Society (ACNS) and served on numerous committees in both organizations. He was a member of the committee of the Accreditation Council for Graduate Medical Education (ACGME), which established the milestones for neurology residency. Besides being certified in general neurology, he is certified in six neurology subspecialties, including EMG, clinical neurophysiology, neuromuscular medicine, headache medicine, vascular neurology, and epilepsy. There are only a few neurologists in the United States certified in this number of subspecialties in neurology.

He has been recognized nationally for his contribution to neurological education and teaching. He was awarded the AB Baker National Teaching Award by the American Academy of Neurology (AAN) in 2002 and the American Academy of Neurology Program Director Consortium Recognition Award in 2010. At an institutional level, he received the UTCOM Teaching Excellence Award in 2012 and the UTCOM Dean's Teaching Excellence Award in 2012. At UTCOM, he has won numerous Golden Apple Teaching Awards from students and Neurology Residents Award for outstanding Neurology Attending from the neurology residents. He has started a YouTube channel, "Neurology Explained," for learners in neurology. He has written numerous abstracts, papers, and book chapters. During his career, he has mentored a large number of residents, fellows, and students; many of them have been recruited as faculty in prominent academic centers.

Noor Ali is married to Yasmin Drabu, who was his classmate at GMC, Srinagar. She is an internist/hospitalist and infectious disease specialist. They have two sons: Adnan, married to Christina; and Farman, married to Emily. They have an adorable granddaughter, Nora, born to Adnan and Christina. They both share an abiding love and sense of loyalty to their homeland, Kashmir, and have passed this on to their children. Both acknowledge with profound gratitude the debt they owe to their homeland, Kashmir, their parents, and their teachers for shaping their lives and making them what they are today.

Twitter: @noorpirzada9

YouTube: https://www.youtube.com/channel/UCL4EDKJA05mMKuzQusaoDoA

Dr. Parvez Ahmad Mir

COVID-19 ripped apart health-care facilities everywhere in the world. It caught the best centers underprepared, unarmed, and in chaos. It brought life to a standstill and death closer to every doorstep. In these times of panic and pain, a Kashmir-born pulmonologist and an intensive care expert led the battle from the front in one of the New York hospitals. He and his team treated around two thousand COVID-19 patients, of whom three hundred, mostly Latino and black with poor health insurance, died. "Dr. Parvez Ahmad Mir is the chief of Pulmonary and critical care at Wyckoff Heights Medical Center (WHMC). Dr. Mir received his first Covid-19 patient, an 82-year-old woman, on March 10, 2020, who later succumbed to the infection after 10 days of her admission to the hospital. She was the first casualty in his hospital and the first death in the pandemic in the whole of New York City, which in a month had a mortality of 30,400. This patient neither had a travel history nor any contact history where she could have come in contact with an infected person In the intensive-care ward, when they received their first patients at WHMC, all they knew that time was what they had come across the various news reports that there was an outbreak in China, which spread to Asia and then jumped to Europe, killing thousands. They had no preparedness like most of the health facilities in America. They just had one room equipped to handle patients with a highly infectious disease.

"WHMC is located in the area dominated by Afro-Americans and Latinos, who mostly belong to the middle class or the lower class setup. So, the hospital staff fearing the spread of the infection, many health workers either went on leave or left the job. But in the intensive care unit of the hospital, none of Dr. Mir's staffers left the job; they worked tirelessly to save the lives of their patients. Dr. Mir worked for six weeks without a day off, updating health officials and colleagues while also trying to come up with an effective mix of drugs and treatments.

"He was probably the first who had his treatment principle simple at first. Instead of medical textbooks, he used the blogs of frontline doctors from other continents to guide him. In late March of the same year, when President Trump was advocating the use of hydroxychloroquine, an anti-malaria drug, Mir gave it to many COVID-19 patients, only to observe that it was impairing their heart function. From autopsy reports, he saw tiny blood clots permeating the bodies of COVID-19 patients, so he ordered patients to get blood thinners. 'I call this disease Russian roulette,' he said. One of the first patients he managed to take off the ventilator was in his 80s. Then he treated two brothers, Miguel and Leobardo Herrera. Leobardo survived. Miguel did not. At WHMC, he was struggling with the virus at multiple fronts like from space crunch to unpreparedness. With no adequate guidelines from the government, the hospital staff was handling the situation on its own with prime responsibility on Dr. Mir.

"With just 350 beds capacity, WHMC treated more than 2000 COVID-19 patients, that included nearly 200 of this facility's staff who got infected while they treated the patients. Getting closer to patients was a risk but the staff took this risk and it was through loudspeakers that they used to connect with the staff inside these wards. At the same time the shortage of masks and disinfectants, resulted in anxiety among the staff, due to which dozens of its healthcare workers, cleaners and technical staff walked off the job, took leave or retired, and by the height of the pandemic, the hospital was operating without 1 in every 4 employees. Among his staff, the first nurse to show symptoms was Amy O'Sullivan. The oxygen levels in O'Sullivan's blood were so low by the time she got tested in early March that colleagues wondered how she was conscious. She was moved to the same isolation room on the 10th floor—Room 11, next door to where the 82-year-old woman was clinging to life. When Dr. Mir asked O'Sullivan if she could breathe without a ventilator and the reply was a 'No.' Through the window of her isolation room, she could see a few of her fellow nurses crying. One of the last things Mir recalls O'Sullivan saying before she went unconscious was, 'Please save me, so I can get back to work.' She was lucky she could fight the virus and survived."

The *Time* team did the above-mentioned elaborate story when they were given access to the health facility starting on April 9, 2020, as the pandemic had reached its apex in the city. The team was witness to how Dr. Mir and his staff were working to improvise with the increased load of patients. As Dr. Mir was managing the crisis from the front, his struggle led him to *Time* magazine's cover story "Contagion of Fear—One Month inside a New York Hospital" as a virus took over the world. Dr. Mir became a hero, a savior, a warrior, giving his best, trying to save lives, and trying to understand a disease that had baffled the world.

The *Times* report also shared some pictures from inside the hospital wards where the COVID-19 patients were getting treated. One of the pictures also showed Dr. Mir leading the prayer with his son. Wearing the PPE, he has reportedly worked tirelessly during the month of fasting as well while keeping his fasts. The faith kept him going, and the fasts of Ramadan kept him strong. When dozens of his patients gasped at the ventilator, he was their only hope; he worked hard to give them a chance to live and prayed hard for them. His pious mother would ask him to recite the verses from the Holy Quran, which would help humankind to tide over the crises.

Dr. Parvez Mir is a proud practicing Muslim who believes the world needs more healers. He is the youngest son of former legislator late Mir Assadullah, a resident of Chareel in Banihal, Kashmir. He graduated from Government Medical College, Srinagar, in 1980 and flew to the US, where he completed his internal medicine residency at Wyckoff Heights Medical Center. After training in pulmonary medicine at Long Island Jewish Medical Center, Northwell, he joined Pulmonary and Critical Care at Wyckoff Heights Medical Center, a department he now heads. He is presently the chief of Bioethics and chairs Critical Care and Information Technology Committee of the hospital. He was awarded notable in health care in the *NY Crain's Business* Magazine (2020). Dr. Parvez is a fellow of the American College of Physicians and American College of Chest Physicians. He has many publications to his credit and supports doctors from Kashmir for short-term training and residency in the US. Dr. Parvez was trained by Dr. Faroque Khan, the messiah for many Kashmiris in his initial years in New York. Dr. Parvez believes that Dr. Khan gave him a chance in life to be where he is now. He has no words to express how grateful he is to him for his inspiration and guidance.

Dr. Parvez has a supportive family. His wife is a highly accomplished geriatrician and a palliative care specialist. She runs a Department of Internal Medicine as chairperson. They support each other's dreams and ambitions. Dr. Parvez has two daughters and a son. The eldest is a lawyer, and the other daughter is a school administrator. His son is an engineer. He stayed away from his affectionate children for many weeks to be there at the front line.

(This profile is mostly based on *Time* magazine's cover story done by Simon Shuster and *Kashmir Life*, June 23, 2020.)

Dr. Prediman K. Shah

Dr. Prediman K. Shah was born and raised in Safa Kadal Srinagar, Kashmir, with seven additional siblings; he came from a middle-class family and lived in an old house with forty relatives. He graduated from DAV High School in 1962 at the top of his tenth-grade class. He aspired to a career as a detective; however, the death of his nineteen-year-old sister from a rare form of lung cancer changed his orientation, and he decided to become a doctor and find cure for the devastating disease. After two years at the SP College, Prediman started Medical School at GMC Srinagar in 1964 (he was one month short of being fifteen years old, although his official records would show him to be seventeen years of age). The medical education was paid for by a loan from the state government, which he eventually paid off in 1978.

At the GMC, Prediman excelled and graduated at the top of the class in 1969, earning multiple honors and distinctions and a Graduate of the Year award. He was greatly influenced by numerous mentors at the Medical College but in particular by the legendary physician Dr. Ali Jan and Dr. Thusoo. After a year at the All India Institute of Medical Sciences, New Delhi, Prediman came to the United States, landing an internship in Milwaukee. While in Milwaukee at the Mount Sinai Medical Center, he was heavily influenced by mentors such as Bud Waisbren and Mortimer Botin and almost decided to pursue his long interest in neurology and was accepted for fellowships in neurology at Johns Hopkins University in Baltimore. However, he declined the neurology fellowship and instead decided to pursue cardiology as a career because of the influence of a senior resident, the late Jorge Levisman from whom he learned much cardiology during internship and residency at Mount Sinai. His further residency training was at Montefiore Hospital of Albert Einstein College of Medicine in New York, where he was offered a second-year residency in medicine because of his outstanding performance and strong letters of recommendations from Mount Sinai. Once at Montefiore, Prediman was completely taken by cardiology largely because of the influence of a great mentor, Dr. James Scheuer, who was then a newly appointed chief of Cardiology at Montefiore.

Dr. Scheuer's grand rounds on ASD convinced Prediman that he needed to become a cardiologist, and so he applied for cardiology fellowships around the nation but really wanted to stay for fellowship at Montefiore because of Dr. Scheuer. After an initial negative response at Montefiore, unexpectedly, he was at the last minute offered a fellowship in cardiology at Montefiore because an additional position had been created; thanks to Jim Scheuer. After completing two years of clinical cardiology training at Montefiore, Prediman moved to Cedars Sinai Medical Center for a research fellowship under the legendary Jeremy Swan, coinventor of the Swan Ganz catheter. After completing a research year, he was offered a faculty position at Cedars and has been at Cedars ever since. Prediman managed the CCU at Cedars for fifteen years before becoming the division director in 1994, a position that he relinquished in 2013 to refocus his attention on clinical work and research. During his stay at Cedars, Prediman took a one-year sabbatical at Massachusetts General Hospital (MGH) in Boston, in 1992 under the tutelage of another living legend and mentor Valentin Fuster, where he developed an interest in vascular biology, atherosclerosis, and inflammation. After returning from MGH,

Prediman set up a basic science laboratory research program in atherosclerosis and vascular biology at Cedars, which has produced some of the most outstanding and seminal work in the field of cardiology.

Prediman K. (PK) Shah, MD, is the director of the Atherosclerosis Prevention and Treatment Center and of the Oppenheimer Atherosclerosis Research Center at Cedars-Sinai, where he leads several studies that focus on heart disease prevention and treatment. Dr. Shah holds the Shapell and Webb Family chair in Clinical Cardiology at Cedars-Sinai and is a professor of medicine and cardiology. He is the immediate past director of Cardiology at Cedars Sinai Heart Institute.

In 1992, Dr. Shah and his colleagues began studying a mutant gene that was found in a small number of inhabitants of a northern Italian town. Compared to the normal gene (apolipoprotein A-1), the mutant gene (apo A-1 Milano) produces a form of HDL (high-density lipoprotein or "good" cholesterol) that provides greater protection against atherosclerosis and vascular inflammation—processes that lead to clogged arteries, heart attacks, and strokes.

In 1994 and 1998, Dr. Shah showed for the first time that intravenous injection of a genetically engineered form of the protein markedly reduced arterial plaque buildup in rabbits and mice fed a high-cholesterol diet. Subsequent animal studies confirmed the potent effects of the apo A-1 Milano protein on the prevention and reversal of plaque buildup, and early clinical trials conducted elsewhere found similar results in humans. Currently, a major pharmaceutical company is doing large-scale clinical trials using recombinant apo A-I Milano protein infusion to reverse arterial plaques.

Dr. Shah's work with the apo A-I Milano protein was the subject of CBS *60 Minutes* in 1994 and 1995. (This is an unprecedented distinction in that CBS *60 Minutes* program is one of the most-watched TV programs in the USA.)

In 2005, Dr. Shah reported that transfer of the apo A-1 Milano gene itself—not just the protein—had been accomplished, also with favorable results. A single injection of a harmless virus engineered to carry the gene enabled mice to manufacture their own supply of the protein produced by the gene. The animals received the protective benefits with a single gene injection rather than repeated protein injections. Safety and efficacy studies are continuing.

Animal studies conducted in Dr. Shah's laboratory and the laboratory of Dr. Shah's longtime collaborator, Swedish scientist Dr. Jan Nilsson, found that a vaccine created from the low-density lipoprotein (LDL, or "bad" cholesterol) molecule significantly reduced plaque buildup in animals that had high cholesterol levels. Experimental studies on this novel vaccine for heart disease continue, and human studies are planned within the next few years.

Dr. Shah is the immediate past-president of the American Heart Association (AHA)—Western States Affiliate and a member of the AHA-Western Regional Board. He is a longtime volunteer with the American Heart Association at the national, regional, and local levels. He was also president of the Los Angeles Chapter of the AHA in 2001 and 2002 and has served as a member of the Los Angeles Board and the Western Regional Peer-Review Group. Dr. Shah has chaired the AHA's Educational Task Force and the Fall Symposium and has been a member of the research committee, national scientific program committee, and Young Investigators Award Group. He is also a member of the Scientific Advisory Board of the Larry King Cardiac Foundation and serves as the national chairman of the Entertainment Industry Foundation's National Cardiovascular Research Initiative (NCRI), which was launched in 2001. He was a member of the Recombinant DNA Advisory Committee (RAC) of the National Institutes of Health and serves on the Data Safety Monitoring Board of the Cell and Gene Therapy

Trials of the National Heart Lung and Blood Institute of the NIH and the Scientific Publication Committee of the American Heart Association. He was also elected to the European Academy of Sciences.

Dr. Shah has edited three books on heart disease and published more than 628 scientific papers, reviews, book chapters, and abstracts. He serves on the editorial boards of the peer-reviewed journals: *Circulation*, *American Journal of Cardiology*, *Journal of the American College of Cardiology*, *Arteriosclerosis, Thrombosis and Vascular Biology*, *International Journal of Heart Failure*, *Indian Heart Journal*, *Journal of Preventive Cardiology*, *Reviews in Cardiovascular Medicine*, *Current Cardiology Reports*, and *Journal of Cardiovascular Pharmacology and Therapeutics.* Well respected by his peers, Dr. Shah has been invited to lecture in many areas of the world and has been a Fulbright visiting professor in Japan, Taiwan, Argentina, Chile, and Brazil. He also has served as visiting professor at highly respected medical and educational centers, including the Cleveland Clinic, Mayo Clinic, Texas Heart Institute, University of Utah, University of Virginia, University of Texas at San Antonio and Medical Branch in Galveston, University of California at San Diego and San Francisco, and Massachusetts General Hospital of Harvard Medical School.

Dr. Shah is a Master of the American College of Cardiology (MACC), a fellow of the American College of Physicians, and the American College of Chest Physicians. He has been a member of the ACC's Annual Scientific Program. Dr. Shah was the program codirector for the Annual Scientific Session of the American College of Cardiology in 2014.

He has won numerous awards, including the Gifted Teacher Award from the American College of Cardiology; an Excellence in Teaching Award from the dean of the University of California, Los Angeles School of Medicine; and two Golden Apple Awards from the school's senior medical students. In 2002, he received a Lifetime Achievement Award from the Los Angeles American Heart Association, and he received the Heart Saver Award from the Save-A-Heart Foundation and Humanitarian Award from the United Hostesses Charities in 1995 and 2006. In October 2007, Cedars-Sinai Medical Center awarded Dr. Shah the Pioneer in Medicine Award, the highest award given at the medical center. In 2008, he received the Annual Distinguished Teaching Award from the Cardiology Fellows at Cedars Sinai. Also in 2008, Dr. Shah received two very prestigious awards from the American Heart Association during its annual scientific sessions in New Orleans: the James B. Herrick Award and the Laennec Society Lectureship Award. In 2012, Dr. Shah was presented with the Steven S. Cohen Humanitarian Award from the Heart Foundation. Dr. Shah received the Distinguished Scientists Award from the American College of Cardiology in 2012 and the Master of the American College of Cardiology in 2015. He was also named the Eliot Rappaport Cardiologist of the Year for 2014 by the California Chapter of the American College of Cardiology.

When asked to recall some key moments from his illustrious career, Dr. Prediman K. Shah stated, "My most fulfilling moment personally was to marry my wife, Kim with whom I developed my family with a wonderful son, Kishore and a terrific daughter, Nisha, who are now grown-ups and living independently pursuing their respective careers. I am grateful to my parents and siblings whose love and support helped me get started. I am grateful to my numerous mentors and professional cheerleaders whose encouragement helped me launch and sustain my career. I am also indebted to my numerous friends and professional colleagues whose support has meant the world to me. I am also grateful to my numerous patients who have kept me professionally challenged and engaged. Most importantly I am grateful to my wife and kids for their unwavering support and love which sustains me."

Dr. Raffit Hassan

Dr. Raffit Hassan received his early education at Burn Hall Higher Secondary School followed by premedical studies at SP College Srinagar. Dr. Hassan followed his father's advice and joined the Government Medical College, Srinagar, in October 1982. He greatly enjoyed his time at the college and was ranked among the top three students in all the exams. Influenced by his brother-in-law Dr. Ghulam Jeelani Mufti, he developed an early interest in medical oncology, and after completing his final MBBS, did his house job in blood banking as well as medicine with Dr. G. Q. Allaqaband.

In 1991, Dr. Khalid J. Qazi, who was the associate program director at Sisters Hospital University of Buffalo, recruited Raffit for residency in internal medicine, which provided an exciting opportunity for Dr. Hassan's introduction to medicine in USA. Dr. Hassan recalls Sisters Hospital as a "wonderful model for medical residency training, incorporating an atmosphere for scholarship, mentorship and made the experience truly enjoyable." Given his interest in medical oncology, he applied for fellowship in medical oncology and was selected for training at the National Cancer Institute (NCI), National Institutes of Health. About the time Dr. Hassan spent at Sisters Hospital, Dr. Khalid Jehangir Qazi recalled, "A graduate of my own alma mater, I have followed Raffit closely since his arrival in the United States. Playing a significant role in his field in the leading cancer research institute of the World, Raffit has gained international recognition for his many achievements. He is an embodiment of commitment, dedication and professionalism. He has set high standard for himself and everyone around him. He has made us all proud and I was very pleased I had him in my training program."

Dr. Hassan joined the NCI in June 1994 and worked in the lab of Dr. Ira Pastan, a world-renowned scientist who has trained a generation of physicians and scientists and two of his students have won the Nobel Prize in Medicine. Joining Dr. Pastan's lab has had a long-lasting influence and shaped his scientific career and has resulted in a productive ongoing collaboration over the years. After completing his medical oncology training at NCI, Dr. Hassan did his bone marrow transplantation fellowship at Georgetown University and joined the faculty at University of Oklahoma in 1998.

In 2002, Dr. Hassan was recruited as a tenure track investigator at NCI and received tenure in 2008 and in 2013 was appointed as co-chief, Thoracic and GI Oncology Branch at NCI, a unique accomplishment and recognition. Dr. Hassan's laboratory and clinical research is focused on developing novel treatments for patients with thoracic cancers including mesothelioma and lung cancer. He has pioneered the development of targeted therapies directed to the tumor antigen mesothelin and has led the development of several drugs currently in clinical trials for treatment of mesothelin expressing cancers. His initial preclinical and early phase clinical trials of the antimesothelin immunotoxin SS1P validated mesothelin as a therapeutic target for cancer therapy, and his work is now focused on increasing the efficacy of SS1P and other drugs targeting mesothelin in patients with cancer. His group has recently shown major and durable tumor responses in patients with treatment refractory mesothelioma by combining SS1P with immunosuppression. This work opens up the field of immunotoxin therapy for solid tumors, and ongoing studies will elevate this approach for treatment of common cancers, including lung adenocarcinoma. In addition, Dr. Hassan and his collaborators will continue to develop less immunogenic immunotoxins for treatment of other cancers. Ongoing efforts are directed to exploiting this approach for treatment of lung and pancreatic cancer as well.

In addition, to conducting clinical trials, he has an active laboratory research program for developing novel treatments for thoracic cancers. Dr. Hassan is a visiting professor at several leading institutions in the US and a frequent speaker at national and international meetings. He is a recipient of several national and international awards for his work on mesothelin, including the American Society for Clinical Oncology Career Development Award, the National Institutes of Health Patient Oriented Research Career Development Award, and the Pioneer Award from the Mesothelioma Foundation, and in 2014 received the Wagner Medal from the International Mesothelioma Interest Group. His studies have been published in reputed high-impact journals—that is, *Cancer* (Hassan R, Alewine C, Mian I, Spreafico A, et al. "Phase 1 study of the immunotoxin LMB-100 in patients with mesothelioma and other solid tumors expressing mesothelin. *Cancer. 2020 15; 126 (22): 4936–4947*) and *J ClinOncol*, 2020 (Hassan R, Blumenschein GR, Moore KN, *et al.* "First-in-Human, Multicenter, Phase I Dose-Escalation and Expansion Study of Anti-Mesothelin Antibody-Drug Conjugate Anetumab Ravtansine in Advanced or Metastatic Solid Tumors." 1; 38 (16): 1824--1835.). His publication "Clinical Response of Live-Attenuated, Listeria monocytogenes expressing mesothelin (CRS-207) with chemotherapy in Patients with Malignant Pleural Mesothelioma" and the associated photo formed the cover page of prestigious *Clinical Cancer Research journal* (2019).

Dr. Raffit Hassan has fond memories from his GMC days, recalling, "The best part of my life was the time spent in Govt.

Medical College Srinagar. It was a fascinating place with great friends and superb teachers both in the pre-clinical sciences as well as in the wards. What stood out for me was the dedication of all our teachers to mentor us and they took great interest in our career development. It is truly a pleasure to see that my young batch mates of Govt. Medical College Srinagar are doing extremely well and many hold senior academic positions at the College as well as SKIMS." Additionally, Dr. Hassan is grateful that GMC has been a place where many of his family members graduated from. "My elder sister, Dr. Faiza Mufti, elder brother Dr. Zubair Hassan, younger sister Dr. Iffat Shah, brothers-in-law Dr. G. J. Mufti and Dr. Parvez Shah, sister-in-law Dr. Rozina Shah, and my wife Dr. Rubina Mattu as well as her brother-in-law Dr. Mudasir Shah are all GMC alumni. We all owe a lot of debt and gratitude to this wonderful institution."

Dr. Riyaz Bashir

Dr. Riyaz Bashir was born and raised in Srinagar, Kashmir, the son of Mr. Bashir ud Din and Rafiqa Bashir and the eldest of three siblings. He attended primary school at the Tyndale Biscoe Memorial School and higher secondary school at DAV Institute. He received his premedical education from Amar Singh College, Srinagar. Childhood for Riyaz was particularly jovial, full of fun and play, both at school as well as at home. He had a passion for playing soccer and swimming, and his childhood dream was to be a farmer and have a cattle farm. Riyaz's grandmother (Hajra), his uncle (Ghulam Qadir Wani), and his friend (Dr. Iqbal-uz-Zaman) were the most influential people in his growing years, and it was Dr. Allama Iqbal's writings that shaped Riyaz's worldview and inspired in him a passion for reading.

In December 1986, he joined Government Medical College, Srinagar, and completed his MBBS in 1992 and was honored with the Best Outgoing Graduate Award. His favorite subjects were anatomy, physiology, ENT, and internal medicine. He attributes his success in medical school to mentoring by several dedicated and sincere teachers like Prof. Mohammad Yousuf, who encouraged him to pursue advanced training in the United States. After completing his MBBS, he met Dr. Faroque Khan, from Long Island, New York, who offered him a research position in his program at Nassau County Medical Center (NCMC). As a research assistant with Dr. Khan, he studied the effect of TNF α monoclonal antibodies in septic shock patients. He also studied the predictors and effects of acute renal failure on ICU mortality and the effects of matrix metalloproteinase inhibitors on atherosclerosis using a mouse model. Riyaz believes that this research experience turned out to be a key asset for his academic career in the US. He then completed his internal medicine residency and later on chief residency at NCMC before starting his cardiovascular fellowship at the Saint Elizabeth's Medical Center in Boston. During his fellowship, he developed an interest in the catheter-based treatment of peripheral vascular diseases and went on to do a dedicated endovascular interventional fellowship with the late Dr. Jeffrey Isner, the father of cardiovascular angiogenesis.

Dr. Riyaz then accepted a faculty position as an assistant professor of medicine at the University of Toledo, in Ohio, where he would work for five years. During this tenure, his main focus was education and clinical training of the house staff in the interventional management of vascular diseases. In 2007, he decided to do a fellowship in interventional cardiology, which he completed at the Mayo Clinic in Rochester Minnesota. The experience at the Mayo Clinic was amazing and has been an enormous asset. He is grateful to the clinic and its teachers, particularly Dr. Chet Rihal and Dr. David Holmes, who inspired him to strive for excellence in academic medicine. Afterward, he took a faculty position at Temple University Hospital in Philadelphia as an interventional cardiologist and the director of Vascular Medicine and Endovascular Interventions. At Temple University, he pioneered many novel therapies in the cardiac catheterization laboratory, including pulmonary balloon angioplasty for CTEPH, percutaneous left ventricular assist devices, laser, orbital and directional atherectomy, and catheter-based treatments of acute and chronic pulmonary embolism and deep vein thrombosis. This work led to the creation of the world-renowned Temple Thromboembolism program and several innovations including the development of a novel device for the treatment of acute pulmonary embolism and deep vein thrombosis called the BASHIRTM endovascular catheter (Thrombolex Inc. New Britain PA USA. https://www.thrombolex.com).

Dr. Riyaz Bashir is interested in outcomes research in interventional cardiology, and his focus has been the catheter-based treatment of venous thromboembolism. He has received numerous awards including the Best Teacher of the Year Award in 2006 and has been listed as America's Top Doctors by Castle Connolly Medical every year since 2014. He has published more than one hundred manuscripts and book chapters and serves as a reviewer for multiple medical journals as well as funding agencies. His work on catheter-directed thrombolysis (CDT) in the treatment of deep vein thrombosis and pulmonary embolism has been featured in regional and national news outlets like Forbes. This research was funded by NIH and has led to the standardization of CDT practices across the country with particular emphasis on improving outcomes in low-volume centers. Riyaz has been involved in organizing and speaking at various national and international cardiovascular conferences like the American College of Cardiology, European Congress of Cardiology, and American Heart Association. He has mentored more than fifty medical students, residents, and fellows during his academic career and has been involved in more than thirty-five multicenter clinical trials like CORAL, ATTRACT, and RESCUE.

Dr. Riyaz currently lives in a Philadelphia suburb with his wife, Najmun Riyaz, and three children. Najmun is also a graduate of GMC Srinagar and is practicing psychiatry. Their family loves to vacation in the mountains. Riyaz enjoys playing soccer with his kids and reading books by M. R. Bawa Muhaiyadeen. He has been a member of the Islamic Medical Association of North America (IMANA) since 1994 and was the vice president of its Greater Toledo chapter from 2003 to 2007. He is passionate about investing in the quality education of Kashmiri youth and is the immediate past president of Kashmir Education Initiative (KEI), a nonprofit charity organization involved in providing need-based scholarships, guidance, and mentoring to bright high school and predoctoral students. He considers himself truly blessed and grateful for a loving family, friends, and great mentors. Among his other mentors include Dr. Abdul Ahad (anatomy), Dr. M. Sayeed (physiology), Dr. Roshan Lal (microbiology), Dr. A. R. Khan (pathology), Dr. Rafiq Ahmad Pampori (ENT), Dr. Yusuf Kanjwal (cardiology), Dr. Farhat Jabeen, and Dr. Rubina Shah (obst/gyn). Riyaz's friends from Kashmir include Arshad Pandit, Javid Ahangar, Arshad Dar, Rauf Baba, Gurpreet Singh, Ghulam Nabi, Ibrahim Masoodi, Yunis Muneer, Anil Kotru, and Bilal Malik.

Dr. Riyaz often has nostalgic memories of Kashmir and its breathtaking scenery, which he had experienced during his weekly boating sessions at the Dal Lake (School Regatta), trekking, cross-country running, and while walking up the stairs of Sultan-ul-Arifeen's shrine. He also reminisces about the last four years of his medical school during the most strife-torn times in the valley.. He remembers the particularly nerve-wracking times he faced in Kashmir. Riyaz says, "These experiences were so distressful that it took 10 years in the United States to get over those nightmares."

Riyaz believes that the greatest joy of the medical profession is the human interaction we have with our patients and our students; it is these interactions that enrich our lives and bring about a paradigm shift from a "life of success" to a "life of significance."

Dr. Romesh Khardori

Romesh Khardori was born and raised in Habba Kadal, Srinagar, Kashmir, in a family where education was a top priority. His sister became a plant physiologist; his brother became an engineer and set up a consultancy firm, and his father practiced law. His earlier schooling was at CMS-Central High School followed by college education (pre-university and premed) from Sri-Pratap College (SP College) Srinagar, Kashmir. He entered Government Medical College, Srinagar (University of Jammu and Kashmir) from where he obtained MBBS with high honors/ distinction and certificates of proficiency (1972). His fondest memories at GMC included his fascination with physiology, and he maintained close contact with the then chair, Prof. B. S. Kahali after he left Kashmir until his death at the age of ninety-eight years. It was that fascination and influence that kindled Romesh's interest in endocrinology.

Dr. Romesh was selected for housemanship in internal medicine at the All-India Institute of Medical Sciences in New Delhi from where he also obtained MD (internal medicine, 1976). He was the first person from clinical sciences to be selected for PhD in experimental medicine/structural physiology. His research work involved the study of neuroendocrine responses in protein-energy malnutrition in rhesus monkeys. While at AIIMS, he was also involved in a project involving fetal surgery under the guidance of the late Dr. Mridula Rohatgi from Pediatric Surgery. Dr. Khardori was adjudged as the Best Outgoing MD

Student and recommended for the newly instituted Glaxo Prize. At AIIMS, he also served as cosupervisor for master of sciences for students enrolled in the Department of Pharmacology.

Following his stay at the AIIMS, he joined as a fellow in endocrinology and metabolism at the Oregon Health Sciences University in Portland, Oregon (USA), where he studied adipocyte physiology under the guidance of Prof. Matthew C. Riddle. The results led to a change in the previously held notion of static adipocyte number (Knittle and Hirsch theory). It was shown for the first time that adipocyte numbers could be manipulated up and down. This was the beginning of a new era in adipocyte biology, and the rest is history (1977–1979).

Upon completion of a fellowship at OHSU, next phase was followed by fellowship at Harvard Medical School in Boston (Joslin-New England Deaconess/Beth Israel Hospital program), where engagements with luminaries such as George Cahill, Alexander Marble, and Sidney Ingbar radically modified his clinical/research interests leading to a long productive academic life. This stint at Harvard was followed by a fellowship in neuroendocrinology under the guidance of the late Dorothy Krieger (MD, DSc) at Mount Sinai Medical Center in New York City. Following the completion of the fellowship, board certifications (ABIM) were obtained in internal medicine and the subspecialty of endocrinology, diabetes, and metabolism.

Dr. Khardori's first faculty appointment was at the Southern Illinois University School of Medicine. During his stay as SIUI-SOM, he served as the director of the Division of Endocrinology, Metabolism, and Molecular Medicine, director of the Endocrinology Fellowship Training Program, and associate chair of the Department of Medicine. He also served as chair of most university/medical school committees, including the Tenure and Promotion Committee, Research Policy Committee, and Clinical Research involving Human

Subjects. While at the SIU-School of Medicine, three major clinical observations were reported:

a) Association between diabetes mellitus and fibrotic breast disease mimicking breast cancer was reported for the first time by N. G. Soler and R. Khardori, sometimes called the Soler-Khardori syndrome.
b) Lymphocytic pneumonitis was reported in patients with lymphocytic thyroiditis.
c) Rationale for high fluid administration in non-ketotic hyperglycemic hyperosmolar state challenged and lower fluid replacement with nuanced insulin replacement recommended, which has drastically improved the outcome in such cases.

In the basic sciences area, his research involved the study of endocrine abnormalities in growth hormone receptor null mice and impact of modulation of cold/warm sensing channels on nociception and the biological role of FGF-21. He participated in a technology transfer mission initiated by the Council of Scientific and Industrial Research—Government of India (CSIR). This resulted in a short stint on faculty in the Division of Endocrinology and Metabolism at the All-India Institute of Medical Sciences, New Delhi (India). Dr. Khardori developed the first comprehensive curriculum for trainees in endocrinology and metabolism in India. The Indian Medical Council adopted this. Following his stay in Delhi, he served as the founding director of the Endocrine Sciences Center at the newly created superspeciality institute—Sanjay Gandhi Postgraduate Institute of Medical Sciences (SGPGIMS), Lucknow, India. This is now India's premier institute in both basic sciences as well as clinical research. It offers DM and PhD in endocrinology and remains a top destination for patients seeking expert opinion in endocrine and metabolic disorders. The first recruit for a PhD is now a senior scientist and the director of the Division of Endocrinology at Central Drug Research Institute (Lucknow, India), and the first DM candidate is now a professor at SGPGIMS.

Dr. Khardori has served on NIH-Study Section as reviewer and provided valuable services to the American Diabetes Association and the Endocrine Society in helping put together annual scientific sessions. He serves as an ad hoc reviewer for over thirty journals of repute (*Lancet*, *Diabetes*, *Diabetologia*, *Diabetes Care*, *Nature reviews*, *Neuroendocrinology*, and many other high-impact journals). He has over 280 publications (manuscripts, editorials, communications, book chapters, and reports). He has been nominated as series editor for *Topics in Endocrinology* (Jay Pee Publishers).

Dr. Khardori serves as coeditor of ASAP (American Association of Clinical Endocrinology Self-Assessment Program) and remains chief editor for content in Endocrinology for WebMD and Medscape, currently serving as professor of medicine: endocrinology and metabolism at Eastern Virginia Medical School in Norfolk, Virginia (USA), and by the time this book is out, he might have taken retirement from this responsibility.

When asked to recall some highlights from his GMC experience, Dr. Khardori stated, "The mentoring and influence of Prof Kahali was priceless, cherish my friends like Afzal Hussain Khan who topped the list in my year. Some Registrars amazed me in my time (MS Khuroo, and Late Dr. Mohi-ud-Din) they enriched our lives through their brilliance. During my SP college years, my best friends were Nazir Gilkar who is a pediatrician in New York, and Ghulam Jeelani Mufti who is a Hematologist/Hematopathologist of repute living in London (UK) now. I met Nancy on the 2nd day of medical school at GMC that led to a happy long lasting union." Dr. Nancy Khardori is profiled elsewhere in the book.

Dr. Shagufta Yasmeen

Dr. Shagufta Yasmeen, a graduate of the Government Medical College in Srinagar, Kashmir, is the clinical professor of internal medicine and obstetrics and gynecology at University of California (UC), Davis. Like many international medical graduates, Dr. Yasmeen came to UC Davis via a long and winding road that began at the University of Kashmir in Srinagar, Kashmir, where she earned a medical degree in 1989. She continued to work in London in the early 1990s and attained membership—not easy for a foreigner—in the Royal College of Obstetricians and Gynecologists. She moved across the Atlantic to begin an internship at the Thomas Jefferson Medical University in Philadelphia in 1994. She then completed residency training at UC Davis, where she has been on the faculty since the late 1990s. She is on the faculty in the Departments of Medicine and OB/GYN, and she put these twin skills to great use in establishing the Shifa Clinic at the Sacramento mosque. This clinic has developed into a model for providing care and at the same time reaching out to members of all faiths.

As the director and founder of the Shifa Clinic (http://www.shifaclinic.org), one of five free student-run clinics (http://www.ucdmc.ucdavis.edu/medschool/clinics/) in the UC Davis Health System, she works with UC Davis medical students and faculty and community physician volunteers to provide much-needed health-care services to uninsured patients in Sacramento. The clinic specializes in serving Middle Eastern and East Indian communities and provides interpretation in Punjabi, Arabic, Farsi, Urdu, and Hindi, the last two of which Dr. Yasmeen speaks, along with Kashmiri and English. I had the pleasure of visiting UC Davis and saw firsthand the remarkable accomplishments of Dr. Yasmeen. Dr. Joseph De Silva, the dean of UC Davis, had only praise for this clinic and told me that the Shifa Clinic was one of the best-run programs at UC Davis. These efforts were recognized nationally when Dr. Yasmeen was honored with the 2007 American Medical Association Foundation Leadership Award. The Leadership Awards are presented annually to medical students, residents/fellows, young physicians, and international medical graduate physicians who have exhibited outstanding leadership in organized medicine and/or community affairs. The awards provide leadership development training for these "emerging leaders" to further strengthen their efforts toward advancing health care in America . . . Establishing a medical clinic on the premises of a mosque represented lots of challenges. Some members of the mosque were not comfortable in having students and staff of all faiths in their midst in the mosque. Dr. Yasmeen overcame these objections with quiet determination and sound arguments based on the teachings of Islam. After convincing the mosque leadership about the importance and significance of having a clinic on premises, she convinced the medical school leadership and obtained an agreement allowing the medical school to send volunteer medical students and faculty to run the clinic, which is located within the premises of the Sacramento mosque.

The Shifa Clinic provides strong training for medical students and UC Davis undergraduate volunteers interested in a career in medicine. Dr. Yasmeen routinely provides one-on-one care to the clinic's patients. She also is the principal investigator on several grants awarded to the clinic. The grant funding has enabled the clinic to implement broader preventive care programs and stronger diabetic nutrition education programs, and to develop more culturally sensitive and linguistically appropriate materials. In 2003, in recognition of her teaching skills, Dr. Yasmeen received the American College of Professors of Obstetrics and Gynecology (APGO) Award for Excellence in Teaching and the Alpha Omega Alpha Honor Medical Society Award in 2006. In 2004, Dr. Yasmeen enrolled in the School of Medicine NIH 'K30/Mentored Clinical Research Training Program', which was developed to provide junior faculty and subspecialty trainees with the didactic training, mentored research, and peer-supported environment needed to launch an innovative clinical and translational research programs. She completed the course work for this program in May 2006. This training from the 'K30 program' equipped Dr. Yasmeen with the foundational concepts of clinical epidemiology, allowing her to undertake an independent research program on the role of screening for breast cancer in elderly women. Dr. Yasmeen was selected as a recipient of the Cancer Prevention, Control, Behavioral and Population Sciences Career Development Award— better known as a 'KO7 career award'—from the National Institutes of Health and the National Cancer Institute. The five-year $600,000 grant enabled Dr. Yasmeen to undertake a research project "Comorbidities and Breast Cancer among Elderly Women in the State of California." In essence, the study evaluated breast cancer screening—or the lack of it—in older women to help answer a much-debated question: When should screening continue, and when should it stop? Dr. Yasmeen received Internal Medicine Outstanding Volunteer Faculty Award from University of California in 2017 and UC Davis Kaiser Teaching Award Ob/Gy in 2021.

Dr. Yasmeen's other research interests include delivery of primary care services to women, cancer screening, and disparities in health outcomes among women, especially among women with breast cancer. Given her interest in cancer screening and prevention, she also sought opportunities to work with cancer registry data. With her department chair, Lloyd H. Smith (MD, PhD), she coauthored an innovative study on the symptoms and diagnostic workups that precede diagnosis of ovarian cancer in elderly women, using data from Medicare provider claims linked to the California Surveillance Epidemiology and End Results (SEER) database. Building on the knowledge and experience she gained working with Dr. Smith, she pursued an independent project (in collaboration with staff from the California Cancer Registry) on thyroid cancer during pregnancy. She analyzed stage at diagnosis, treatment, and survival among pregnant women, and the impact of treatment on maternal and perinatal outcomes. She completed several studies using the California Office of Statewide Health Planning Development's (OSHPD) Patient Discharge Data Set, which has been linked with birth certificates and fetal death certificates. Through these studies, they focused on specific problems of pregnancy such as systemic lupus erythematosis, grand multiparity, and thyroid cancer. Her primary mentor, Dr. Patrick Romano (MD, MPH) has a longstanding interest in the use of administrative data to assess the quality of hospital care. She collaborated with him on the validity of using risk-adjusted postpartum maternal readmission rates and perineal laceration rates as measures of obstetric performance. This work resulted in three excellent manuscripts.

Dr. Yasmeen was a member of Medicine in Action,- a mission-based nonprofit organization that provided gynecological surgeries and medical care to women. In 2007, she, along with residents, other faculty members and nurses from UC Davis Department of Obstetrics and Gynecology, performed approximately fifteen gynecological surgeries and provided medical care to more than five hundred women in Kingston, Jamaica. This was a unique cross-cultural learning experience to work alongside local medical professionals, engaging in mutually beneficial learning exchange while providing valuable care and support to hospitals and clinics within the local communities. Since Dr. Yasmeen was the only internist on the team, it was rewarding for her to educate and treat patients with medical problems. With the same organization (Medicine in Action), she traveled to Tanzania in 2009 for a three-week medical mission. The team conducted women health clinics, medical clinics, and performed gynecological surgeries. Dr. Yasmeen recounts an unforgettable experience from her medical mission. She says, "During this trip I successfully climbed Mount Kilimanjaro. During our ascent to Mount Kilimanjaro one of our Sherpas, 18 years old developed chest pain and shortness of breath at approximately at 3000 meter elevation. Being an internist helped me again and I diagnosed patient with mitral stenosis and pulmonary edema. Arrangements for his descent were made and I followed the patient, on my return in a local hospital in Arusha where he was treated and was doing well." Dr. Yasmeen has done volunteer work in Cambodia also through Catholic Church. And what does Dr. Yasmeen get out of this volunteer experience? To hear her tell it is a pure bliss. "At the end of the day seeing patients- gives me a lot of joy," she said. "It has made me a different person. I just thank God I was able to help people."

Dr. Yasmeen organized a grass roots effort to start Shifa COVID vaccine clinic. Under her leadership, an infrastructure for vaccine storage was launched, and protocol for vaccine educational outreach, vaccine training, and administration was developed prior to vaccine availability in Sacramento County. Shifa Community Clinic became one of the sites for COVID vaccination in partnership with Sacramento County Clinic. She organized a COVID vaccine team of medical students, undergraduate students, and volunteer physicians. In partnership with mosque administration and UC Davis volunteers, eleven thousand vaccines were administered in diverse greater Sacramento. Shifa Clinic vaccine program has been one of the most successful vaccine clinics in Sacramento. To promote vaccination in vulnerable refugee community, an educational campaign was organized with local religious leaders to demystify vaccine hesitancy. Additionally, vaccines were provided on site in the mosques close to underserved population to promote vaccination and prevent barriers (transportation/ language).

Shifa Clinic is a comprehensive medical center focused on spiritual, sociocultural, and language-specific medical care for every individual irrespective of race, ethnicity, religion, and gender. Over the past ten years, total number of patients has doubled from 1,710 to 3,543. Alongside the increase in patient population, there has also been an increase in demographic diversity that includes an increase of Hispanic patients from 8 percent to 24.56 percent. According to Dr. Yasmeen, "To best address the health care needs of our diverse under-served community, I believe healthcare needs to be transformed, not only by improving access to care, but by developing an educational approach that empowers and engages patients to improve their health and help to transform their lives. Shifa Clinic has developed a promoter based, sustainable, culturally competent, language specific, comprehensive health education program design, helping people to identify, address, and overcome barriers to achieve health and wellbeing."

Dr. Yasmeen has been an active participant in IMANA. During the annual convention IMANA, held in San Francisco in 2005, Dr. Yasmeen and her colleagues from the Shifa and the UC Davis School of Medicine were present in full force. JIMA profiled Dr. Shagufta Yasmeen as a young, energetic physician who, through her actions, has developed a great reputation within her circles at UC Davis and now has been recognized by the American Medical Association, the National Institutes of Health, and the National Cancer Institute. In the post-September 11 atmosphere, Dr. Yasmeen has done a great job in winning the hearts and minds of many, presented a real face of Islam and Muslims and set an example for all of us. She is a true example of "faith in action." Her greatest achievement has been transforming the lives of students and families. Over the past twenty years, more than three hundred undergraduate students have successfully launched careers in health care.

(A part of Dr. Shagufta Yasmeen's profile was taken from *JIMA*: volume 39, 2007, page 127, by Dr. Faroque Ahmad Khan, MB, MACP.)

Dr. Suhail A. Shah

Born in Srinagar to a family of doctors, Dr. Suhail Shah has been an exceptionally talented and gifted individual right from his childhood. He always topped his class even as a child right through primary and high school. He topped the entire state of Jammu and Kashmir in 1981 in eleventh grade. He graduated from Government Medical College in 1989 and was the best outgoing graduate/valedictorian of his medical school class.

Dr. Suhail moved to the US for his residency training in internal medicine and rapidly distinguished himself in his residency program and was promoted to chief residency. He was the primary author of multiple articles in a national medical journal and copresented many posters in the prestigious annual APDIM meeting in San Francisco. He chose to work in the prestigious North Shore University Hospital (NSUH) at Manhasset as a hospitalist attending in its burgeoning Hospitalist Program. Not surprisingly, he was promoted to the chief of the Hospitalist Program in less than a year. He led the program from its initial four to more than eight physicians.

Suhail then left North Shore employment to pursue his dream of self-ownership of a successful private hospitalist practice. Once again, he demonstrated foresight, and he has been extremely successful in this endeavor. Many practitioners have since emulated him once he set the pace. He runs a busy inpatient practice and still finds time to be a wonderful husband and a devoted father.

Suhail has always been concerned with the issues that confront his fellow physicians in practice, and, by logical progression, he was inducted into the NSUH physician leadership. As a result of his diligence, hard work, and perseverance, he was elected president of the more than three thousand physicians of North Shore University Hospital in 2013. No mean feat, especially in a very competitive physician system. Suhail is the first nonwhite/Asian American to be the secretary, treasurer, and then president of the prestigious NSUH Staff Society, breaking that particular ceiling. Of course, he is part of more than a dozen other committees that the hospital needs him for and now has been honored with the post of chair of the North Shore/LIJ Credentialing Committee, responsible for credentialing over six thousand physicians.

Suhail has also been involved in Kashmiri community affairs and, during the devastating floods of 2014 in Kashmir, personally donated and was responsible for raising thousands of dollars for the flood victims. Suhail, using his influence and position, was able to generate money for flood victims from his fellow physicians and contributed to the relief and rehabilitation of flood victims in Kashmir.

Suhail is a nondenominational giver and has consistently supported global charity organizations like MSF by personal monthly donations and soliciting his colleagues. Suhail has considerable experience of being involved in medical student and medical resident teaching in NSUH and LIJ Medical Center. Even now, he is regularly scheduled for ongoing lectures for PAs and NPs in the system.

On a personal note, Suhail is a giver in more ways than one. He is a leader; he has been a torch-bearer for the beleaguered Kashmiri community, especially its physicians. He has many more dreams, many more goals to accomplish. He is always eager for more accomplishment and was granted prestigious NSUH Medical Ethics Fellowship for 2015/2016.

Dr. Tanveer P. Mir

Dr. Tanveer Mir is a highly accomplished physician who has received local, regional, and national recognition for her work in geriatric medicine, palliative care, end-of-life issues, and innovative contributions to health-care policy. From 1999 to 2001, she served on the board of governors of the American College of Physicians. She represented the Long Island region of New York. In April 2009, she was elected as a regent of the American College of Physicians (ACP), making her the first Muslim woman physician to serve on its board. She served as the chair of the American College of Physicians Board of Regents from 2015 to 2016, the year of ACP's centennial celebration.

The ACP is the largest medical specialty organization and the second-largest physician group in the United States. Its members include 148,000 internal medicine physicians (internists), related subspecialists, and medical students. Internists specialize in the prevention, detection, and treatment of illness in adults. The board of regents is the main policymaking body of ACP. Regents may serve two three-year terms (www.acponline.org).

Dr. Tanveer P. Mir graduated valedictorian from Government Medical College in Srinagar, Kashmir, and was judged the best graduate from the University of Kashmir in 1981. She came to the United States from Kashmir after marriage and pursued her training in internal medicine at Long Island Jewish Medical Center and served as the chief medical resident at Nassau University Medical Center in New York. She is board certified in the internal medicine, geriatrics, hospice and palliative medicine, and bioethics. She was on the staff at Nassau County Medical Center (NCMC) in New York as associate program director and chief of Geriatrics. She was judged the best teacher by the medical house staff on several occasions, and her innovative work in redesigning the training program resulted in New York State granting NCMC more than $3 million. Over the ensuing years, Dr. Tanveer Mir became active in the New York chapter of the ACP (NYACP), served as interim governor for the ACP in New York for several years, and remained active in NYACP chapter (resident and teaching activities). In 2002, she was awarded the very prestigious NYACP Laureate Award. During the 2009 Internal Medicine Convocation ceremony, ACP honored Dr. Mir with advancement to master. This distinction from the ACP Board of Regents recognizes outstanding and extraordinary career accomplishments, exhibiting preeminence in practice or medical research. Of the 126,000 ACP members globally, only 648 (0.5 percent) have become masters, indeed a very unique and rare honor.

Dr. Tanveer Mir's area of interest and expertise includes hospice and palliative care services, end-of-life care, bioethics, geriatrics education and practice models, bioethics, and pain management. Dr. Mir was also instrumental in obtaining a substantial grant for the cancer center in Kashmir from the Indo-American Cancer Society. This grant has funded the staff—a physician, a social worker, and a nurse—for the much-needed palliative care program in Kashmir. Dr. Mir's other achievements include serving as the senior medical director at the Hospice Care Network, an affiliate of North Shore Long Island Jewish Healthcare System in New York. She is the recipient of the George W. Frank Chairman's Award for Humanitarian Services in Hospice (2009), the Nargis Dutt Foundation Award for Palliative Care in 2012, and the Distinguished Palliative Services Award from AAPNA (2020).

She has served as an associate professor of Medicine at New York University (NYU) School of Medicine, an associate professor of Medicine at Hofstra University, and professor of Medicine at the University of Florida College of Medicine. Dr. Mir is currently the chairperson of the Department of Medicine and president of the Medical Board at Wyckoff Heights Medical Center in Brooklyn, New York. Dr. Mir has been an active member of IMANA, having participated at several national conventions, both as a member and as faculty.

When asked what advice she has for her younger and upcoming colleagues, in particular, to reflect on while combining professional and family obligations, Dr. Mir commented, "Work-family balance. A woman physician cannot put off family for work or work for the family. A successful balance of both these roles is possible. I find that planning, efficient time management; prioritizing work and home schedules and identifying problems and attention to detail are some of the skills that are common to both roles. How to juggle a parent-teacher meeting, teaching rounds, and office hours on the same day is an achievable task. In addition, community involvement is important. Establishing open communication with growing children and being involved in their activities and accomplishments is important for work-family balance as well."

Dr. Tanveer is married to Dr. Parvez Mir, an internist-pulmonologist, and they are blessed with three children: two daughters, Tanya and Natasha, and a son, Nabil (*JIMA*: volume 41, 2009, page 83, July 2009).

Dr. G. M. Din

One of my relations got into a government job immediately after graduation. She was bright and wanted to pursue postgraduation in a discipline for which the facilities were not available in the valley. She had a "hunger" for more education but did not want to leave her job. She applied for permission to go outside the state for further education. She was allowed to go but with a condition that she would not get any salary for three years (the period of her study). The girl was from a family who could not afford to educate her outside. Sad and facing the dilemma of whether to go or not to go for postgraduation, she came to know about a "trust" run in the name of Dr. Mohi-ud-Din at Poloview, Srinagar. The girl, ventured into the trust, expecting a "refusal." Hearing her unique story, the person in charge of the scholarship gave a nod to the scholarship for the young girl. The scholarship continued for three years till the girl completed her postgraduation. I was told that hundreds of poor boys and girls pursuing studies outside the state were beneficiaries of this scholarship. The amount was enough to cater to their day-to-day expenses and their college fees. This was way back in the '90s, and the trust was created much earlier than this in the 1970s by a great son of the soil—Dr. Ghulam Mohi-ud-Din, popularly known as Dr. G. M. Din. The concept of financial help for studies was unique in that era, and I know how many people benefited from this endeavor.

It seems many people in Srinagar are familiar with Dr. Din and his efforts to pay back to his own community. Dr. Gulzar Mufti has written in detail about him in his book *Kashmir in Sickness and Health.*

Dr. G. M. Din was the son of Mufti Saad-ud-Din, a revered Islamic scholar who was born on January 1, 1903. He was nominated for MBBS to Lahore, like many of his contemporaries, and he completed his MBBS from King Edward Medical College in 1930.

Dr. Din returned to Kashmir from Lahore and was appointed as the doctor in charge of the traveling dispensary in Kashmir. He did wonderful work during the cholera epidemic of 1931 and was appointed as assistant surgeon in-charge of epidemics. He traveled to the United Kingdom in 1937 for further studies. He completed MRCP (Edinburgh) in 1942. Dr. Din was actively involved in volunteer work during wartime in the cities that were bombed by Germans during World War II. He was appointed as a consultant physician at Kingston General Hospital, Hull.

Dr. Din was elected as a Fellow of the Royal College of Physicians of Edinburgh (FRCP) in 1965. He retired from service in 1968. His wife, Jean Mitchell, who married him in 1955, calls him "Mohi" and, according to Dr. Gulzar, lives in Yorkshire, England. He would provide help and guidance to many doctors from the subcontinent who would come to UK for job and further studies.

Dr. Din died in Hull in 1984 at the age of eighty years. He was buried in Hull in a piece of land that he had purchased and was donated to the Islamic community of Hull to be used as a cemetery. Dr. Gulzar Mufti talks about the philanthropy that Dr. Din was interested in. He contributed to Oxfam, Mother Teresa's Fund, and Salvation Army.

His trust, erstwhile Mohi-ud-Din Trust, which took care of poor but bright students, provided financial aid for the marriage of daughters to deserving poor and also for the funeral expenses of the poor, is almost defunct now. There is a need to revive this legacy of his, and, in this endeavor, all of us need to participate.

Dr. Muzaffar, ex-director of Health Services, Kashmir, recalls Dr. Mohi-ud-Din's contribution in the form of a large number of books donated to the library of GMC Srinagar, and there was a photo of Dr. Din hung on GMC Srinagar's walls as a tribute to what he had done ("Returning the Debt," *Kashmir Life*, May 13, 2023).

Dr. Ghulam Jeelani Mufti

Prof. Ghulam Jeelani Mufti is a world-renowned driving force for the research, diagnosis, and treatment of blood cancers. He is one of the most renowned physicians of Kashmiri origin who has left an indelible mark in the field of hematology and contributed significantly to the treatment and management of blood cancers. He has published over 450 papers (H Index 95) and chapters in scientific journals and textbooks on leukemia and myelodysplastic syndromes (MDS). He retired from his roles as head of King's College London's Department of Hematological Medicine and the Hematology Institute director (academic lead) for King's Health Partners on September 7, 2020.

Dr. Ghulam Jeelani is a pioneer who radically changed the way blood cancers were treated at King's College Hospital NHS Foundation Trust and across the world. Professor Mufti has dedicated thirty-five years of his career to his clinical work and research. As the head of Hemato-oncology at King's College Hospital, his team, in collaboration with the Institute of Liver Studies, carried out the first-ever combined liver and bone marrow transplant at King's in 1985. With his leadership, the hospital now has one of the largest bone marrow transplant programs in the UK and performs over two hundred transplants a year.

Working with leukemia charities including Leukemia UK and Blood Cancer UK, Professor Mufti tirelessly pressed for enormous expansions to the services and resources of his department, transforming it from one that initially had two inpatient beds to one with sixty—creating four new specialist hematology wards, including the Derek Mitchell ward.

Over time, he expanded his department—which originally had no research laboratories—to house 180 researchers and a new dedicated research facility for finding game-changing new treatments. As a result, his department went on to become a renowned international center for the diagnosis and treatment of blood cancers. It is a center of excellence for Leukemia Lymphoma Research and the only gene and cell-based therapies center for myeloid leukemia and allied diseases. It is also a national center for several hematological disorders such as aplastic anemia or thalassemia, and an exemplar center for clotting disorders and sickle cell disease. Under Professor Mufti's oversight as the Pathology director, the department was the largest pathology hub in the UK and the first to have a single track for pathology.

Professor Mufti has devoted much of his time to roles across King's Health Partner organizations as the head of the Department of Hematological Medicine at King's College London and King's College Hospital NHS Foundation Trust (since 1997), nonexecutive director at King's College Hospital NHS FT (since 2012), Hematology Institute director (academic lead) for King's Health Partners (since 2015), professor of hemato-oncology, King's College London School of Medicine at Guy's, King's and St. Thomas' Hospitals (since 1995), clinical director of Pathology, King's College Hospital NHS FT (1995–2005), clinical director of Hematology (1995–2002), head of Division of Clinical Laboratory Sciences, GKT School of Medicine, chair of several committees at King's College Hospital NHS FT, including the Pathology Management Board, Hematology Consultants' Committee, and the Hematology Laboratory Senior Staff Committee, and at King's College

London chair of the BAME Steering Group and the Promotions Committee.

Over the course of Professor Mufti's distinguished career with King's and King's Health Partners, he has driven many significant and impactful clinical achievements, changing the lives of many patients across London and beyond. His specialist work in myelodysplastic syndrome (MDS), acute myeloid leukemia, and stem cell transplantation has helped to transform the detection and treatment of many cancer cells, resulting in improvements in the diagnosis, treatment, and life expectancy of people with leukemia. Dr. Jeelani contributed to the first international prognostic scoring system of myelodysplastic syndromes published in 1997. This was a landmark paper that standardized the treatment of myelodysplastic syndromes.

Dr. Ghulam Jeelani Mufti was awarded an OBE (the Order of the British Empire) in 2017 for services to hematological medicine, which include:

- significant research achievements focused on molecular aberrations in MDS/AML and the identification of novel therapies that include gene and cell-based therapies;
- leading the development of a potential new vaccine for acute myeloid leukemia—the first of its kind in the world;
- leading the team at King's that developed the first immune gene therapy program for leukemia to be approved by the Gene Therapy Advisory Committee (GTAC);
- opening the Leukemia UK Ambulatory Care Unit at King's College Hospital, which allowed patients to receive stem cell transplants as outpatients for the first time ever;
- leading the research groups at King's working on the molecular genetics of MDS/aplastic anemia/acute

myeloid leukemia, and sitting on the working group that produced national and international guidelines on the treatment and prognosis of MDS;

- being a founding member and chair of the UK MDS Forum;
- being a member of the European Bone Marrow Transplantation Group and a founding member of the Board of the International Myelodysplastic Foundation, for which his department at King's College Hospital is a recognized center of excellence;
- being awarded the Lifetime Achievement Award from the Turkish government, awarded by the Turkish minister of health, for advising on the setting up of hemato-oncology services and BMT programs in Turkey;
- championing the Mind and Body Team at King's College Hospital NHS Foundation Trust, funded by the charity Leukemia UK, which became the first in the country to offer integrated physical and mental health care to people living with blood cancer;
- being the founding institute director for KHP Hematology, working as part of the program board to take the institute from concept to reality, to establish a wide-ranging clinical academic portfolio of projects, to improve care and outcomes, to develop education and training of future generations, and to secure significant commercial partnership grants to drive forward leading research, including one of the AHSC's largest commercial partnerships with Celgene.

Prof. Sir Robert Lechler, the outgoing senior vice president (Health) at King's and executive director of King's Health Partners, said, "Prof. Mufti's contribution to blood cancer research and treatments is unparalleled, and his work will have a lasting impact on the lives of so many of our patients across the country. We have been extremely fortunate to have had his expertise and leadership in our Haematology Institute, and his support was instrumental for our Mind and Body team to offer whole body care to those with blood cancer. All of us at King's Health Partners wish him the very best as he continues his research and clinical practice."

Prof. Richard Trembath, the incoming senior vice president (Health) at King's and executive director of King's Health Partners, said, "Prof Mufti's commitment and enthusiasm has impacted on so many staff across the King's College community together with the broader King's Health Partnership. We are as a consequence so well placed to build on his legacy and thrive. Prof Mufti's research across a number of areas of haematology not least in leukaemia and MDS, has advanced the science base but also led to significant advancement in clinical practice, including the development of guidelines that have improved outcomes from disease for patients across the world. I personally wish him much gratitude and wish for his continued success, as Ghulam charts this next and exciting new chapter in his career."

Prof. Clive Kay, chief executive of King's College Hospital NHS Foundation Trust, said, "Prof Mufti has been a part of history for hematology, particularly at King's College Hospital. He performed our first combined liver and bone marrow transplant in 1985, and since then our department has gone from strength to strength with his incredible expertise and passion. His services to hematological medicine are unrivalled and have helped so many of our patients and staff at King's. All of our staff join me in wishing him the very best as he continues his research and clinical practice."

Besides being a member of many international societies and foundations, Dr. Mufti has been the founder member of the MDS International Symposia and senior executive board member of the International MDS Foundation. He has been a member of the scientific team to Moscow and Minsk following the Chernobyl disaster. He is an invited speaker to many internal conferences and adviser, Bone Marrow Transplantation Program, of many reputed hospitals in East and West.

Dr. Mufti has been an examiner for membership examinations of the Royal College of Pathologists (Hematology), King Saud University Hematology Fellowship Finals—for which Professor Mufti was given an award. He has been an examiner for final MB examination in pathology and examiner for PhD and MD degrees in hematology in universities through UK and Europe. Professor Mufti is the advisory board chair and member for Celgene, GSK, Novartis, Amgen, among other pharmaceutical companies. Professor Mufti will continue to focus on his Celgene program research, fundraising, and his clinical practice.

Postscript: I and Prof. Faroque Khan requested Dr. Ghulam JeelaniMufti for his bio, but he politely refused, saying he considered doctors working in Kashmir more deserving to be in the list of one hundred outstanding ones than he himself. To be fair to the readers of this book, we got his achievement profile from King's College, where he did his work, which we reproduce with thanks. Dr. Mufti's achievements make all of us proud. His trajectory has been the same as has been for all the doctors who are performing so well in UK and US, being born in Kashmir, graduating from GMC Srinagar, getting into UK, and doing an amazing work. One of my classmates working as a hematopathologist at MD Anderson US, says, "Books can be written on the achievements of Dr. Geelani Mufti. He is the most accomplished physician that Kashmir has ever produced. In fact one of the most accomplished hematologists in the entire world." When I emailed this abridged draft to Dr. Mufti and asked for his consent to publish it in our book, he was kind enough to agree to my request.

Dr. Ghulam Rasool (Gulzar) Mufti

Dr. Ghulam Rasool or Dr. Gulzar Mufti as he is popularly called is an outstanding clinician who has served in various capacities in the UK and done a commendable job as a surgeon and urologist and helped to launch the careers of many doctors from Kashmir in the UK. Born in Downtown Srinagar, he did his MBBS from GMC Srinagar and was the first batch alumnus of GMC Srinagar. He did his MS (general surgery) from MP Shah Medical College, Gujarat, India, and MCh (urology) from All India Institute of Medical Sciences (AIIMS), New Delhi, India, in 1978. He was the first qualified Muslim urologist from India. After serving in Kashmir for some time, he moved to Iran and later flew to the UK and did his FRCS (the Royal College of Surgeons of Edinburgh).

Dr. Gulzar Mufti served as registrar and senior registrar in London Hospitals from 1981 to 1985. He was a consultant urological surgeon, Walsgrave Hospital, Coventry; Glasgow Royal Infirmary, Glasgow (Scotland); and Cumberland Infirmary, Carlisle, England (1987–1990). He served as a consultant urological surgeon, Medway Maritime Hospital Gillingham, Kent, from 1990 to 2011 (twenty-one years).

Beginning with a small center for urology in 1990, in two decades, Dr. Gulzar established a comprehensive Urology Department at Medway, which is now the Urological Cancer Center for West Kent. His speciality interest was urological cancer, and he performed hundreds of radical cystectomies and pelvic exenterations, radical prostatectomies, and radical nephrectomies. He established Medway as one of the centers in the country that offered patients orthotopic bladder reconstruction (neobladder) after radical cystectomy.

He was the deanery trainer for junior as well as senior urological trainees for more than fifteen years. Many of his trainees are working in senior positions in various departments in the UK and abroad. Medway gave him an opportunity to head the Department of Urological Sciences.

Dr. Gulzar later served as a clinical director and chairman, Division of Surgery Medway NHS Trust Gillingham, Kent, England (2000–2004). As the clinical director of Surgery, he streamlined emergency and elective surgical pathways by remodeling team structures and established the Surgical Assessment Unit, one of the first such centers in the UK. This was the feature article in the "Hospital Doctor" issue of June 2005. He separated the elective and emergency surgical commitments of surgeons by remodeling their timetables, which led to consultant-led emergency surgical services. The Royal College of Surgeons England and the Department of Health set the model as an example for other hospitals. This was a new concept then, but the model is currently in vogue in most hospitals in the UK.

Dr. Gulzar Mufti also changed the "on-call" duties for surgeons from 5:00 p.m. to 5:00 p.m. the next day instead of the traditional 9:00 a.m. to 9:00 a.m. model. Over the years, many UK hospitals have adopted this model. He received B Distinction Award by the Department of Health England for his services to health care in 2003. He was awarded Clinical Excellence Silver Award in 2007 by the UK Department of Health for services to National Health Service (NHS) in England.

Medway NHS FT Board is responsible for the management of Medway Maritime Hospital (MMH)—a six-hundred-bed associate teaching hospital affiliated with the University of

London and GKT Medical School. He was a member of the executive team that transformed the organization from a no-star trust to a foundation trust—the first hospital in Kent, Sussex, and Surrey to achieve that. MMH was listed as one of the top forty hospitals in CHKS ratings and the most improved hospital in 2009. As medical director, Dr. Gulzar was responsible for leading on patient safety and conceived the action plan that led to a substantial reduction in Hospital Standardized Mortality Ratio (HSMR) at MMH. He conceived and led the Trust's Quality and Safety Agenda with the development of the Trust Risk Register, Quality Assurance Framework, Clinical Governance Strategy, Patient Safety Strategy, Clinical Audit Strategy, and introduced the concept of Quality Accounts. He also introduced the two-monthly medical director's grand rounds under the banner "Reflection with Education." He led on the development of tertiary services in cardiology, oncology, and vascular surgery and established West Kent Urology Cancer Services at MMH and conceived and led the merger of urology departments at Medway and Dartford. He turned around poorly performing orthopedic services through joint work with the National Orthopedic project team and through performance management of medical staff.

As medical director of Medway NHS Foundation Trust (executive director, FT Board), he led the development of job planning guidelines, yearly appraisal and performance management strategy, and other policies for medical staff. He led the "High Dependency Care Strategy" with the establishment of Surgical and Medical High Dependency Units at MMH. He set up the Emergency Department teaching rotation between MMH and Aga Khan Medical School in Karachi, Pakistan. Plans to set up a similar program with AIIMS New Delhi, India, fell victim to bureaucratic hurdles in both countries. As chairman Medical Advisory Committee (MAC), SPIRE Alexandra Hospital, he introduced and developed the concepts of clinical governance in a private UK hospital at a time when these concepts were beginning to evolve.

Dr. Mufti's services were commissioned (through the UK Department of Health) by the Government of Barbados (2011–2012) to advise on the reorganization of health services, in particular, the organizational restructuring at QEH—the teaching hospital affiliated to Barbados Medical School (University of West Indies). He authored and presented to the Health Minister the paper entitled "QEH—Agenda for Change," which incorporated the "Hub and Spoke Model" for health services, a long-term strategic plan for QEH and Clinical Directorate Model for hospital services. The Ministry of Health accepted the proposal and implemented most of the recommendations enlisted in the paper.

Dr. Gulzar served as the medical director for Care UK since 2013. Care UK is the largest private health-care provider in England and manages more than twenty hospitals and daycare centers across England. The organization does not treat private patients but provides services to NHS patients for which it is paid by UK Health Commissioners. As a medical director, Dr. Gulzar implemented a number of systems changes in the organization. He introduced and developed the "Quality and Safety Action Plan" (including quality accounts), led the job planning and appraisal of senior and junior medical staff, introduced a governance structure, and streamlined clinical audit and incident management processes.

Dr. Gulzar served as IRM reviewer for RCS England and specialist advisor Care Quality Commission England (2013). In this role, he was deputed by the Royal College to undertake a review of a hospital, a department, or a doctor and suggest systems, processes, or practice changes, which are then implemented. Care Quality Commission (CQC) is the regulator of health care in England. The organization conducts inspections of health-care institutions in the country on a cyclical basis and makes a judgment on whether a hospital or a clinic is "safe, caring, responsive, effective and well-led." Dr. Gulzar has been involved with several inspections and has completed the review of services of many UK hospitals. These two roles have provided him with the opportunity to gain expertise and experience in the regulation of health-care institutions.

Dr. Gulzar is a panelist of Fitness to Practise Tribunals for the GMC—the regulator of doctors in the UK, and adjudicates on issues related to the professional and/or personal conduct of doctors. He has delivered judgments on tens of such cases. This role has provided him with insight into the professional regulation of doctors.

A number of overseas doctors, some from Kashmir, were trained in his urological unit. Some of these doctors from Kashmir Valley are working in urological centers in the UK in senior positions. When he left the department, he was happy to see that the person appointed in his place was also a Kashmiri. He was appointed by Dr. Gulzar as a senior house officer and worked his way up to be appointed to the top position. On leaving the department, it was a personal triumph for him. He also assisted many Kashmiri doctors to secure placements in various specialities in the UK. Many of them are working in responsible positions across UK.

Dr. Gulzar has authored about fifty papers in peer-reviewed scientific journals. He has given more than forty presentations at prestigious international urology meetings such as the British Association of Urological Surgeons (BAUS), European Association of Urology (EAU), American Urological Association (AUA), Societe Urologie International (SUI), Urological Society of India (USI), Association of Surgeons of India (ASI), etc. Several presentations were judged as the best paper or poster at some of these meetings. He also gave a number of invited lectures in the UK and abroad and participated as a guest speaker in a number of urology meetings in Srinagar. Most of these were under the auspices of the Urological Society of India. Dr. Gulzar has the membership of distinguished organizations—that is, full member, British Association of Urological Surgeons (BAUS); full member, Section of Oncology at BAUS, and full member, Section of Endourology at BAUS. He is the founding secretary, Asian British Urological Society, and trustee, British Kashmir Medical Association (BKMA).

The place of his birth (Kashmir Valley) is close to his heart; its health-care scenario is closer. He enjoys writing and wrote a few newspaper articles regarding health-care issues in the valley. Examples include "Is There a Stone in Your Bladder" (*Greater Kashmir* June 11, 2007) and "A Journey from Heaven to Hell" (*Greater Kashmir* July 16 and 23, 2007). He contributed a book chapter in the multiauthor book entitled *Kashmiriyat through the Ages*, published in 2011 by Gulshan Books, Srinagar. He authored and published a booklet entitled *Shah-i-Hamadan and Khanqah-i-Moalla* in 2002. To introduce the beautiful booklet of supplications to the generation not familiar with Arabic, he translated *Aurad-i-Fathiya* into English. This book was published by Ali Mohammad and Sons in 2022.

After several years of research involving many days spent in dark and dusty rooms of the Directorate of Archives Jammu and Kashmir at Old Secretariat Srinagar and at Sri Pratap Singh Library Srinagar, he authored his three-hundred-page book entitled *Kashmir in Sickness and in Health*, which was published in 2013 (Partridge Publications). *Kashmir in Sickness and in Health* juxtaposes the last 150 years of Kashmir's turbulent history with its educational and social development, from the start of Dogra rule in the mid-nineteenth century until the present time. To illuminate specific aspects of the story, the narrative interweaves with his own experiences of growing up in Downtown Srinagar. It also provides an insight into the role of the British in the development of Kashmir's health-care infrastructure and its social and intellectual upbringing. I have read his book and quoted it extensively especially when writing about the Kashmiri doctors who introduced the allopathic system of medicine in Kashmir.

Dr. Gulzar Mufti's second book, entitled *Under the Knife: Surgical Stories from All Over the World*, is centered on the world of surgery in general and surgeons in particular—their feelings and emotions, their strengths and weaknesses, their joys and sorrows, and much more. Importantly, the book is about patients who put their life into the hands of a surgeon. The stories have been used to lace together and bolster the narrative. The book has been published by the Book Guild Company Ltd., UK, in 2016. It has been reviewed by Mark J. Speakman, president, British Association of Urological Surgeons.

About his personal and professional achievements, Dr. Gulzar says, "I had the pleasure of working in a rural dispensary, a health centre, a sub-district hospital, a district hospital and two teaching hospitals in Jammu and Kashmir State. Following that, I had the privilege of working and visiting many renowned healthcare institutions in the world—in India, Iran, Europe, the USA, and of course the UK. I am a clinician at heart but concurrent winds of fate moved me into healthcare management, which I enjoy too. With time I was steered into healthcare regulation—of doctors who deliver care on the front line and of hospitals where care is delivered."

Dr. Mohamed Abdullah Sofi

Born in the pristine surroundings of majestic mountains and freshwater streams that sprawl across vast paddy fields, Dr. Mohamed Abdullah Sofi completed his elementary school education from Ganderbal High School, Kashmir, in 1960. His extensive academic profile includes graduating with an MBBS from Prince of Wales Medical School in Patna, 1970; MD, 1973; MRCP (UK), 1980; MRCP (Ireland), 1981; FRCP (London), 1990; FRCP (Edinburgh), 1991; and FRCS (Edinburgh), 1991. One of Dr. Sofi's most notable achievements was being selected for inclusion in the thirteenth edition of the *Who's Who in the World* publication. His broad profile of professional assignments at Prince Sultan Military Medical City in Riyadh Saudi Arabia, have included advisor/consultant of Academic Affairs and Training (2010–2014); director of Health Studies (2008–2010); and dean of Medical Studies (1987–1990).

During his professional tenure, Dr. Sofi has been an active member of eleven national and international scholarly societies in the field of medical education and neurosciences. In addition, he has presented multiple papers in fifty national and international scientific meetings and peer reviewed several medical journals for scientific deliberations. In pursuit of promoting excellence in training and education, Dr. Sofi has been the principal author of several periodicals and manuscripts for postgraduate medical teaching and instruction. The training manuals outlined the course specific curriculum, training structure, skills and learning objectives, rotations, and methods of evaluation as were deemed appropriate for learning outcomes under the auspices of the Saudi Commission for Health Specialties. Since there was no precedence for postgraduate medical training in the Kingdom of Saudi Arabia in the early '80s, Dr. Sofi undertook the challenge of establishing residency and fellowship training at Riyadh Al Kharj Hospital. This was successfully achieved with an unrivalled commitment to hard work and meticulous attention to the finest detail in the training structure, which has now successfully evolved into a program that exemplifies excellence to those of the highest international standards.

The Prince Sultan Military Medical City today is a premier institute for higher professional training and postgraduate medical education in the Middle East. Dr. Sofi was integrally involved with the institution, which has excelled beyond expected scope in its endeavors to establish strong foundations that were laid with meticulous planning and a strategically organized training structure in the early '90s. Today, the center boasts twenty-one established residency training programs and an equal number of fellowship training programs under the auspices of the Saudi Commission for Health Specialties. Dr. Sofi was involved in initiating and establishing dialogues with internationally reputed institutions of excellence such as the Royal College of Surgeons of Edinburgh, the Royal College of Physicians London, and the Royal College of Surgeons of Ireland, as well as the Royal College of Physicians of Australasia for promoting higher professional training and advancing postgraduate medical and surgical examinations on their behalf for the Kingdom of Saudi Arabia. Aside from structured residency and fellowship training, the focus on continuous professional development was put in place with thoughtful planning for all levels of professional staff to advance continuing medical education for excellence in patient care.

Outside the remit of medical education and training, Dr. Sofi has professionally contributed towards the highest quality of clinical service in the field of neurosciences. Supported by state-of-the-art facilities, he was able to contribute to the excellence of patient care with active participation in the research of neurological disorders. As a major teaching hospital, accredited for board certification in residency and fellowship training programs, Dr. Sofi actively participated in all teaching activities of clinical, didactic, seminars and symposia, and scientific conferences. The teaching also included nursing staff, neurophysiology technologists, and paramedical staff affiliated with service structure or an accredited training course. He has been to other university hospitals and teaching hospitals in the Kingdom of Saudi Arabia as an invited faculty member panelist. Dr. Sofi has also been involved in organizing courses for neurology residents for written and clinical examinations including Organized Structures Clinical Examinations (OSCE).

Dr. Sofi's contributions to the community are widespread and include raising funds for orphanages, victims of natural disasters and human tragedies culminating in loss of innocent lives, and sources of income for the noncombatant people in armed conflict zones. Dr. Sofi retired as the associate professor of Medicine at Al Maarefa Medical College Riyadh, Saudi Arabia.

Dr. Noor Ul Owase Jeelani

Craniopagus twins (CPT) are two independent children connected to each other with fused skulls, intertwined brains, and shared blood vessels. Fifty such sets of twins are estimated to be born around the world every year, of which it is thought only fifteen survive beyond the first thirty days of life. This is the most difficult surgery and requires months of planning and a huge team effort. A world-renowned Kashmiri-origin pediatric neurosurgeon in the UK has helped a group of Israeli doctors to successfully operate on a pair of twins conjoined at the head, with the babies now likely to lead normal lives. Dr. Noor Ul Owase Jeelani, who works at London's Great Ormond Street Hospital, agreed to carry out such a surgery outside the UK when contacted by doctors at Israel's Soroka Hospital, according to a report in the *Times of Israel* (TOI). He and his colleague, Prof. David Dunway, are globally seen as experts on such cases. "The fact that a Kashmir-born Muslim doctor scrubbed up alongside an Israeli team to help a Jewish family was a reminder of the universal nature of medicine," the report quoted him as saying so. Dr. Jeelani reminded the world that medicine transcends all divisions. "From a doctor's point of view, we're all one," he said. "All children are the same, whatever color or religion," he was quoted as saying. "The distinctions are man-made. A child is a child. From a doctor's point of view, we're all one," he emphasized. The doctor found the family's delight at the success of the operation "deeply moving."

"There was this very special moment when the parents were just over the moon. I have never in my life seen a person smile, cry, be happy, and be relieved at the same time. The mother simply couldn't believe it, we had to pull up a chair to help her to calm down," Dr. Jeelani told the news portal. It is also a major achievement for the medical team at Israel's Soroka Hospital that managed this complex operation despite having never performed such a surgery. It involved complicated on-the-spot decisions regarding which blood vessel to give to which twin and assessing in real time the impact that immediate decisions were having on the functioning of the brains, the report said (*Times of Israel*, September 12, 2021).

Dr. Owase Jeelani has received international recognition for separating craniopagus twins, including Sudanese twins Rital and Ritag in 2011 and then Pakistani twins Safa and Marwa in 2019 (BBC News coverage of Safa and Marwa ranked as the sixth most-read news item globally in 2019), Turkish twins Yigit and Derman in 2020, and a set of Israeli twins in 2021. Earlier, in 2020, when he separated Turkish twins after twenty hours of tiring surgery, his team reached a point when the retractor went in and one brain could be separated neatly from the other, and Dr. Owase called it a "Moses moment"—as the Red Sea parted and the path could be seen as a ray of light. His personal involvement with conjoined twins started in 2017 when a neurosurgeon from Peshawar, Pakistan, asked him to operate on identical conjoined twins Safa and Marwa, born three months earlier to a woman from rural northern Pakistan. He raised the money for the surgery from a Pakistani oil trader called Murtaza Lakhani and, with Dr. Dunaway, successfully operated after hundreds of hours of preparation. In 2019, he cofounded "Gemini Untwined," a global charity dedicated to supporting research and the treatment of CPT twins as well as other complex craniofacial and neurosurgical conditions. In 2021, the charity is supporting three further sets of craniopagus twins, their families, and medical teams to secure the treatment they need. Dr. Owase Jeelani is a codirector and leader of FaceValue, a research team of scientists and biomedical engineers based at the Institute of Child Health, UCL. The research focus is on defining craniofacial morphology in the normal and affected populations and developing techniques and distractors to achieve this change in a less invasive and more predictable manner.

Time magazine ranked Dr. Owase among the top one hundred surgeons in the UK in 2011 and the top one hundred pediatric specialists in the UK in 2012. His endeavors are designed around optimal prediction algorithms that increase efficiency, limit errors, and improve outcomes.

Dr. Owase Jeelani was born in Srinagar, Kashmir, in a well-to-do family in 1974. His father, Mr. Manzoor Jeelani, was an engineer, and his mother, Mrs. Razia Saif, has been one of the first woman engineers in Kashmir. She lives with Owase presently in London. He received his early education from Burn Hall School, Srinagar, and then went to the UK to study medicine. Dr. Jeelani holds a BMedSci from the University of Nottingham. He also holds an MPhil in Medical Law from the University of Glasgow, studying medical ethics and the legal dimension of practicing medicine on the Internet, and an MBA from INSEAD (ranked among the top ten global MBA schools), and majored in strategic health-care planning. He studied in France, Singapore, and the Wharton Business School in Philadelphia. About his many degrees and diverse interests, he says, "I often get asked why I undertook these extra degrees whilst simultaneously undertaking my Neurosurgical training at a considerable personal cost in time and money. I now answer with a rhetorical question; I was asked to take a world-class Neurosurgery department and make it better; how does one do that? I undertook these degrees some 12 to 17 years ago and whilst I did not know what the future would hold, I remained convinced that armed with the above, I would be better able to serve my patients. Super-specialization at the expense of a breadth of knowledge is a modern-day fallacy." He undertook basic surgical training in Nottingham and Southampton, neurosurgical and craniofacial training in the UK and Canada, and fellowships in pediatric neurosurgery and craniofacial surgery at GOSH and Sick Kids, Toronto. He is a consultant pediatric neurosurgeon and craniofacial surgeon at Great Ormond Street Hospital (GOSH).

Dr. Owase has worked at Great Ormond Street Hospital (GOSH) part time since 2000 and full time since 2009, and he undertakes two hundred to three hundred pediatric neurosurgical and craniofacial surgeries annually. His subspecialty interests are craniofacial reconstructive surgery, craniopagus separation surgery, surgery for brain tumors, and cerebrospinal fluid and intracranial pressure pathologies.

Dr. Owase Jeelani was head of the Department of Neurosurgery at GOSH from 2012 to 2018. He established it as a flagship service and one of the largest pediatric neurosurgery services in the world. During his tenure, four new consultant neurosurgeons were appointed to the service, the annual surgical case load increased to 1,100 cases, and operating revenues increased circa 14 percent year-on-year. Owase Jeelani is an honorary associate professor at the Institute of Child Health at University College London (UCL). Dr. Owase Jeelani has mentored dozens of surgeons from across the globe and regularly receives outstanding reviews from colleagues and students.

Combining medical and entrepreneurial aptitude, Owase Jeelani is a principal investigator of FaceValue, a UCL-based research team of doctors, scientists, and biomedical engineers that design surgical devices and machine-learning algorithms to predict and improve surgical outcomes; the inventor of CranioXpand, a cranial distractor system; and part of the team behind Klay Biotech, an AI-driven 3D VR platform.

The Klay Platform uses proprietary hardware and software to plan, visualize, develop, and execute procedures. It offers an unprecedented level of predictability for craniofacial surgeries, patient control, and informed consent. In 2013, Owase Jeelani cofounded the London Craniofacial Unit to benefit patients with craniofacial and neurosurgical issues globally and replicate GOSH's standard of care in the private sector.

Dr. Owase Jeelani also provides strategic counsel through a medical consulting company, Interface Health Solutions (IHS). IHS assisted in launching the Moorfield's Eye Hospital in Dubai in 2007, undertook a national review of all neurosurgical services for the government of Kuwait in 2010, and helped to establish the neurosurgery and craniofacial service at Sidra Hospital in Qatar in 2018.

Dr. Owase is a young sensation, and it would be interesting to follow his career as he accomplishes newer heights and bigger goals. Nothing seems impossible for this neurosurgeon of immense skill and patience.

Dr. Rizwan Romee

Rizwan Romee is a bright star and an upcoming sensation at Harvard known for his research on Natural Killer (NK) cells. Presently an associate professor of medicine at Harvard Medical School, he has been a brilliant alumnus of GMC Srinagar. I have known him from his GMC days as an inquisitive, highly focused, and a bright student. Presently, he is the principal investigator of Romee Lab for NK Cell Gene Manipulation and Therapy (https://romeelab.dana-farber.org).

Dr. Romee was born in Srinagar, Kashmir, to Mr. Shafi Shauq and Feroza Beg; however, he spent most of his childhood in a small village named Kaprin in the district of Shopian, where he did most of his early schooling. He has very fond memories of their ancestral house in Kaprin surrounded by beautiful apple orchards and paddy fields. While growing up, he was strongly influenced by his paternal uncle Naji Munawar (Sahitya Akademi awardee Kashmiri writer), who taught him the importance of being passionate about following your dreams without fearing failure and striving to make a difference in the lives of people. While he was surrounded by literary giants in his own family where the aroma of poetry prevailed, he was attracted towards scienceWhile growing up in his native village, Romee fell in love with science; as a matter of fact, he built his first laboratory in his ancestral home in Kaprin, naming it Romee Lab (the same name he has chosen for his current lab at Harvard).

As he moved to Srinagar for pursuing studies, he says moving to Srinagar from his native village was a bigger cultural shock for him than moving to the US! At GMC Srinagar, he was strongly influenced by teachers like Prof. Taffazull Hussain (biochemistry) and Dr. A. R. Khan (pathology). He says it was Professor Taffazull who got him interested in molecular biology and studying the role of the innate immune system in tackling cancer. He credits Prof. Taffazull Hussain for teaching him how to think big in life and pushing his ideas to transform science.

After graduating from medical school in 2003, he spent some time at SKIMS Srinagar as an internal medicine postgraduate student. During those few months, he greatly enjoyed working with Dr. Sheikh Aijaz (oncology) and Dr. Parvez Koul (medicine, currently director SKIMS), whom he gives credit for advising him to pursue his academic career in the US. Dr. Romee moved to the US in 2005 and did his internal medicine residency (2008) and a hematology-oncology fellowship (2011) from the University of Minnesota. Afterward, he did an advanced BMT Fellowship at Washington University in Saint Louis (2012). At the University of Minnesota, Dr. Romee also did a postdoctoral fellowship in Dr. Jeffrey S. Millers's laboratory, where his work helped describe the CD16 shedding mechanism in NK cells. At Washington University, his research work helped discover human memory-like NK cells with enhanced antitumor function (now being evaluated in multiple clinical trials). He stayed as a junior faculty at Washington University until 2018, when he was recruited by Dana Farber Cancer Institute, Harvard Medical School, in Boston to lead the NK cell program.

At Harvard Medical School, he leads the NK cell therapeutics initiative and is the director of the haploidentical stem cell transplant program at Dana Farber and Brigham and Women's Hospital. His laboratory is working on developing novel TCR-like CAR NK cells against liquid and solid malignancies with otherwise limited tumor-specific antigen expression on the cell surface. Furthermore, using CRISPR and other advanced gene-editing technologies; his lab is generating gene constructs aimed at overcoming the highly immunosuppressive tumor microenvironment, particularly in malignancies like pancreatic and ovarian cancer. His team discovered human memory-like NK cells, and Dr. Romee has led several studies assessing the safety and efficacy of these cells in advanced malignancies. He has received awards from the Leukemia and Lymphoma Society (LLS Clinical Scholar Award, 2021), the American Society of Hematology (ASH) Scholar Award (2015), the American Society of Clinical Oncology (ASCO) Career Development Award (2015), Barnes Jewish Hospital Foundation Team Science Award (2014), and Barnes Jewish Hospital Foundation Award (2014). His research is funded through various foundations, philanthropy, industry, and the National Institutes of Health (NIH).

Rizwan is married to Dr. Saba Beg (rheumatologist and a 2004 GMC Srinagar graduate), and they have two children, Myra Romee (fourteen) and Arsh Romee (eleven), who were both born in Minnesota, though they consider Kashmir as their second home. Outside of his work, he greatly enjoys traveling and exploring nature. He is also passionate about bird photography and loves to spend most weekends exploring various wildlife sanctuaries in Massachusetts and neighboring states. He says he is extremely lucky to meet and become close friends with some of the brightest minds during his medical school. His close friends from GMC include Dr. Sheikh Hilal (currently a neurology consultant at GMC Srinagar), Dr. Sheikh Zahoor (surgical oncology consultant at SKIMS), Dr. Gowhar Mufti (pediatric surgery consultant at SKIMS), Dr. Umar Amin (pediatrician consultant at GMC Srinagar), Dr. Basharat Andrabi (endocrinology consultant in NHS UK), and Dr. Zahoor Ahmad (surgical oncology consultant at GMC Srinagar). He dearly misses spending time with his friends and sipping tea with freshly baked samosas at the old GMC cafeteria. "My career was strongly shaped by my experiences at the medical school and close bonding with some of my teachers and friends there."

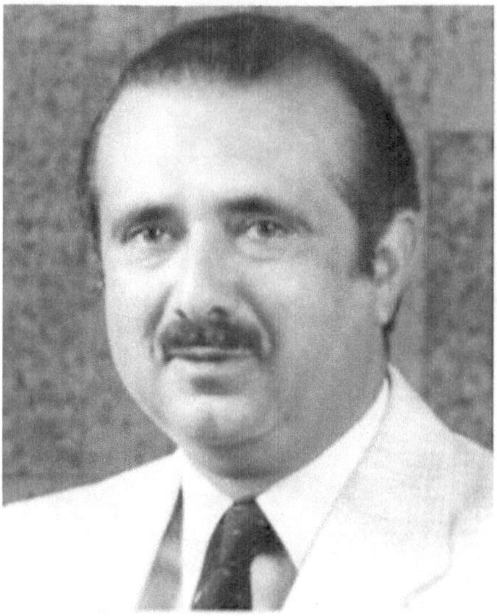

Dr. Mian Mohammad Ashraf—one of the first Kashmiri doctors to achieve success in US established himself as an acclaimed cardiac surgeon and one of the first bypass surgeons in Boston.

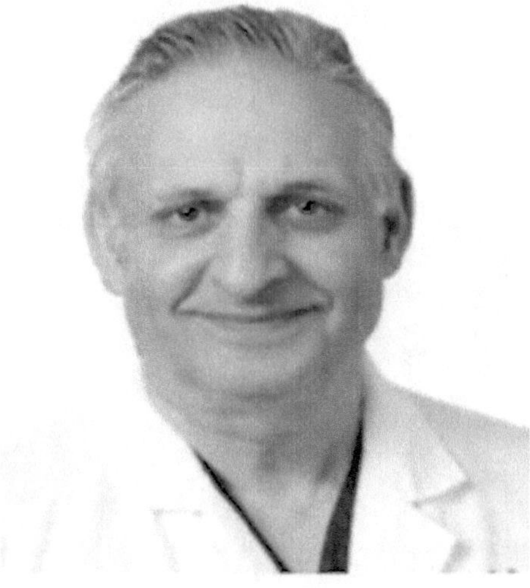

Dr. Fayaz Shawl—the world-famous innovative interventional cardiologist who introduced percutaneous technique called "Shawl's technique"

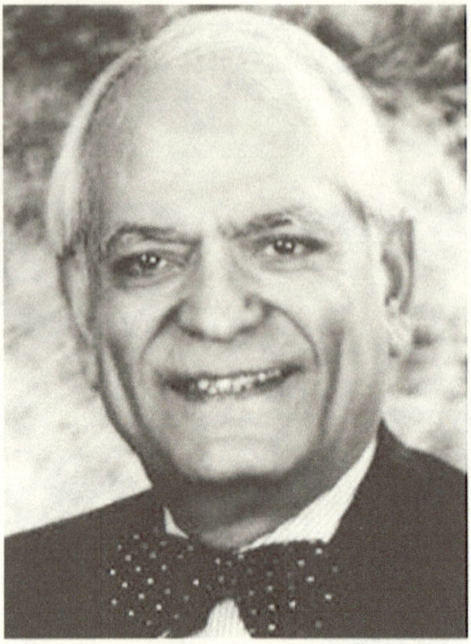

Dr. K. J. Qazi, the alumnus of GMC Srinagar, served chair of Medicine and program director for Internal Medicine (Buffalo)

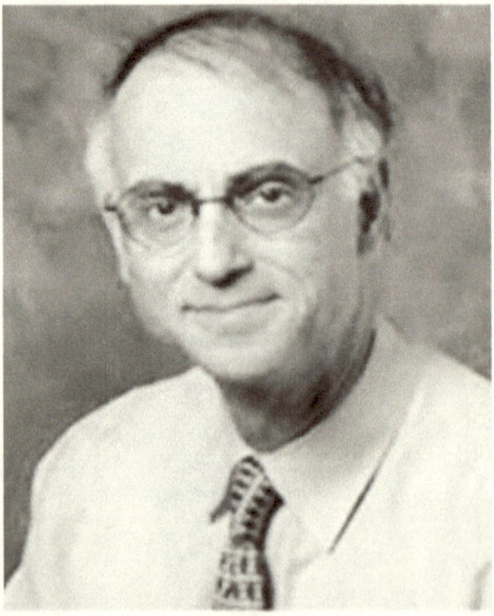

Dr. P. K. Shah—director of the Atherosclerosis Prevention and Treatment Center and Oppenheimer Atherosclerosis Research Center at Cedars-Sinai.

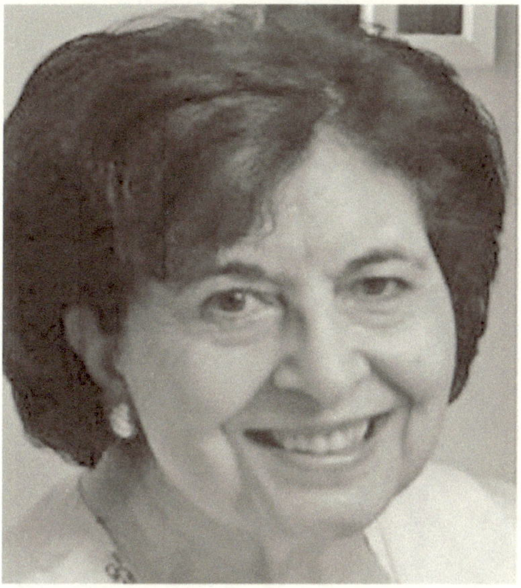

Dr. Arfa Khan—professor emeritus, Zucker School of Medicine at Hofstra/Northwell, former chief of Thoracic Radiology, LIJMC.

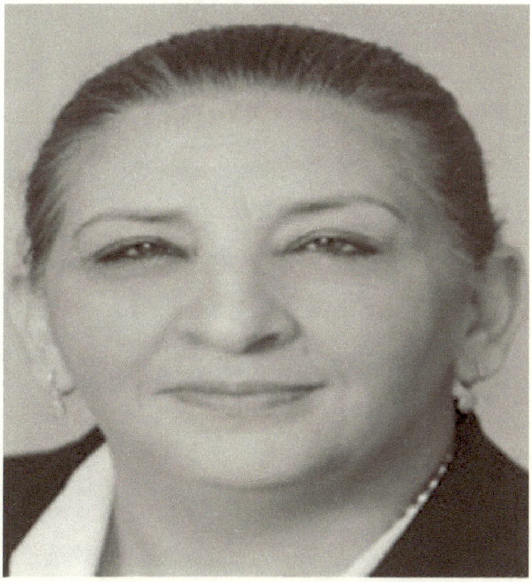

Dr. Tanveer P. Mir, geriatrician—served as chair of the American College of Physicians (2015–2016)

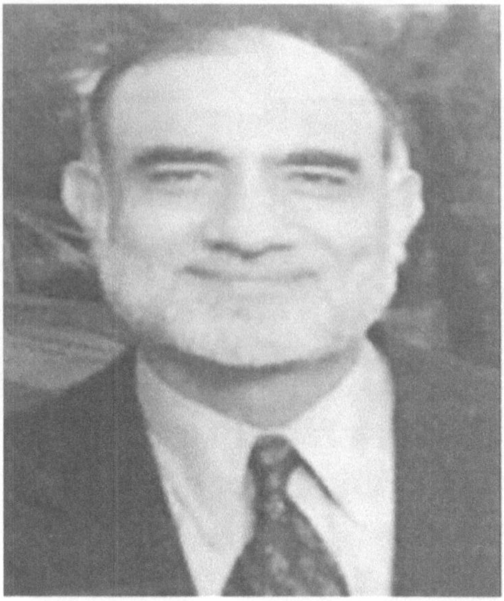

Dr. A. R. Mir—eminent nephrologist and
a founding member of IMANA.

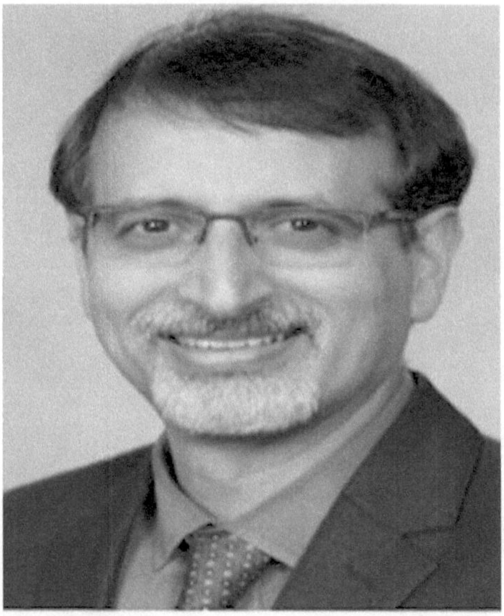

Dr. Iftikhar J. Kullo, cardiologist and genetic
epidemiologist at Mayo Clinic, Rochester.

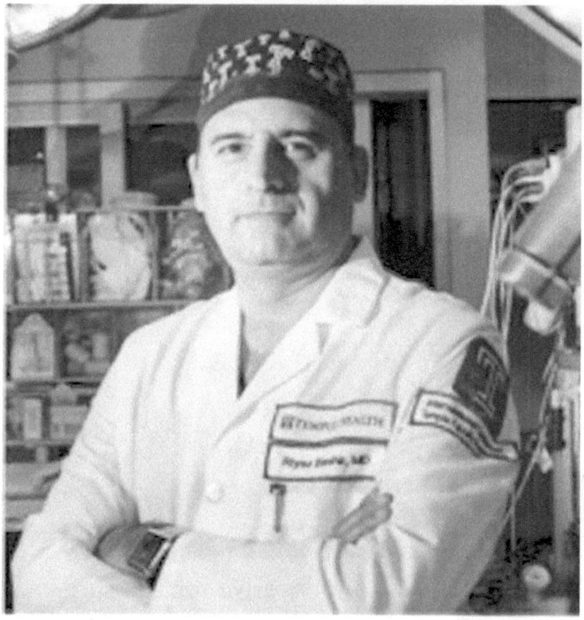

Dr. Riyaz Bashir—interventional cardiologist and professor of medicine at Temple University, Philadelphia.

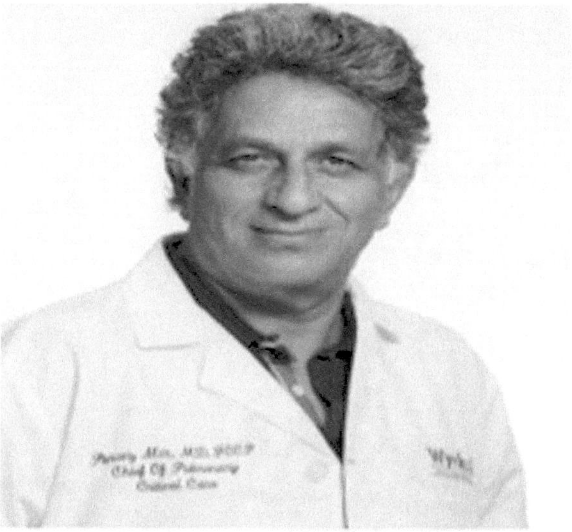

Dr. Parvez Mir—listed by *Time* magazine as a hero in COVID-19 pandemic.

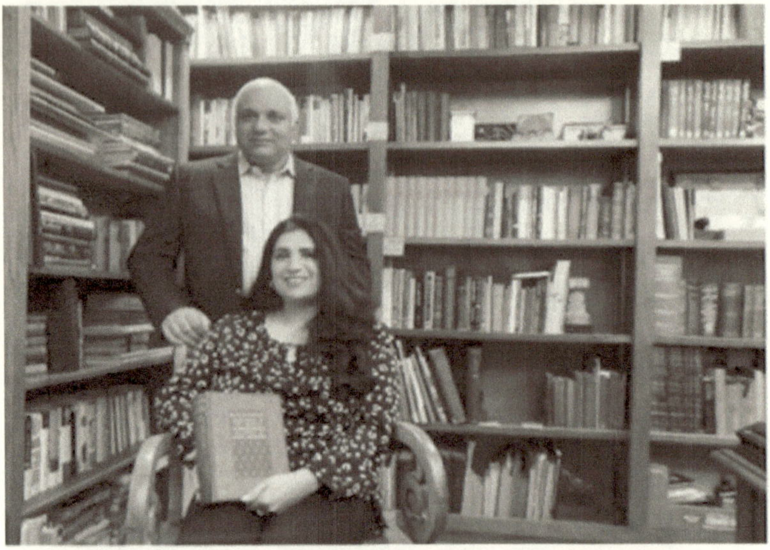

Dr. Khurshid Guru, an innovative robotic surgeon from Buffalo who, with his wife, Dr. Lubna, created a museum near Niagara Falls depicting Kashmiri art, crafts, and history.

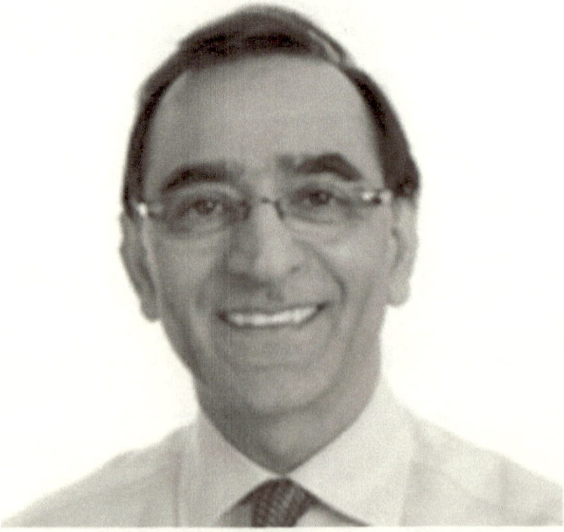

Dr. Ghulam Jeelani Mufti—hemato-oncologist awarded Order of the British Empire (OBE).

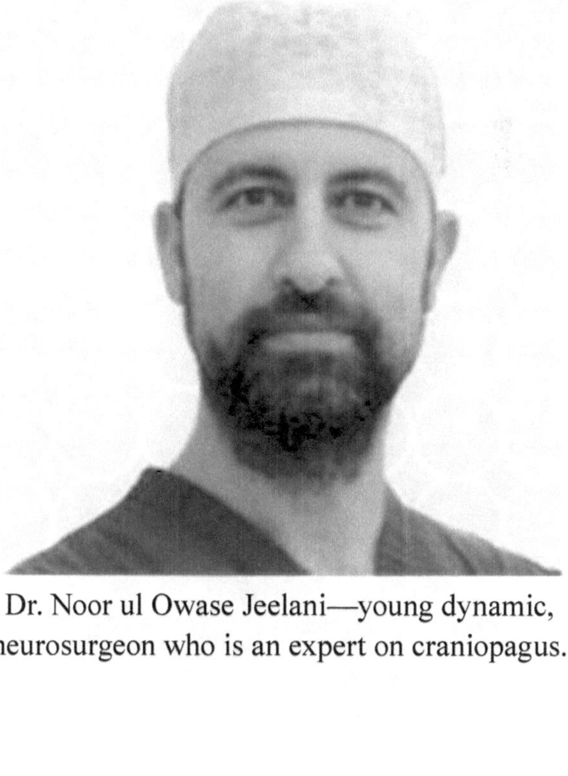

Dr. Noor ul Owase Jeelani—young dynamic, neurosurgeon who is an expert on craniopagus.

Tribute

While closing this book, I realized there were many non-Kashmiri doctors who contributed immensely to health care and medical education in Kashmir and left their visible imprints on the health landscape of Kashmir. The contribution of Neve brothers—namely, Arthur Neve and Ernest Neve—is tremendous. They witnessed and treated large goiters, disfiguring leprosy, advanced cancers, and crowds with every type of surgical ailment. They also treated accidents that included fall from fruit trees and bear mauls. Tuberculosis was rampant, so were the deficiency diseases. They wrote books and excellent papers in *Lancet* about their experience in Kashmir. I do not want to take away the credit from Dr. Gulzar Mufti, who has done an in-depth analysis of their work in Kashmir and written elaborate descriptions about their role as excellent and busy surgeons in Kashmir Mission Hospital. I would refer the readers to his book *Kashmir in Sickness and in Health* (Partridge Publishing 2013) not only for the role of Neve brothers in tackling the epidemics of surgical and medical diseases but also for the minute details about the hospital, the wards, and the wide variety of patients they treated. These heroes should not be forgotten. Their role as "father surgeons" of Kashmir is unquestionable. They provide a conduit between a primitive place called Kashmir and an advanced power of the times the United Kingdom. Their love for God translated so well into their love for the sick and ailing in Kashmir. Here is a brief sketch of some legendary figures in addition to Neve brothers whom we should not forget.

The Madhouse at the Lotus Lake (Dr. Erna M Hoch)

In an era when immigration to the West was a norm with doctors who were trained in the subcontinent, there was a curious case of "reverse migration." A psychiatrist trained in the best institutions of Zurich chose to work at AIIMS New Delhi and thereafter came to work in Srinagar as a professor of psychiatry and transform the rather backward "madhouse" into a "modern psychiatry hospital." Before she came to Srinagar, she was the deputy head of Psychiatry at the AIIMS New Delhi. She wanted to take up a job that would offer more opportunities for development and pioneering work. On a chance visit to Srinagar, she saw an opportunity for herself to build a psychiatry hospital' and a department from nothing. Not many would have at that point of time dared to venture into those "backward conditions."

Erna M. Hoch was born in 1919, grew up in Basel, and trained in medicine and psychiatry. She lived in India from 1956 to 1988. She arrived in Srinagar in September 1969 as a visiting professor of psychiatry to organize the teaching of psychiatry for the medical students in Srinagar's newly constructed medical college and at the same time to set up a Psychiatry Department for the college. Dr. Hoch was handed over the charge of an "old-fashioned lunatic asylum" that only served the protective and nursing functions and was far from being a hospital.

Dr. Hoch sums up her experience as she built up a hospital where there was none for mental diseases in a land too far away—for a people socially, culturally, and geographically too distinct and too different, in her book titled *The Madhouse at the Lotus Lake*. Eager to know how she did that, I read her priceless book written by her in 2000, wherein she describes her struggle to convert a "*Pagal Khana*" (as she calls it) into a "hospital for psychiatric diseases." Call it a review, a short extract, or a leaf from our medical history, these lines of mine are a tribute to this great doctor who worked with utmost dedication to set up a facility for mental diseases in the heart of a beautiful land.

The "mental hospital," where Dr. Hoch worked was an appendage to a prison. It was surrounded by barred cells to keep "intolerable mental patients" prone to violence in safe custody. For her residence, Dr. Hoch chose the vicinity of the hospital and gave up her job as a warden in the girls' hostel that was first assigned to her. She chose a small two-room house that was not even walled when she moved in. When Dr. Hoch took over, the cell complex was still part of the hospital, and many of the cells were still occupied with old chronic patients who had never come out of them for years.

In her book, Dr. Hoch gives a detailed overview of the part of Srinagar where the mental hospital is located. She talks about its serene surroundings, the blossoming almond trees, the temples, the fort, and the graveyard. The layout of the hospital and the rooms where patients were housed gives goose bumps to the reader. She describes the hospital, the inmates, and the building of the hospital in detail. She talks about a room for patients who had destructive tendencies and who were incapable of observing even the most primitive rules of cleanliness and hygiene. This room was furnished with a layer of straw. While other halls had an annex with bathing cubicles and latrines, this straw hall had no sanitary facilities at all. Dr. Hoch counts it as one of the greatest deeds of her life that she managed to demarcate a small compartment in one corner of this room behind which the patients could defecate in a recess in the floor. Through an opening in the wall, the excrement was flushed away by a cleaning crew into the sewers outside the building. Until then, the dirt had to be wiped up from the floor and removed from the straw and at times scraped off the walls.

Some of the changes that were introduced were dramatic whereas she treaded cautiously to bring out the other changes in a slow and steady manner. The staff had to be reaccustomed, reeducated, and the budget allocations steadily increased. Initially, there was resistance from staff, the neighborhood, and the people to a change to which they were unaccustomed. She realigned the budget for medicines that was used by her predecessors to run a small general medical polyclinic and supplied expensive medicines free of charge to employees and the neighborhood. She drastically reduced the expenditure on general medicines and spent it on psychotropic drugs not only for hospital inmates but also for outpatients. This resulted in uproar in neighborhood because their right for free medicine had been curtailed. This uprising and uproar was very skillfully handled, and the Psychiatric Disease Hospital continued to provide first-aid medical services to the neighborhood but reserved drugs for patients only. The polyclinic also provided a "triage point" for psychiatric patients so that physical diseases would be excluded.

With time, the faith of people in the hospital increased. The population realized that help was available not only for desperate cases of mental derangement and confusion but also for disorders like anxiety, depression, hysterical manifestations, attacks of possession, etc. There was help available for children with learning difficulties, behavioral disorders, people with seizure disorders and unspecified physical complaints. There was a tremendous increase in the patients visiting the hospital, especially ones with milder diseases. Seventy percent of the clientele to the hospital was from the recommendations of other patients who were already cured. The first part of the battle that included "goodwill of patients and population" had already been won.

Gradually, the staff had to be expanded, nurses to be employed, supervisors and assistants to be recruited. Nothing came about without effort. The unskilled had to be trained;

those without zeal had to be stimulated. The kitchen staff, the electricians, the compounders, the laboratory assistants, the tailors, the gardeners, the launderers—Dr. Hoch gives details of each one and how she used their services to make a "hospital" out of a prison cell. She was bothered by the leisurely attitude of the employees who misused "casual leave" option to the maximum; however, she controlled nearly eighty employees very well. When she joined the hospital, a very rough tone prevailed among the employees for the patients, but, gradually, her presence brought up a change in their behavior towards these "social outcasts." There were chronic patients in the hospital, vegetating anonymously, and it was her endeavor to help them regain the human dignity to which they were entitled. No medical records had been kept on these inmates. Many patients had been hospitalized for more than twelve years and many for more than a year. For inpatients, there were only one hundred beds, which served a population of 2.5 million and thus were usually occupied. The hospital was overcrowded, as active efforts were not made to discharge patients after they were admitted. In her desire to know about these chronic inmates, Dr. Hoch writes, "I tried to find something about the origins of these chronic patients and reasons for their hospitalization. These figures that were staring at dirt mostly naked and wrapped only in ragged woolen blankets—I wanted to assess whether there was any hope of rehabilitation. Unaccustomed to such human attention some hid as we approached them, others ran away in fright; still, others burst into tears when they heard friendly voices and concerned questions about their welfare. Many, however simply remained closed, not trusting such astonishing interest or perhaps too hopeless to once again dismantle the walls of protection and defense they had erected inside and then perhaps be disappointed again. Even today, I remember quite a number of them especially of course those who continued to remain under our care in the following years and some of whom we were able to bring back to life."

Dr. Hoch developed interest in the traditions of Kashmiris, their fears, their concerns, their idiosyncrasies, their positive points, their negative aspects and struggled to make a decent space for patients with psychiatric diseases on the banks of a lake. She struggled as a *pagalmeem*, an outsider, an imposer, but was focused on her goal to care for a community forgotten in the backyards of a backward place.

Dr. Hoch heeded to the advice of a patient in Delhi and implemented his advice in Srinagar. The patient once told her, "There are times when everything and especially all human contact, seems to be poisoned. Only the Earth, the sky, the wind, trees, flowers, mountains still have a healthy beneficial effect. And it is precisely from these that we are cut off when we are put in a psychiatry hospital." In the hospital at Srinagar, she exposed patients to these elements as whole-day patients moved in and out of the wards breathing fresh air, looking at the open sky and the beautiful garden in the middle. They could enjoy the sun, the rain, the breeze, and the wind, and this kept them happy. She took extra care of the nearby garden and ensured that it was well maintained.

Dr. Hoch had an eye for detail. She studied the customs of Kashmiris and applied them in the hospital for the benefit of patients. The chill of winter bothered her, and it was not possible to have the "central heating system" as in SMHS Hospital installed; however, she was impressed by "Hamam" concept, and she applied it to her hospital. The Hamam eased the suffering of shivering patients for whom winter signified an added calamity.

Dr. Hoch has contributed a lot to the psychiatric care in Kashmiri population. Her dedication, commitment, and zeal to work have no parallel. She was a doctor, a nurse, a psychologist, a physician, a landscapist all rolled into one. She did not fight to get through her point but reasoned in a beautiful manner for the right of people who had no rights. She lived for a cause, and she realized it.

The book is a tribute to her work and is a must read for all the psychiatrists practicing psychiatry in Kashmir. She has carefully chosen many index cases that tell a lot about the apathy towards the problems confronting patients with mental ailments. I close this with a description that she gives of herself: "On one occasion, it was mainly my arrogance that caused me to fall: I had just received a letter asking me to provide a short curriculum vitae and photograph for the publication of a *Who is Who Encyclopedia* of the 7000—or may be it was 700—most famous women in Asia. On the way home from Medical college to the hospital, I was smugly gloating over the honor of belonging to this select circle of prominent ladies, forgetting to pay attention to my path in the rain-soaked old town alley. Suddenly, one of the 7000 most famous women in Asia was sitting in the mud, exposed to the ridicule of the street urchins and only concerned about whether the rain jacket would cover the patch of excrement on the back of her skirt. After this disillusionment and literal humiliation-the English 'humiliation' indicates even more clearly that it means 'coming back to Earth' or becoming Earth itself—I naturally made no effort to reply to this letter." Women of her caliber do not strive for medals and honors but work for a cause in most unfamiliar of the surroundings delivering what they can amid all the odds that they face.

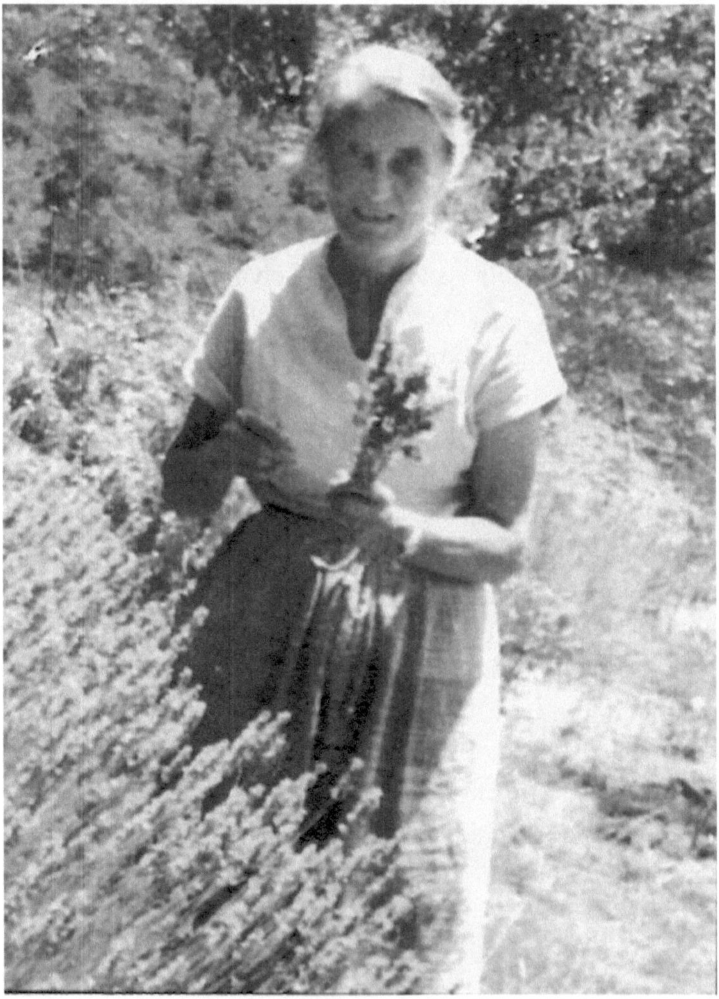

Dr.Erna M Hoch-the legendary Swiss psychiatrist who contributed immensely to psychiatric care in Kashmir.

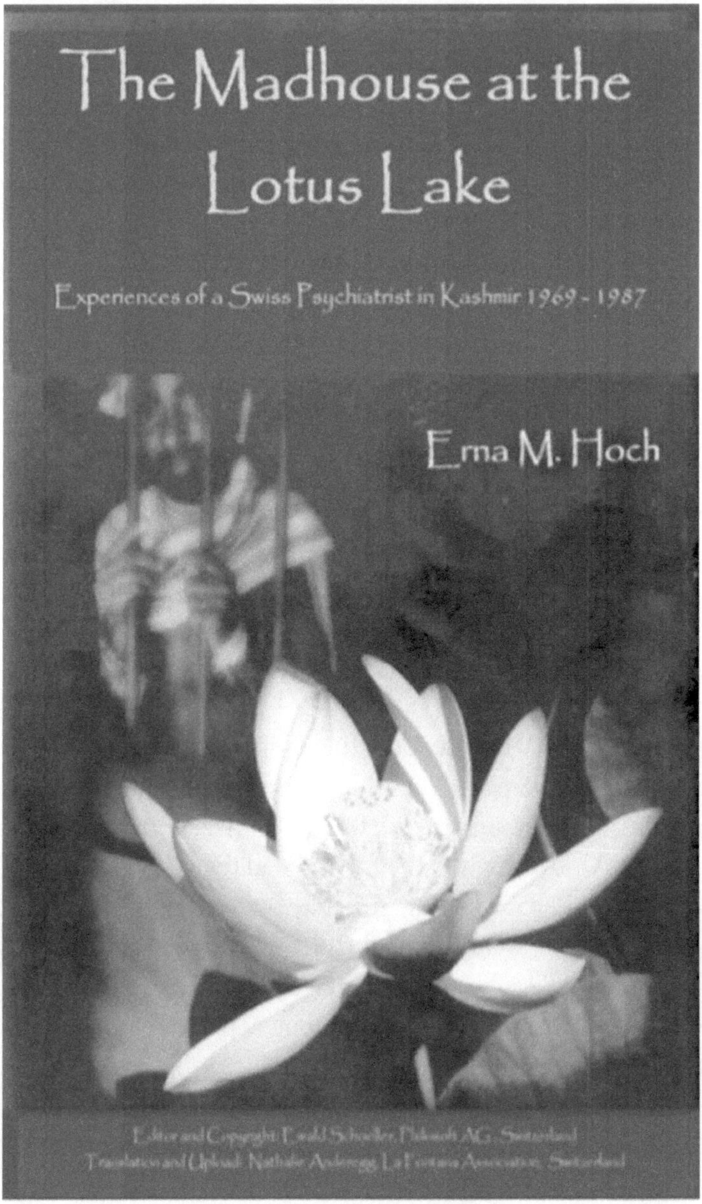
The Madhouse at the Lotus Lake
Experiences of a Swiss Psychiatrist in Kashmir 1969 - 1987
Erna M. Hoch

Dr. B. S. Kahali

Professor Kahali headed the Department of Physiology, Government Medical College, Srinagar, in its formative years. According to Dr. M. S. Khuroo, "he taught the subject with great passion. His weekly quiz of ten MCQ's with ten marks is reminiscent of modern methodology widely practiced in East and West."

Dr. Kahali, according to Dr. Ghulam Jeelani, was "a combination of strictness and knowledge." The system of in-house timely examinations called "stages" was his novel idea of regular checkups of students' knowledge. Dr. B. S. Kahali was an honest and impartial teacher from Bengal.

According to Dr. Altaf Hussain, "Prof. Kahali of Physiology department displayed fair-minded approach, fearlessness and precision in his dealings with students."

Dr. C. L. Ahluwalia

Professor Ahluwalia headed the Department of Social and Preventive Medicine in the initial years of the creation of GMC Srinagar. He created the best SPM museum in the country. Professor Ahluwalia was the most loved teacher, and the exotic beauty of college was his gift. No one would pluck flowers from the Government Medical College lawns. He had imposed a fine on anyone who would dare to do so. In the morning, he would take the round of whole campus with head *Mali* to ensure that the plants and the flowers are well kept in the lawns like a specialist floriculturist. Without exaggeration, the GMC campus was the best college campus, and Dr. Ahluwalia would proudly say, "I don't think my students need to go to Mughal gardens in view of the beauty of the GMC campus" ("Nostalgic GMC in '60s," Prof. Ghulam Jeelani, *KASHMED* 2011). Students would remember him as a futurist who was far ahead of his time. He would take students to Oberoi Hotel and show them the waste disposal system (Dr. Qadiri).

Dr. P. S. Sikand

Dr. P. S. Sikand served the Department of Surgery GMC Srinagar as the professor and head of the department. He was a surgeon of great skill and an excellent teacher. Dr. Pankaj Kaul, his student and a CVTS surgeon, writes in his praise the following: "I would be a second or third Assistant to him and never first. Even from that distance, however, watching him perform surgery was pure joy. All movements were unhurried but fast. There was a flow and rhythm and economy of movement, a calm demeanor signifying confidence and control, and a sense for the assistant that one was witnessing something special. My surgical experience was too rudimentary to deconstruct it beyond that. But, once, looking at me, across two assistants, or so I imagined, he said, 'It should look good, whatever you do. If it doesn't look good, it, probably, isn't good.'"

His reputation had been constructed on operating on patients most surgeons may not have had the skill or confidence to operate, and a folklore and legend had built around his name. To be operated by PS was to be assured of success and cure, no matter how sick one was. Dr. Sikand is believed to be a fun-loving surgeon who enjoyed Harrissa parties with his staff frequently.

Dr. Jagat Mohini

Dr. Jagat Mohini was born in Lahore Punjab (Pakistan) on January 11, 1921. She was the daughter of Mr. Rajendra Prasad Atal. She did her MBBS from King Edward Medical College, Lahore. She came to Kashmir in 1945 as a young bride and a young lady doctor, in a culture different from hers. She settled down quickly and adopted the Kashmiri culture to become an integral part of it. Since then, she dedicated her entire life to the service of the people of Kashmir Valley. She and her husband, the late Dr. Onkar Nath Thussu, a renowned pathologist, started the Rattan Rani Hospital at Barbarshah, Srinagar, named in memory of Dr. Omkar Nath's late first wife. It was the very first hospital in Kashmir based on modern treatment and is now a century-old heritage site. Dr. Jagat Mohini worked selflessly for the people of Kashmir at a time when there were very few doctors and hardly any specialists. She treated all types of patients and battled all diseases deftly, but the most important contribution to society was as a champion fighting for issues of women, like discrimination, violence, dowry, health issues of women, etc. She was widely known for her generosity and charity.

Dr. Jagat Mohini not only treated patients medically but also put a healing touch on their socioeconomic ailments also. She became a champion for the cause of women of the valley. She worked hard her entire life, totally dedicated to her profession. She saved, treated, and cured countless patients. As time passed, people looked up to her as a mentor, guardian, and a savior. She earned the nickname "Mummy" from her staff and all her patients. She was literally a mother to all as she brought endless many to this world as a gynecologist. She was truly the "Florence Nightingale" of Kashmir or the "Mother Teresa" of the valley. The national newspaper the *Hindustan Times* wrote on its front page an article about her achievements, and it was titled "The Supermom of Kashmir." Her work was also recognized and complimented by many other national papers.

Dr. Jagat Mohini worked as a social reformer and a philanthropist, doing a lot of charity work without looking for any reward. She was a social worker who fought all evils of society and became a source of inspiration to many. She was instrumental in employing many people, both directly in the hospital, as well as by opening vocational centers. A multitalented woman, she used her knowledge of stitching, sewing, and knitting to open centers to train women from the weaker sections of society so that they could live a life of dignity. The vocational training camps and centers started and run by her provided a source of livelihood to countless women in Kashmir. She was successfully running a nursing school, which enrolled many students from many parts of the country and provided a source of livelihood to women of the state and other parts of the country.

A bold upright woman, she stood for justice and never wavered in spite of all odds. Whenever and wherever a person needed help, she was there for them. She opened a school, Viswa Bharati, which from a two-room set up became a college, later having a branch in NOIDA near Delhi. She had the foresight to acquire land for the school at NOIDA and then converted it into a successful school. She organized and conducted health camps in and around the city for the benefit of poor and needy people of the state.

She was a brave and a fearless soul who never deserted the people of the valley. She stood tall and courageously faced both the good and bad times of the valley. A simple and good human being, she never faltered to help a Kashmiri.

Dr. Ajit Kumar Nagpal

The hero who built SKIMS!

Dr. Nagpal is the founding director of Sher-i-Kashmir Institute of Medical Sciences, who was handpicked to carry out the task of building up a health-care facility on the banks of Aanchaar Lake, which would cater to the tertiary care needs of the people of the valley and discourage referrals to the outside institutions. Dr. Nagpal is a graduate of the All India Institute of Medical Sciences and Harvard University with preparation in medicine, hospital administration, and health policy and management.

He created an institution that not only became well known for its beauty, cleanliness, and landscape but also provided state-of-the-art health-care facilities to the people of the state. It was his dream project, and he put all his faculties into it. He braved all the difficulties that came up while the institution was being built and ensured that the institution was built in record time and had the best infrastructure, best equipment imported from all over the world, and a trained staff to run it. A team of fifty-six doctors from Jammu and Kashmir was sent outside to get trained in various specialities. At the same time, a group of reputed doctors from all over the country was sent for heading faculties like neurosurgery, anesthesia, and cardiac surgery. To create a dependable health-care facility, bright girls and boys interested in science were sent to various reputed institutions of the country to get trained as technicians and technologists and perform sophisticated tests and handle delicate instruments. This workforce at SKIMS made SKIMS a leader in diagnostics not only in Kashmir but also at the national level. For instance, electron microscope was introduced in SKIMS when there were just three throughout India.

Dr. Nagpal is credited with removing the taboo associated with the nursing profession in Kashmir. People in Kashmir were hesitant to send their daughters in this profession. They would choose to become doctors or teachers, which were more sought after professions and easily available. Subsequently, the government relaxed norms for the Kashmir girls to undertake nursing courses. A scholarship of Rs 600 per month was offered to attract girls towards the nursing profession and strengthen medical assistance staff at the SKIMS.

Dr. Nagpal created a model institute that had no parallel when it was created. It had strong foundations, and it withstood the test of the times very well. It did not tremble, shake, or waver in the toughest of the times and maintained the label of being a "brand." Besides being the founder director and CEO of Sher-i-Kashmir Institute of Medical Sciences, Srinagar, Dr. Nagpal has been the convener of the Task Force on Health Sector Reforms for Jammu and Kashmir engaged in the development and implementation of public policy to incentivize investment in health care and foster public private partnerships to achieve the laudable objective of universal and equitable access to health care.

Dr. Nagpal's principal interests include global and national health policy, financing of health services, regional health planning, and hospital development. His lifetime endeavors have been focused on optimizing the use of technology and human skills in achieving the highest standards of technical efficiency, clinical effectiveness, and quality in the delivery of health care. In public domain, he is also the founder trustee and member, Governing Board of the Apka Swasthya Bima Trust of the Government of NCT, established to provide social health insurance to over two million population living below poverty line. Formerly, Dr. Nagpal was the principal advisor on health policy and hospital affairs, Ministry of Health, United Arab Emirates; chairman of Scientific Advisory Council, Welcare World Health Systems; chairman, Executive Council, Batra Hospital and Medical Research Center; chairman, Hospital

Planning Sectoral Committee, Bureau of Indian Standards; and member of the Medical Council of India.

Dr. Nagpal has delivered over seventy-five invitational guest lectures at the professional conferences and renowned European and North American academic medical centers and has chaired over twenty-five international conferences and seminars on topical issues concerned with health sector reforms, health-care financing, and hospital planning and development.

Dr. Nagpal has published extensively and has authored many policy papers, project reports, and feasibility studies. Dr. Ajit K. Nagpal is the chairman of Amity PACIFIC Forum, an instrument to foster partnership with corporate and social sectors of the industry for education, research, and innovation through the medium of National Federations of Commerce and Industry.

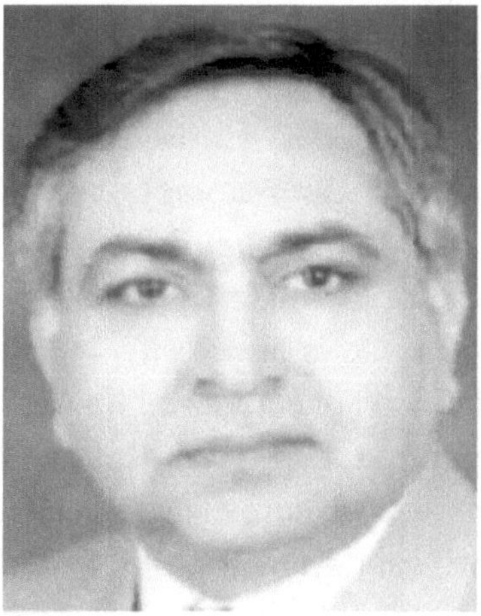

Dr. Ajit K Nagpal—the founder director of SKIMS.

Not the forgotten ones!

The following profiles would have been mentioned, but I could not contact the family members or those alive did not wish to be included in the book:

1. **Dr. Jahan Ara Naqshbandi,** professor of gynecology and obstetrics, GMC Srinagar who has been a favorite teacher and a skilled surgeon having taught generations of doctors at GMC Srinagar and Lal Ded hospital. A pioneering name in gynecology and obstetrics GMC; lives with her daughter. Dr. Allaqaband tried to reach her to give her CV, but I could not get it.
2. **Dr. Ghulam Hassan Hajini,** professor and ex-HOD, Department of Dermatology, GMC Srinagar. He is the father of dermatology in Kashmir and served the Department of Dermatology with great dedication and commitment. He is an excellent clinician and a great teacher. I could not convince him to give his CV to me.
3. **Dr. Mohammad Afzal Wani,** professor and ex-head, Department of Neurosurgery,dean medical faculty SKIMS Srinagar. Known as the "father of neurosurgery" in Kashmir; is the first qualified neurosurgeon from Kashmir and is credited with starting neurosurgery at SKIMS. Efficient, energetic, and bold, he has inspired many to pursue neurosurgery. Tried to contact him but could not get his CV
4. **Dr. Mohammad Shafi Misgar,** professor and ex-head, Department of Surgery, SMHS Srinagar. One of the quick and able surgeons. I tried my best to reach out to his family for his CV but could not manage to get it.
5. **Dr. Farhat Hamid,** professor of gynecology and obstetrics, GMC Srinagar. A very dedicated and sophisticated gynecologist and obstetrician who served

at Lal Ded Hospital for a long time and contributed greatly to patient care and teaching. Nowadays lives with her son in the US.

6. **Dr. Sheikh Jalal,** professor and ex-head, Department of Cardiology, SKIMS Srinagar; ex-dean and director, SKIMS Srinagar. Dr. Jalal is remembered for his work as the director of SKIMS who set right the system post turmoil and reclaimed a space for SKIMS as the best health-care institution of Jammu and Kashmir. He unfortunately fell a victim to the bullets from an unknown source.
7. **Dr. G. R. Mir**, professor and ex-head, Department of Orthopedics, GMC Srinagar; and ex-principal, GMC Srinagar. An innovative orthopedic surgeon who worked in very difficult times and was one of the pillars during the initial years instrumental in establishing orthopedics as a separate speciality.

Epilogue

I am wise today. My story is incomplete. All my stories are incomplete. I am able to hold just a drop from the ocean and put it in this book. That drop hasn't quenched my thirst, and that won't quench yours too. I have not touched the ocean that is waiting to be explored. Happy exploring!

Further reading

1. *Kashmir in Sickness and in Health*; Gulzar Mufti 2013 Partridge Publication Penguin Books, India Pvt Ltd.
2. *Stories from K. L. Chowdhury's "My Medical Journey"*—compiled by M. K. Raina.
3. Erna M Hoch. *The Madhouse at the Lotus Lake: Experiences of a Swiss Psychiatrist in Kashmir.* 1967–1987.
4. *KASHMED.* 2011, Golden Jubilee Issue—editor Dr. Zaffar Abass.
5. *When My Valley Was Green; Kanwar K. Kaul 2017, Notion Press.*

About the authors

Dr. Rumana Makhdoomi is a professor of pathology at Sher-i-Kashmir Institute of Medical Sciences Soura. She has graduated from GMC Srinagar and done her postgraduation in pathology from the same institution. She has received fellowship in neuropathology from NIMHANS and training in oncopathology from Kidwai Memorial Institute Bengaluru. She is a prolific writer whose passion for healthcare related issues shines through her work. Beyond her contributions to the world of medicine, Dr. Rumana habitually shares her insights on sociocultural issues through her writings in local newspapers. She is a very sensitive writer whose essays have won her many awards. Her first book, *White Man in Dark*, described the work done by the doctors in Kashmir during turmoil. It was received well by the readers. This is her second book. This book, focuses on the top 100 Kashmiri doctors, is a testament to her dedication to the medical field and her commitment to recognizing excellence within it. Her ability to bridge the gap between the medical and social realms demonstrates her multifaceted approach to creating positive change in her community. Dr. Rumana's work not only elevates the profiles of exceptional medical professionals but also serves as a powerful voice in addressing the broader societal issues that impact us all. She lives in Srinagar with her husband and daughters and is greatly attached to the culture and traditions of downtown Srinagar.

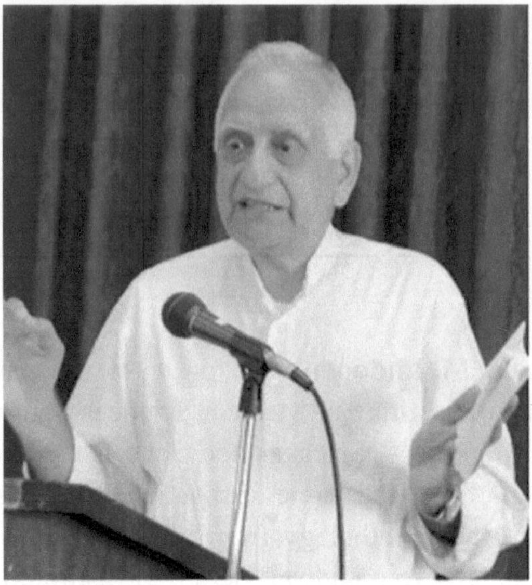

Dr. Faroque Ahmad Khan

Dr. Faroque Ahmad Khan is a Kashmir-born US doctor who graduated from Government Medical College in Kashmir, India, and moved to the United States in 1966. Dr. Khan served as chairman of Medicine at Nassau University Medical Center (NUMC) in New York from 1987 to 1999. He held the rank of professor of medicine for twenty-one years at the State University of New York at Stony Brooke and has held numerous leadership positions. He was the first Muslim awarded mastership in American College of Physicians (ACP). Dr. Khan helped launch the Interfaith Institute of Long Island. Dr. Khan serves as the chair of the board of trustees at the Interfaith Institute. In September 2013, the Long Island Press elected Dr. Khan as one of the Fifty Most Influential People of Long Island, New York. Even though Dr. Khan lives away from Kashmir, his heart beats for it, and he leaves no occasion to render his services for providing help to Kashmir's ailing health-care system. He has authored three books and been a part of multiple discussions, debates, and associations aimed to promote harmony among the followers of various religions. He lives with his radiologist wife and children in New York. He not only compiled the list of outstanding doctors of Kashmiri origin from US but also helped to motivate others in Kashmir and elsewhere to contribute to the book.

www.ingramcontent.com/pod-product-compliance
Lightning Source LLC
Chambersburg PA
CBHW020719180526
45163CB00001B/32
* 9 7 8 1 5 4 3 7 0 9 2 6 1 *